PLASTIC SURGERY

VOLUME 7
THE HAND
Part 1

1990
W.B. SAUNDERS COMPANY
Harcourt Brace Jovanovich, Inc.
Philadelphia ■ London ■ Toronto
Montreal ■ Sydney ■ Tokyo

W. B. SAUNDERS COMPANY
Harcourt Brace Jovanovich, Inc.

The Curtis Center
Independence Square West
Philadelphia, PA 19106

Library of Congress Cataloging-in-Publication Data

Plastic surgery.
    Contents: v. 1. General principles—v. 2–3.
The face—v. 4. Cleft lip & palate and craniofacial
anomalies—[etc.]
    1. Surgery, Plastic.   I. McCarthy, Joseph G., 1938–
[DNLM: 1. Surgery, Plastic. WO 600 P7122]

RD118.P536   1990   617'.95   87–9809

ISBN 0–7216–1514–7   (set)

25/7/94

Editor: W. B. Saunders Staff
Designer: W. B. Saunders Staff
Production Manager: Frank Polizzano
Manuscript Editor: David Harvey
Illustration Coordinator: Lisa Lambert
Indexer: Kathleen Garcia
Cover Designer: Ellen Bodner

Volume 1 0–7216–2542–8
Volume 2 0–7216–2543–6
Volume 3 0–7216–2544–4
Volume 4 0–7216–2545–2
Volume 5 0–7216–2546–0
Volume 6 0–7216–2547–9
Volume 7 0–7216–2548–7
Volume 8 0–7216–2549–5
8 Volume Set 0–7216–1514–7

Plastic Surgery

Last digit is the print number: 9   8   7   6   5   4   3   2   1

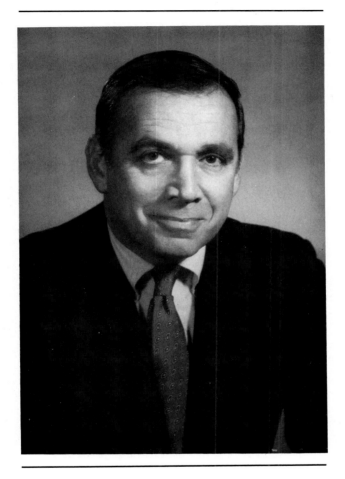

Richard J. Smith, M.D.
(June 13, 1930–March 30, 1987)

The Hand Surgery volumes are dedicated to Richard J. Smith.
A family man, a scholar, a teacher, and a surgeon of the hand,
whose professional life transcended specialty boundaries.

Contributors

STEPHAN ARIYAN, M.D.
Professor of Surgery and Chief of Plastic and Reconstructive Surgery, Yale University School of Medicine; Chief of Plastic Surgery, Yale–New Haven Hospital, New Haven; Consultant in Plastic Surgery, Veterans Administration Hospital, West Haven, Connecticut.

ROBERT W. BEASLEY, M.D.
Professor of Surgery (Plastic Surgery), New York University School of Medicine; Director of Hand Surgery Services, Institute of Reconstructive Plastic Surgery, New York University Medical Center, New York, New York.

PAUL W. BRAND, C.B.E.-M.B.-B.S., F.R.C.S.
Clinical Professor of Orthopaedics and Surgery, Louisiana State University Medical School; Senior Consultant, Gillis W. Long Hansen's Disease Center, Carville, Louisiana.

GARRY S. BRODY, M.D.
Clinical Professor of Surgery (Plastic Surgery), University of Southern California School of Medicine; Chief of Plastic Surgery Research, Rancho Los Amigos Hospital; Attending Surgeon, Downey Community Hospital, Downey, California.

EARL Z. BROWNE, JR., M.D.
Chairman, Department of Plastic and Reconstructive Surgery, Cleveland Clinic Foundation, Cleveland, Ohio.

HARRY J. BUNCKE, M.D.
Clinical Professor of Plastic Surgery, University of California, San Francisco, School of Medicine; Director, Department of Microsurgical Transplantation and Replantation, Davies Medical Center, San Francisco; Consultant, San Francisco General Hospital, Fort Miley Veterans Administration Hospital, and Oak Knoll Naval Hospital; Attending Surgeon, Mills Hospital, San Mateo, and Peninsula Hospital, Burlingame, California.

ROBERT A. CHASE, M.D.
Emile Holman Professor of Surgery Emeritus, and Chairman, Division of Anatomy, Stanford University Medical Center, Stanford, California.

BENJAMIN E. COHEN, M.D.
Clinical Assistant Professor, Division of Plastic Surgery, Baylor College of Medicine; Academic Chief and Director, Plastic Surgery Residency Program, and Director, Microsurgical Research and Training Laboratory, St. Joseph Hospital, Houston, Texas.

MATTHIAS B. DONELAN, M.D.
Assistant Clinical Professor of Surgery, Harvard Medical School; Chief, Plastic and Reconstructive Surgery, Shriners Burns Institute, Boston; Assistant Surgeon, Massachusetts General Hospital, Boston, Massachusetts.

RAY A. ELLIOTT, JR., M.D.
Clinical Professor of Plastic Surgery and Associate Clinical Professor of Orthopedics (Hand), Albany Medical College; Attending Surgeon, Albany Medical Center, Albany Memorial Hospital, and Albany Veterans Administration Hospital, Albany, New York.

G. GREGORY GALLICO III, M.D.
Assistant Professor of Surgery, Harvard Medical School; Assistant Surgeon, Massachusetts General Hospital, Boston.

VINCENT R. HENTZ, M.D.
Associate Professor of Surgery, Stanford University School of Medicine; Chief, Division of Hand and Upper Extremity Surgery, Stanford University Hospital, Palo Alto, California.

MICHAEL E. JABALEY, M.D.
Clinical Professor of Plastic Surgery, University of Mississippi School of Medicine; Attending Sur-

geon, St. Dominic/Jackson Memorial Hospital, Mississippi Baptist Medical Center, River Oaks Hospital, Women's Hospital, and Doctors Hospital; Consultant in Plastic Surgery, Jackson Veterans Administration Hospital, Mississippi Methodist Rehabilitation Center, and University Hospital, Jackson, Mississippi.

LYNN D. KETCHUM, M.D.

Clinical Professor of Surgery, University of Kansas Medical Center, Kansas City; Attending Surgeon, Humana Hospital, Overland Park, Kansas.

MALCOLM A. LESAVOY, M.D.

Associate Professor of Surgery, Division of Plastic Surgery, University of California, Los Angeles, School of Medicine; Chief, Plastic & Reconstructive Surgery, Harbor/UCLA Medical Center, Torrance, California.

GRAHAM D. LISTER, M.B., Сн.B., F.R.C.S.

Professor of Surgery and Chief, Division of Plastic Surgery, University of Utah School of Medicine; Attending Surgeon, University Hospital, Latter Day Saints Hospital, Primary Children's Hospital, and Shriners Hospital, Salt Lake City, Utah.

J. WILLIAM LITTLER, M.D.

Senior Attending Surgeon, St. Luke's–Roosevelt Hospital Center, New York, New York.

JOHN W. MADDEN, M.D., F.A.C.S.

Clinical Professor of Orthopedics, University of New Mexico, Albuquerque; Director, Tucson Hand Rehabilitation Program, Tucson, Arizona.

RALPH T. MANKTELOW, M.D.

Professor and Head, Division of Plastic Surgery, University of Toronto Faculty of Medicine; Head of the Division of Plastic Surgery, Toronto General Hospital, Toronto, Ontario, Canada.

IVAN MATEV, M.D.

Professor of Orthopaedic Surgery, The Medical Academy; Head, Department of Upper Extremity Surgery, The Institute of Orthopaedics and Traumatology, Sofia, Bulgaria.

JAMES W. MAY, Jr., M.D.

Chief of Plastic and Reconstructive Surgery and Hand Surgery Service, Department of General Surgery, Massachusetts General Hospital; Associate Clinical Professor, Harvard Medical School, Boston, Massachusetts.

ROBERT M. McFARLANE, M.D.

Professor of Surgery and Head, Division of Plastic Surgery, University of Western Ontario Faculty of Medicine; Head, Division of Plastic Surgery, Victoria Hospital, London, Ontario, Canada.

MARY H. McGRATH, M.D.

Professor of Surgery and Chief, Division of Plastic and Reconstructive Surgery, George Washington University School of Medicine and Health Sciences; Chief of Service, University Hospital; Attending Surgeon, Children's Hospital National Medical Center, Washington, D.C.

NANCY H. McKEE, M.D.

Associate Professor of Plastic Surgery, University of Toronto Faculty of Medicine; Attending Surgeon, Mount Sinai Hospital, Toronto General Hospital, and Hospital for Sick Children, Toronto, Ontario, Canada.

WYNDELL H. MERRITT, M.D.

Assistant Clinical Professor, Medical College of Virginia, Richmond, Virginia.

ERIK MOBERG, M.D., Ph.D.

Professor Emeritus of Hand Surgery and Orthopaedic Surgery, University of Göteborg Medical School, Göteborg, Sweden.

WAYNE A. MORRISON, M.B., B.S., F.R.A.C.S.

Associate, Department of Surgery, University of Melbourne; Assistant Plastic Surgeon and Deputy Director, Microsurgery Research Centre, St. Vincent's Hospital, Melbourne; Plastic Surgeon, Repatriation Hospital, Heidelberg, Melbourne; Consultant Plastic Surgeon, Geelong Hospital, Victoria, Australia.

JAMES F. MURRAY, M.D.

Professor Emeritus, Department of Surgery, University of Toronto Faculty of Medicine; Attending Surgeon, Sunnybrook Medical Center, Toronto, Ontario, Canada.

ALGIMANTAS O. NARAKAS, M.D.

Associate Professor, Medical School of the University of Lausanne; Surgeon-in-Chief and Head of the Longeraie Clinic; Consultant, University Hospital and Children's Hospital, Lausanne, Switzerland.

HENRY W. NEALE, M.D.

Professor of Surgery and Director, Division of Plastic, Reconstructive and Hand Surgery, University of Cincinnati College of Medicine; Attending Surgeon, University Hospital, Children's Hospital Medical Center, and Shriners Burns Hospital, Cincinnati, Ohio.

MICHAEL G. ORGEL, M.D.
Associate Professor of Surgery (Plastic), University of Massachusetts Medical School at the Berkshire Medical Center; Attending Surgeon, Berkshire Medical Center and Hillcrest Hospital, Pittsfield, Massachusetts.

ANDREW K. PALMER, M.D.
Professor of Orthopedic Surgery, State University of New York Health Center at Syracuse College of Medicine; Coordinator of Hand Service, State University of New York Health Science Center at Syracuse; Consultant and Director of Hand Service, Veterans Administration Hospital, Syracuse, New York.

CHARLES L. PUCKETT, M.D.
Professor and Head, Division of Plastic Surgery, University of Missouri–Columbia School of Medicine; Attending Surgeon, University of Missouri–Columbia Hospital and Clinics, Harry S Truman Memorial Veterans Administration Hospital, Boone Hospital Center and Ellis Fischel State Cancer Hospital, Columbia, Missouri.

ROBERT C. RUSSELL, M.D.
Professor of Surgery, Division of Plastic and Reconstructive Surgery, Southern Illinois University School of Medicine; Chairman of Plastic Surgery, St. John's Hospital, Springfield, Illinois.

ROGER E. SALISBURY, M.D.
Professor of Surgery and Chief of Plastic and Reconstructive Surgery, New York Medical College; Director, Burn Center, Westchester Medical Center, Valhalla; Consultant, Plastic and Reconstructive Surgery, Castle Point Veterans Administration Hospital and Glythedale Children's Hospital; Chief of Plastic and Reconstructive Surgery, Metropolitan Hospital Center, New York, New York.

ROBERT C. SAVAGE, M.D.
Clinical Instructor in Surgery, Division of Plastic Surgery, Harvard Medical School; Associate Surgeon, Massachusetts General Hospital; Attending Surgeon, Faulkner Hospital, Boston, New England Deaconess Hospital, Boston, and Mount Auburn Hospital, Cambridge, Massachusetts.

LEONARD A. SHARZER, M.D.
Clinical Professor of Plastic Surgery, Albert Einstein College of Medicine; Attending Surgeon, Montefiore Medical Center, Bronx, New York.

NATHANIEL M. SIMS, M.D.
Instructor in Anesthesia, Harvard Medical School; Assistant in Anesthesia, Massachusetts General Hospital, Boston, Massachusetts.

RICHARD J. SMITH, M.D. (deceased)
Clinical Professor of Orthopaedic Surgery, Harvard Medical School, Boston; Director of Hand Surgical Service, Department of Orthopaedic Surgery, Massachusetts General Hospital, Boston, Massachusetts.

JOSEPH UPTON, M.D.
Assistant Professor of Surgery, Harvard Medical School; Active Staff, Division of Plastic Surgery, Department of Surgery, Beth Israel Hospital and Children's Hospital, Boston, Massachusetts.

ALLEN L. VAN BEEK, M.D.
Clinical Assistant Professor of Surgery, University of Minnesota Medical School; Director of Microsurgery, North Memorial Medical Center, Minneapolis, Minnesota.

PAUL M. WEEKS, M.D.
Professor of Surgery (Plastic and Reconstructive), Washington University School of Medicine; Chief of Plastic Surgery, Barnes Hospital and St. Louis Children's Hospital, St. Louis, Missouri.

ANDREW J. WEILAND, M.D.
Professor, Department of Orthopaedic Surgery, Division of Plastic Surgery, and Department of Emergency Medicine, Johns Hopkins University School of Medicine, Baltimore, Maryland.

E. F. SHAW WILGIS, M.D.
Associate Professor of Plastic Surgery and of Orthopaedic Surgery, Johns Hopkins University School of Medicine; Chief, Division of Hand Surgery, Union Memorial Hospital, Baltimore, Maryland.

R. CHRISTIE WRAY, JR., M.D.
Professor of Surgery, University of Rochester School of Medicine and Dentistry; Plastic Surgeon in Chief, Strong Memorial Hospital, Rochester, New York.

EDUARDO A. ZANCOLLI, M.D.
Professor of Orthopaedics and Traumatology, Medical School of Buenos Aires; Chief of Orthopaedic Surgery of the Rehabilitation Center of Buenos Aires, Buenos Aires, Argentina.

ELVIN G. ZOOK, M.D.
Professor of Surgery and Chairman of the Division of Plastic Surgery, Southern Illinois University School of Medicine; Attending Surgeon, Memorial Medical Center and St. John's Hospital, Springfield, Illinois.

Preface

Were it not for the continuing expansion of knowledge, experience, and change, older textbooks would need no replacement. These two Hand Surgery volumes represent nearly one-fourth of the material contained in this edition of *Plastic Surgery,* a testament to the enormous contribution made by the subspecialty of hand surgery to the contemporary field of Plastic Surgery. It is of particular interest to compare this work of over 1300 pages with the 30 pages devoted to the hand in *Plastic Surgery,* the first American textbook on the subject by Dr. John Stage Davis, published in 1919.

The authors for these chapters were considered and selected with two criteria in mind: first, their personal experience of treating a large number of patients with hand problems related to their assigned topic, and second, their devotion to teaching and their accomplishments relative to the subject. The fact that the authors spent many hours of essential time in pursuit of this endeavor reflects a special will in making their expertise available in these comprehensive volumes. Each chapter is single authored and offers the undiluted experience of world class contributors; to them the credit and value of this work is due.

The content of the volumes on The Hand is organized into topic related chapters with an outline at the beginning of each one. This format should orient the reader throughout each volume of the book and within each chapter. Although no single part can be wholly comprehensive, each author has worked toward a sound basis for understanding the topic being discussed and has provided an extensive bibliography to assist in the pursuit of further information.

The opportunity to guide, contribute to, and edit a text in one's chosen field comes to few and is cherished by those who are selected. We thank Dr. Joseph McCarthy for the opportunity he provided by inviting us to edit these two volumes within this edition of *Plastic Surgery.* We also join our valued contributors in hoping that the content and organization of Hand Surgery will benefit and aid those physicians and surgeons who treat with knowledge, compassion, and precision the many patients of all ages with hand afflictions.

JAMES W. MAY, JR., M.D.
J. WILLIAM LITTLER, M.D.

Contents

Volume 7

The Hand (Part 1)

Volume *8*

The Hand (Part 2)

PLASTIC SURGERY

89

Robert A. Chase, M.D.

Examination of the Hand and Relevant Anatomy

During the Renaissance Vesalius corrected early misconceptions and brought gross anatomy into proper focus. Since that time many investigators have embellished the basic structural studies with functional, physiologic, and philosophical observations. The forearm and hand have been prominently included in those observations. Sir Charles Bell (1834), in his thought-provoking little volume *The Hand—Its Mechanism and Vital Endowments as Evincing Design,* presented a concept of hand anatomy that places it in proper context with man's position in the animal kingdom. Frederick Wood-Jones (1920) probed more extensively into comparative anatomy and anthropology in his excellent work *The Principles of Anatomy as Seen in the Hand.* Duchenne (1867) carried out detailed analysis of muscular function by isolated electrical stimulation, described in his classic volume *Physiologie des Mouvements.*

Allen B. Kanavel (1925) published his monograph *Infections of the Hand,* which reported detailed analysis of the spaces and synovial sheaths. *Surgery of the Hand* by Sterling Bunnell (1944) became an indispensable reference during World War II. Emanuel B. Kaplan (1953) produced the nicely illustrated, detailed volume *Functional and Surgical Anatomy of the Hand.* Detailed studies of the integration of the intrinsic and extrinsic muscles operating the polyarticular digits may be found in the work of Landsmeer (1949, 1955, 1958, 1963), Kaplan (1953), Eyler and Markee (1954), Stack (1963), Tubiana and Valentin (1963), and others.

As a functional puppet, the hand responds to the desires of man; its motor performance is initiated by the contralateral cerebral cortex. The conscious demands relayed to the hand and forearm from the central nervous controlling mechanism are sent as movement commands. At the subconscious levels, such a movement command is broken down, regrouped, coordinated, and sent on as a signal for fixation, graded contraction, or relaxation of a specific muscular unit. The degree of contraction or relaxation is then modified by relayed evidence that the motion created is that desired by the person. The modifying factors arrive centrally from a multiplicity of sensory sources such as the eye, peripheral sensory end organs, and muscle or joint sensory endings. The surgeon planning reconstructive surgery on the upper extremity must be aware not only of the complex anatomy of the hand and arm, but also of the physiologic interplay of balanced muscular functions under the influence of complex central nervous coordination. The maintenance of physiologic viability by the central and peripheral circulatory and lymphatic systems must also concern the reconstructive surgeon.

SKIN, SUBCUTANEOUS TISSUE, AND FASCIA

There is great disparity in the character of the integumentary envelope covering the dorsum of the hand and that covering the palm. Dorsal skin is thin and pliable, anchored to the deep investing fascia by loose, areolar tissue (Fig. 89–1). These characteristics, coupled with the fact that the major venous and lymphatic drainage in the hand courses dorsally, serve to explain that hand edema is first evident dorsally regardless of its cause. The prominent, visible veins in the subcutaneous tissue make it the standard site in which to evaluate venous filling and limb venous pressure on physical examination. The same characteristics make the dorsum of the hand vulnerable to skin avulsion injuries.

Palmar skin by contrast is characterized by a thick dermal layer and a heavily cornified epithelial surface. The skin is not as pliable as dorsal skin, and it is held tightly to the thick fibrous palmar fascia by diffusely distributed vertical fibers between the fascia and dermis. Stability of palmar skin is critical to hand function. At the same time, if scar fixation or loss of elasticity occurs in palmar skin, contractures and functional loss result. The skin of the palm is laden with a high concentration of specialized sensory end organs and sweat glands, the diagnostic importance of which is discussed under Peripheral Nerves (p. 4277).

The surgeon must understand the relationship of skin creases and the underlying joints in order to plan precise placement of skin incisions for exposure of joints and their related structures (Fig. 89–2).

Examination of hand skin during normal ranges of motion in various planes is important in planning incisions or geometrically rearranging lacerations that might result in disabling scar contractures. Absent a significant loss of skin from the dorsum of the hand and fingers, most loss of elasticity and some longitudinal shortening is compensated for quite adequately by mobility and elasticity of the uninjured dorsal skin. On the palmar aspect, however, scar shortening and inelasticity of the skin alone may result in contracture. The nature of palmar skin, its stabilizing fixation to the palmar fascia, and its position on the concave side of the hand are the bases for such contractures. Littler (1974) outlined the specific sites in the palm where longitudinal scar will impede extension (Fig. 89–3). For example, in each digit the geometry has been worked out by noting each joint

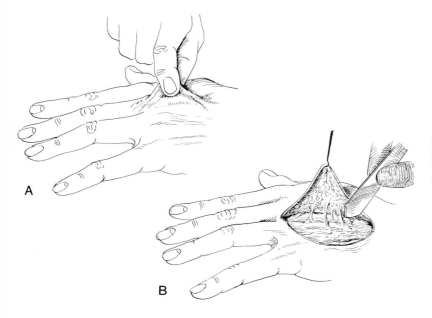

A

B

Figure 89–1. *A, B,* Dorsal skin is mobile as a result of the loose areolar subcutaneous fascia. It may be bluntly dissected and is subject to avulsion injuries.

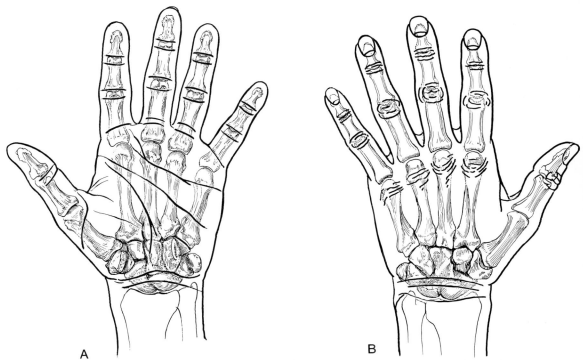

Figure 89–2. *A, B,* Palmar and dorsal skin creases and relationship to underlying joints. Note the fixed palmar creases resulting from skin fixation to the underlying palmar fascial plate by numerous vertical fibers. (From Chase, R. A.: Atlas of Hand Surgery. Vol. 1. Philadelphia, W. B. Saunders Company, 1973.)

axis and the kissing surfaces of the palmar skin in full flexion. These diamond-shaped skin surfaces should not be shortened and rendered inelastic by longitudinal scars if limitation of extension is to be avoided.

A host of systemic diseases are reflected in integumental findings in the hand (Bradburn and Chase, 1962). These signs may include ecchymosis, calcium depositions, circulatory and temperature changes, and alterations in skin texture.

Examination of the integument may also show evidence of tumor (see Chap. 133). Epithelial tumors are not infrequently complicated by the inflammatory signs of secondary infection. Tumors of the deep structures may be manifested by distortion of the integumental contour. They are readily palpated and their relation to the skin may cause fixation. Color changes are characteristic of some vascular tumors. Arteriovenous intercommunications elevate the temperature of the area and discolor and distort the surface; often a thrill can be felt and a bruit heard over the lesion.

In hand injuries and during transfer of composite tissues either by pedicle techniques or by free transfer with immediate revascu-

larization, the skin may be the best monitor site for evaluation of vascular perfusion. The examination is enhanced and is made more objective through use of pulse oximeter technology, intravenous fluoroscein and Wood's lamp, or electronic fluoroscanning devices (Graham and associates, 1984).

Palmar Fascia

The palmar fascia consists of resistant, fibrous tissue arranged in longitudinal, transverse, oblique, and vertical fibers. The longitudinal fibers concentrate at the proximal origin of the palmar fascia at the wrist, taking origin from the palmaris longus when it is present (in about 80 to 85 per cent of individuals). The fascia at this level is separable from the underlying flexor retinaculum, being identified by the longitudinal orientation of its fibers in contrast to the transverse fibers of the retinaculum. The palmar fascia fibers fan out from this origin, concentrating in flat bundles to each of the digits. Generally, the fibers spread at the base of each digit and send minor fibers to the skin and the bulk of fibers distal into the fingers, where they at-

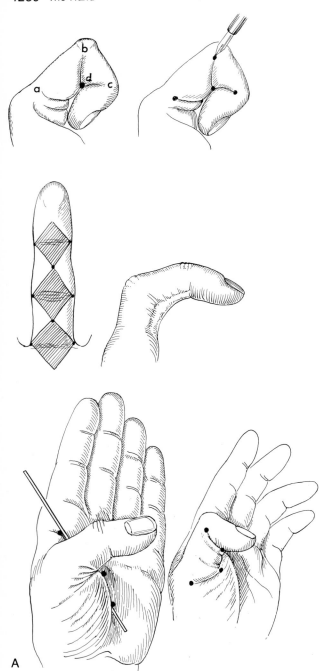

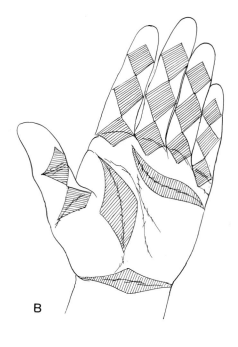

Figure 89–3. A, B, Schematic representation of the joint axes. The longitudinal dimensions in the midpalmar and middorsal aspect of the digits change maximally. The midaxial line through the three joint axes does not change in length with flexion and extension. Palmar incisions placed longitudinally produce contracture if they pass across the palmar diamonds delineated by lines joining the joint axes (after Littler). Transverse incisions avoid the occurrence of flexion scar contractures. The same principle applies at the wrist. (From Chase, R. A.: Atlas of Hand Surgery. Vol. 1. Philadelphia, W. B. Saunders Company, 1973.)

tach to tissues making up the fibrous flexor sheath of the digits. There are attachments of the fascia to the palmar plate and intermetacarpal ligaments at each side of the flexor tendon sheath at the level of the metacarpal heads.

Transverse fibers are concentrated in the midpalm and the web spaces. The midpalmar transverse fibers, although intimately asso-

ciated with the longitudinal bundles, lie deep to them and are inseparable from the vertical fibers that concentrate into septa between the longitudinally oriented structures passing to the fingers. This system of palmar transverse fibers makes up what Skoog (1967) called the transverse palmar ligament. In fact, the transverse fibers form the roof of tunnels at this point that act as pulleys for the flexor

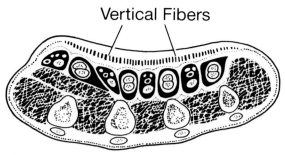

Figure 89–4. The palmar fascia with its longitudinal, transverse, and vertical fibers. The longitudinal fibers take origin in the palmaris longus (when present). Transverse fibers are concentrated in the distal palm supporting the web skin and in the midpalm as the transverse palmar ligament. Vertical fibers extend superficially as multiple, tiny tethering strands to stabilize the thick palmar skin. The deep vertical components concentrate in septa between the longitudinally oriented structures to the fingers.

tendons proximal to the level of the digital pulleys. Longitudinal fibers pass toward the palmar surface of the thumb, but these fibers are generally less numerous and sometimes difficult to identify. The thumb fibers blend into the deep fascia overlying the thenar muscles. The ulnar extreme palmar fascia blends with the hypothenar fascia. The prox-

imal one-third of this border is the attachment site of the palmaris brevis muscle. Laterally, the muscle attaches to the hypothenar skin and hypothenar fascia.

The vertical fibers of the palmar fascia, which lie superficially to the tough triangular membrane made up by the longitudinal and transverse fibers, consist of the abundant vertical fibers to the palm skin dermis. Deep to the palmar fascial plate, the vertical fibers coalesce into septa, forming compartments for flexor tendons to each digit and separate compartments for the neurovascular bundles together with the lumbrical muscles. There are eight such compartments, which extend proximally to about the midpalm. Proximal to this, there is a common central compartment (Bojsen-Moller and Schmidt, 1974). The marginal septa extend more proximally than the seven intermediate septa closing the central compartment laterally and medially. The major septum between the index flexor tendons and the neurovascular and lumbrical space to the third interspace attaches to the third metacarpal, dividing the thenar or adductor space from the midpalmar space (Fig. 89–4).

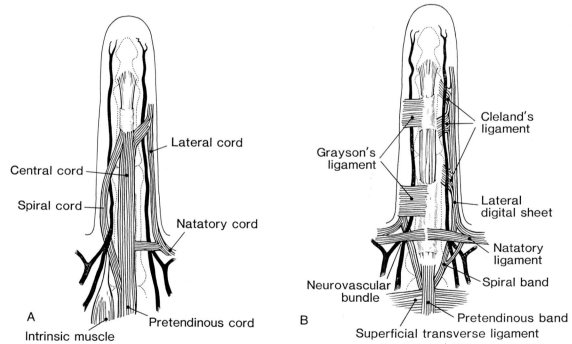

Figure 89–5. A, B, The components of the digital fascia that help to anchor the axial plane skin are Grayson's ligaments palmar to the neurovascular bundles and Cleland's ligaments dorsal to the bundles. These fibers, as well as the web or rotatory ligaments and the spiral bands of palmar fascia, may become involved with Dupuytren's contracture. Spiral cords may extend from the pretendinous band at the metacarpophalangeal joint level to pass dorsal, then palmar to the neurovascular bundle before inserting at the midphalanx level. (Modified from McFarlane.)

Fibers extending into the fingers arrive at points of attachment to the fibrous flexor sheath and digital fascia by several routes. The central cord remains pretendinous and passes distal to the proximal interphalangeal (PIP) joint to attach to the thick fibrous flexor sheath, usually at the A_4 pulley. Rarely, fibers pass beyond the distal interphalangeal joint.

At the level of the metacarpophalangeal (MCP) joint, fibers extend down each side of the flexor tendon sheath as spiral bands passing superficially or deep to the proper digital artery and nerve. Frequently these bands extend dorsally to the neurovascular bundle at the base of the finger, then curl back around the bundle before crossing the proximal interphalangeal joint. They are referred to as spiral cords (Fig. 89–5) (McFarlane, 1974, 1982). Isolated digital cords may become prominent as a cause of proximal interphalangeal joint contracture in Dupuytren's contracture (Strickland and Bassett, 1985).

BONES AND JOINTS

The ability of the hand to resist and create powerful gross action, combined with its capacity to perform intricate fine movements in multiple planes, reflects the masterful construction of its supporting architecture. Reducing the hand to its supporting skeleton and its restraining ligaments reveals the architectural basis for its varied function. A study of the range of joint motions in the hand and forearm with all motor elements removed discloses the full range and limitations that the skeleton imposes on hand function.

The hand skeleton is divisible into four elements, in descending order of specialization (Fig. 89–6):

1. *The thumb* and its *metacarpal* with a wide range of motion at the carpometacarpal joint. Five intrinsic muscles and four extrinsic muscles are specifically influential on thumb positioning and activity.

2. *The index digit* with independence of action within the range of motion allowed by its joints and ligaments. Three intrinsic and four extrinsic muscles allow such digital independence.

3. *The third, fourth, and fifth digits with the fourth and fifth metacarpals.* This unit functions as a stabilizing vise to grasp objects for manipulation by the thumb and index

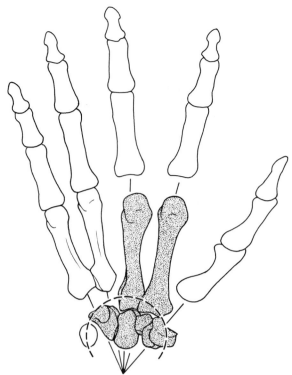

Figure 89–6. Exploded view of functional elements of the hand. The hand is a composite of four elements of descending order of specialization: (1) the thumb with its metacarpal with wide range of motion at the carpometacarpal saddle joint; (2) the index digit with its independence of function in several planes; (3) the third, fourth, and fifth digits with metacarpals 4 and 5, which work as a unit on the ulnar aspect of the hand; and (4) the fixed unit or backbone of the hand, consisting of the carpals with the fixed transverse carpal arch and the central, second, and third metacarpals forming a fixed longitudinal arch projecting from the carpus.

finger, or in concert with the other hand units in powerful grasp.

4. *The fixed unit of the hand* consisting of *the second and third metacarpals and the distal carpal row.*

FIXED UNIT OF THE HAND

The distal row of carpal bones forms a solid architectural arch with the capitate bone as a keystone. The articulations of the distal carpals with one another, the intercarpal ligaments, and the important volar carpal ligament (flexor retinaculum) maintain a strong, fixed transverse carpal arch. Projecting distally from the central third of this arch are the fixed central metacarpals, the second and third. Littler called this "the fixed unit of the is a lot of slack in the joint capsule, allowing a wide range of motion, including joint distraction of up to 3 mm (Kuczynski, 1974).

A detailed study of the dynamic contribution of various muscles producing the range of motion of the metacarpotrapezial joint within the constraints imposed by the joint surfaces and the capsular ligaments was presented as a doctoral thesis by Chin Jen Ou (1980).

Ligaments Surrounding the Metacarpotrapezial Joint

An important stabilizing capsular ligament is the anterior oblique carpometacarpal ligament referred to above (Fig. 89–11). It extends like the leg of a person seated in the trapezial saddle extending from the "beak" of the first metacarpal to the anterior crest of the trapezium and adjacent intercarpal ligaments. It retains the fragment of bone fractured free from the base of the metacarpal as the metacarpal displaces radially in Bennett's fracture. In advanced metacarpotrapezial joint arthritis it weakens and attenuates, as also does the intermetacarpal ligament, allowing radial subluxation of the metacarpotrapezial joint (Dahhan, Fischer, and Alliey, 1980; Tubiana, 1985).

The ligament at the radial border of the joint is like a radial collateral ligament and is referred to as the dorsoradial or anteroexternal ligament. Thus, the radial side of the joint support is the right anteroexternal ligament, which inserts close to but beneath the insertion of the abductor pollicis longus on the radial base of the first metacarpal. It

forms part of the joint capsule and then attaches to the anterior crest of the trapezium. Dorsally, one sees the posterior oblique ligament crossing the dorsal joint capsule from the radially positioned posteroexternal tubercle of the trapezium to attach to the ulnar base of the first metacarpal.

There is a stout intermetacarpal ligament between the base of the first metacarpal and the adjacent base of the second metacarpal, and good evidence that this ligament together with the anterior oblique or deep ulnar ligament is a key to prevention of radial subluxation of the metacarpotrapezial joint, as seen in arthroses of the joint (Pagalidis, Kuczynski, and Lamb, 1981).

Function and range of motion within the limits imposed by these ligaments is influenced by the extrinsic and intrinsic muscles of the thumb and the external forces applied to the thumb.

Metacarpophalangeal Joint

(Harris and Joseph, 1949; Joseph, 1951; Kaplan, 1966) The first metacarpophalangeal joint is in most respects similar to the other metacarpophalangeal joints. It differs in several respects, however, in both anatomic make-up and function. Generally, the first metacarpophalangeal joint range of motion in flexion and extension, as well as abduction and adduction, is less than that in the finger metacarpophalangeal joints. The metacarpal and proximal phalanx are more stout in order to accommodate to greater forces normally borne by the thumb in pinching and grasping. The head of the first metacarpal is different

Figure 89–11. Palmar view shows the (1) anterior oblique carpometacarpal ligament, (2) dorsoradial or anteroexternal ligament, (3) joint capsule, and (4) intermetacarpal ligament. Dorsal view shows the (1) posterior oblique ligament and (2) joint capsule.

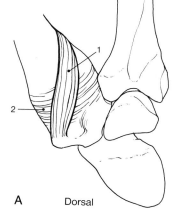

A   Dorsal

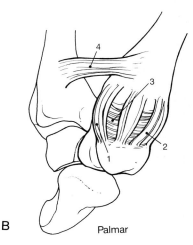

B   Palmar

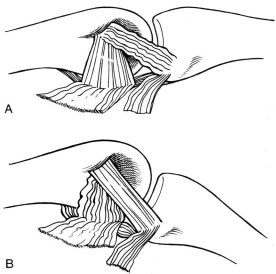

Figure 89–12. *A, B,* Metacarpophalangeal joint collateral ligaments. With the joint extended, the metacarpophalangeal joint component of the collateral ligament is loose, and that from the metacarpal to the palmar plate is taut. Lateral movement is possible in extension. In flexion, the metacarpophalangeal joint collateral ligament is taut, and that to the palmar plate is loose. Thus, no lateral movement is possible in metacarpophalangeal flexion. (Redrawn from Aubriot, J. H.: The metacarpophalangeal joint of the thumb. *In* Tubiana, R. (Ed.): The Hand. Philadelphia, W. B. Saunders Company, 1981, p. 187.)

because the radial articular prominence is larger than the ulnar. The articular surface of the proximal phalanx is fashioned reciprocally to match.

The collateral ligaments are similar to those of finger metacarpophalangeal joints. The metacarpophalangeal portion is taut in flexion and looser in extension. In extension the portion of the fanlike collateral ligaments to the palmar plate is taut; thus, adduction and abduction is limited in both extension and flexion (Fig. 89–12) (Aubriot, 1981). Some pronation but no supination is allowed at the metacarpophalangeal joint when it is in extension. In supination the joint locks into a stable position for secure grasping.

The sturdy fibrocartilaginous palmar plate (the glenoid ligament) of the metacarpophalangeal joint extends from the palmar base of the proximal phalanx to the neck of the metacarpal. It regularly incorporates two sesamoid bones, one medial and one lateral to the flexor pollicis longus (Fig. 89–13).

Interphalangeal Joint

The nature of the condyle of the proximal phalanx of the interphalangeal joint is such that upon flexion of the joint, pronation of the distal phalanx occurs.

THE WRIST

The wrist joint is the site for major postural change between the arm beam and the working hand end piece. It has a multiarticulated architecture that creates a potentially wide range of motion in flexion, extension, radial deviation, ulnar deviation, and circumduction. The most extensive range of motion occurs at the radiocarpal joint. The distal radius presents a shallow articular surface that is concave from radial to ulnar extremes, as well as in the dorsal to palmar projection. Its articular junction with the distal ulna presents a concave surface in a third plane that allows rotation of the radius around the ulna in supination and pronation. The hand rotates with the distal radius.

The navicular and lunate bones of the proximal carpal row form the convex articular counterparts of the concave distal radius for the major wrist articulation.

All four of the bones in the distal carpal row present articular surfaces for junction with the metacarpals. The distal carpal row forms a solid architectural arch with the central capitate as the keystone. The nature of the articulations of the distal carpals with one another, and of the carpal ligament (flexor retinaculum), is such that they make up a strong and fixed transverse carpal arch.

The wrist is a very complex series of joints, the anatomy and function of which have been under intense study during the last decade. The enormous amount of data and the detailed morphologic information form the basis for a number of books devoted exclusively to the wrist. It is beyond the scope of this volume to describe the details of wrist morphology and function; interested readers should explore the monograph by Taleisnik (1985).

EXAMINATION OF THE SKELETAL SYSTEM

Examination of the skeletal system is concerned with bones, joints, and the related fascial investments. Chronic disorders are to a great extent related to secondary joint disease. Persistent osteomyelitis and nonunion, in contrast to malunion, are uncommon in metacarpals and phalanges. In any acutely injured patient with a closed wound, painful swelling, ecchymosis, crepitation, and pos-

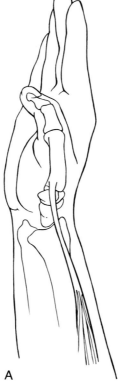

Figure 89–18. *A, B,* The abductor pollicis longus radially abducts the first metacarpal and aids in radial deviation of the wrist. It often sends a band or two into the fascia of the abductor pollicis brevis. (Redrawn from Chase, R. A.: Atlas of Hand Surgery. Vol. 1. Philadelphia, W. B. Saunders Company, 1973.)

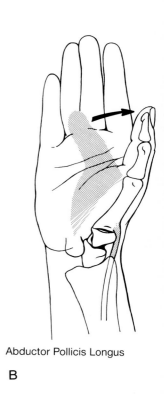

Abductor Pollicis Longus

A

B

sheath that has thickened areas (see Retinacular System, p. 4265). The tendons at this level are surrounded by synovial sheaths (Fig. 89–22). The flexor pollicis longus is the interphalangeal flexor of the thumb equivalent to the finger profundi.

The flexor digitorum profundus is the only muscle that flexes the distal interphalangeal joint. Testing for profundus function requires observation of active flexion of the distal interphalangeal joint.

Selected flexion of one or more of the metacarpophalangeal joints, or either the proximal or distal interphalangeal joint, depends on stabilizing fixation of the remainder by flexor-extensor interplay. Elimination of any single motor element reduces the selective adaptability of a finger (Fig. 89–23).

As noted above, a muscle may positively influence any joint between its site of origin and its insertion. The flexor digitorum profundus muscle originates in the forearm, and its tendon therefore bridges the wrist joint, the metacarpophalangeal joint, the proximal interphalangeal joint, and the distal interphalangeal joint before it inserts on the distal phalanx. It may flex any of these joints, depending on the dynamic fixation of the

others. Fixation of the distal interphalangeal joint converts the profundus tendon into a functional superficialis tendon by recessing its prime site of action to the proximal interphalangeal joint. By combined fixation of any of the joints, the profundus tendon may primarily flex any selected one.

It is intriguing to realize that under certain conditions the flexor profundus may accentuate extension of the proximal interphalangeal joint. The profundus pulling primarily at the distal interphalangeal joint may flex it acutely. In flexing the distal interphalangeal joint, the insertion of the extensor mechanism is advanced distally. This advancement, combined with either a contraction or fixation of the lateral bands, results in extension of the proximal interphalangeal joint. This effect is easily aborted by the intact flexor superficialis, whose prime flexion function is exerted on the proximal interphalangeal joint. Absence of the superficialis, whether occasioned by injury or by tendon graft replacement of the profundus only, results not infrequently in flexion of the distal interphalangeal joint with recurvatum deformity at the proximal interphalangeal joint. This can be corrected by fusion of the distal

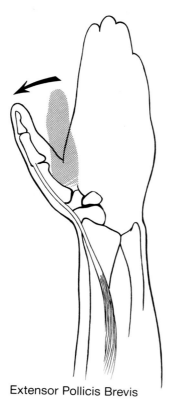

Extensor Pollicis Brevis

Figure 89–19. The extensor pollicis brevis travels with the abductor pollicis longus and inserts into the proximal phalanx, thus acting as an extensor of the metacarpophalangeal joint in addition to aiding the abductor pollicis longus. (Redrawn from Chase, R. A.: Atlas of Hand Surgery. Vol. 1. Philadelphia, W. B. Saunders Company, 1973.)

interphalangeal joint, making the profundus a functional superficialis, or by tenodesis or capsulodesis of the proximal interphalangeal joint in mild flexion. It is wise to keep in mind the innumerable functional circumstances that can be created by selective interplay of multiple motor forces exerted through a series of interdependent joints (Stack, 1963).

FLEXOR TENDONS AND ASSOCIATED RETINACULA

The gross anatomic configuration and function of the extrinsic digital flexor tendons have been known since antiquity. The great growth in our knowledge and understanding of functional biomechanics, muscle physiology, tendon nutrition, and blood supply has influenced the management of problems involving these important flexor tendons.

The long flexor tendons cross multiple joints. The tendon-muscle unit has an effect on each joint it crosses, which is altered by the positioning of the other joints in the linkage system. Thus, the influence of the long flexor tendon on one joint in the system is augmented by the function of its antagonists at each of the other joints it crosses. For example, a digital flexor tendon aids in flexing the wrist, but its flexion capability within the digit at the metacarpophalangeal joints and interphalangeal joints is increased by wrist extension using wrist extensors, which in fact are antagonists to the digital flexors at the wrist. This is the simplified definition of synergistic function—finger flexion augmented by wrist extension, and vice versa.

Synergistic and antagonistic groups of muscles in hand function must be considered when functional substitution by tendon transfers is contemplated. Obviously, certain

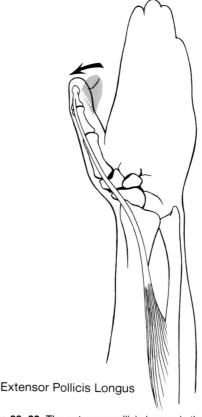

Extensor Pollicis Longus

Figure 89–20. The extensor pollicis longus is the primary extensor of the interphalangeal joint of the thumb. Secondarily, it may extend and dorsally abduct the metacarpophalangeal joint and the metacarpotrapezial joints. (Redrawn from Chase, R. A.: Atlas of Hand Surgery. Vol. 1. Philadelphia, W. B. Saunders Company, 1973.)

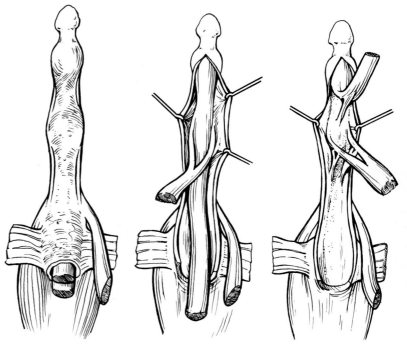

Figure 89–21. The profundus and superficialis flexors lie within the digital sheath. The superficialis divides to allow passage of the profundus, then decussates and inserts on the middle phalanx. The profundus continues and inserts on the distal phalanx. (Redrawn from Chase, R. A.: Atlas of Hand Surgery. Vol. 2. Philadelphia, W. B. Saunders Company, 1984.)

groups of muscles have developed functional synergism, which makes readjustment natural when one group is transferred to take on the function of the other. Examples of such natural synergism are the united functions of the wrist flexors and digital flexors or the wrist extensors and digital flexors.

In its course from forearm to fingers, the digital profundus flexor crosses the palmar aspect of the wrist joint, the metacarpophalangeal joint, and the interphalangeal joints. The relationship of the tendon to the joint axes is maintained by retinacular structures, or pulleys. This prevents the bowstring effect, which would allow the tendon to move away from the joint axis, changing the moment arm and therefore the force exerted at that joint by the flexor tendon. The finely balanced relationship between the flexor muscle-tendon unit at each joint in the series may be disrupted by such a change. Such alterations can be compensated for, to some extent, by graded, proportional changes in the controlled power of antagonists, but the physiologic balance may be interfered with.

Retinacular System

Wrist Pulley. The large, restraining pulley at the wrist, which serves all the long digital flexors, is the transverse carpal ligament (Fig. 89–24). It bridges the volar surface of the carpals from the pisiform and hook of the

Figure 89–22. The extrinsic flexor tendons of the fingers lie within fixed fibrous tunnels at the wrist and within the digit. (From Chase, R. A., and Laub, D. R.: The hand. Therapeutic strategy for acute problems. Curr. Probl. Surg., *1*:64, 1966.)

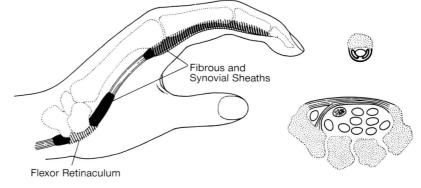

Fibrous and Synovial Sheaths

Flexor Retinaculum

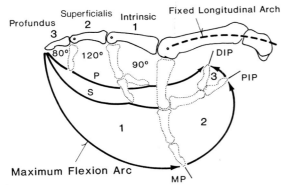

Figure 89–23. The flexion arc. In isolated injuries to the flexor profundus in which the flexor superficialis is fully functional, the greatest part of the flexion arc is maintained (denoted by areas 1 and 2 at bottom of illustration). Restoration of active profundus function provides only that portion of the arc denoted by the small area 3 (right center). (Redrawn from Littler, J. W.: The physiology and dynamic function of the hand. Surg. Clin. North Am., *40*:259, 1960.)

hamate medially to the navicular tuberosity and trapezium laterally. It confines the long flexor tendons and median nerve within the carpal tunnel, and prevents bowstringing of the long flexor tendons at the wrist.

Thumb Pulleys. Three pulleys housing the flexor pollicis longus within the thumb are regularly present (Fig. 89–24). The proximal annular pulley is at the level of the metacarpophalangeal joint arising from the volar plate and base of the proximal phalanx. The distal annular pulley is located over the volar plate of the interphalangeal joint. Between the two is a single oblique pulley that originates proximally on the ulnar side of the middle phalanx, where it also gains fibers from the adductor pollicis before it extends to the middle one-third of the radial palmar surface of the middle phalanx.

Finger Pulleys. Four or five discrete annular pulleys and three cruciate bands are ordinarily present in the fingers (Fig. 89–24). The most proximal pulley (A_1) begins 0.5 cm proximal to the metacarpophalangeal joint. It is anchored to the volar plate and the proximal phalanx. Just distal to it is the second annular band (A_2), which is the largest pulley, extending to nearly the proximal one-half of the proximal phalanx. The first cruciform band (C_1) lies distal to A_2 and well proximal to the proximal interphalangeal joint. The third annular pulley (A_3) lies over the proximal interphalangeal joint arising from its volar plate. The second cruciate ligament (C_2) is at the base of the middle pha-

lanx. The fourth annular pulley (A_4) lies over the middle one-third of the middle phalanx, and just distal to it is the third cruciate (C_3). Often it is possible to identify thickening of the sheath over the distal interphalangeal joint, which, when present, is designated the fifth annular pulley (A_5).

The pulleys are strategically placed to maintain the relationship of the flexor tendons to the axis of each finger joint, thus preventing the bowstring effect. The gaps between pulleys allow unrestrained flexion and extension of the joints by folding and pleating of the thin sheath between pulleys. Note the wrinkling of the darkly stained synovium between the pulleys in Figure 89–24D. The gaps also allow dynamic change in the moment arms when the finger is actively flexed against resistance (Doyle and Blythe, 1975, 1977; Hunter and associates, 1980). Strauch and Maura (1985) noted variations in standard pulley and blood supply patterns, and suggested a change in nomenclature.

Synovial Sheaths (Fig. 4–1A)

The synovial sheaths are closed sacs around the tendons composed of a visceral layer on the tendon surface and a parietal layer on the fibrous sheath surface. The thumb synovial sheath is continuous from the wrist to the distal extreme of the flexor pollicis longus. The digital synovial sheaths for the index, long, and ring fingers usually start at the level of the distal palmar crease and extend to the distal interphalangeal joints. Often the little finger sheath extends more proximally to communicate with a common sheath around the finger flexors and then across the wrist to the distal forearm, where tendons pass through the carpal tunnel.

Mesotenon and Vincula

During embryonic development, synovial sacs form where the flexor tendons are subject to restraint by retinacula. The tendon invaginates into the sac, creating a two-layered, closed synovial membrane around the tendon. The tendon carries its segmental nutrient vessels, and thus with invagination a mesentery-like mesotenon is formed. As time passes, and where the tendon has great excursion in relationship to adjacent bone, the

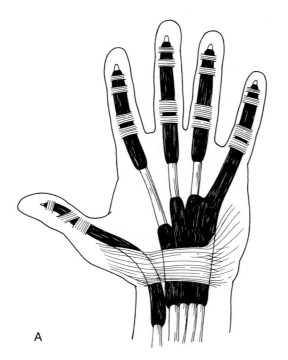

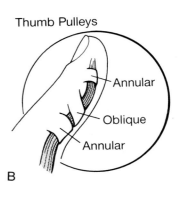

Thumb Pulleys

Finger Pulleys

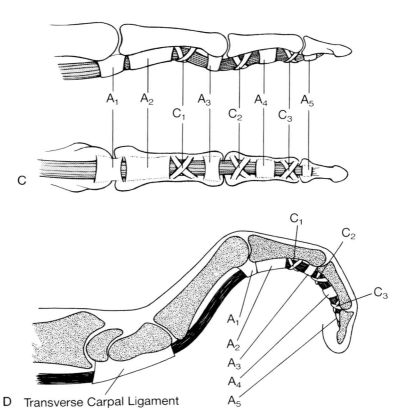

D   Transverse Carpal Ligament

Figure 89–24. *A to D,* The flexor tendon pulley system for fingers and thumb. (From Chase, R. A.: Atlas of Hand Surgery. Vol. 2. Philadelphia, W. B. Saunders Company, 1984.)

Vincula

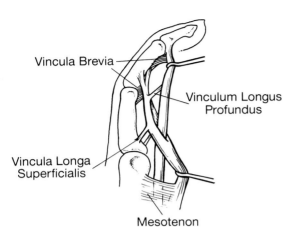

Figure 89–25. The common configuration of the vincula. (From Chase, R. A.: Atlas of Hand Surgery. Vol. 2. Philadelphia, W. B. Saunders Company, 1984.)

mesentery refines itself to tiny, flexible bands, or vincula (Fig. 89–25). At the sites of insertion, where differential motion between the bone and tendon is least, the mesenteric configuration persists, as it does for flexor tendons in the hand outside the confining tunnels. The vincula brevia form the residual mesotenon at the sites of insertion of the profundus and superficialis tendons on the phalanges. The vincula longa are the flexible, vessel-carrying bands to each tendon in the area where the complete mesotenon has disappeared.

Tendon Nutrition

Because the cell population of tendons is sparse, metabolic demand is low and cells can survive with minimal nutritional support. The longitudinal blood supply to a tendon comes from its musculotendinous junction and its insertion site into bone. The segmental blood supply derives from the mesotenon where a mesotenon exists and from the vincula within the digital sheaths.

It is now clear that synovial fluid within the sheath supplies nutrition to the tendon much as synovial fluid in a joint supports cartilage. This fact has altered thinking about the necessity for adhesion formation to ensure cell survival within a lacerated tendon stripped of blood supply or within tendon grafts.

FLEXOR TENDON ZONES

On the basis of the anatomy of the flexor tendons and the associated synovial and fibrous sheaths, the area traversed by the tendons is divided into clinically important zones (Fig. 89–26).

Zone 1. Zone 1 is the area traversed by the flexor digitorum profundus distal to the insertion of the flexor digitorum superficialis on the middle phalanx.

Zone 2. Zone 2 extends from the proximal end of Zone 1 to the proximal end of the digital fibrous sheath. It is subdivided into distal, middle, and proximal components.

Distal. The distal portion extends from the insertion of the superficialis on the middle phalanx deep to the profundus to the proximal end of the A_3 pulley.

Middle. The middle component extends from the proximal end of the A_3 pulley to the distal end of A_2. The roof of the sheath in this zone consists only of synovial sheath and the C_1 cruciate ligament.

Proximal. The proximal portion extends from the distal end of A_2 to the proximal end of A_1, a tunnel covered by the tough A_1 and A_2 pulley system.

Zone 3. Zone 3 is the area traversed by the flexor tendons in the palm and is free of

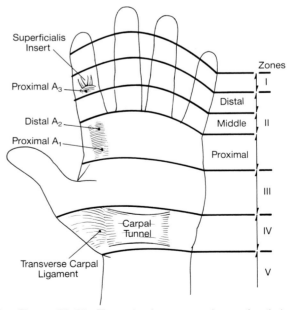

Figure 89–26. Flexor tendon zones chosen for their relevance to flexor tendon injuries. (Redrawn from Chase, R. A.: Atlas of Hand Surgery. Vol. 2. Philadelphia, W. B. Saunders Company, 1984.)

fibrous pulleys. It extends, therefore, from the proximal end of the finger pulley system (A₁) to the distal end of the wrist retinaculum, the transverse carpal ligament.

Zone 4. Zone 4 is the carpal tunnel. It extends from the distal to the proximal borders of the transverse carpal ligament.

Zone 5. Zone 5 extends from the proximal border of the transverse carpal ligament to the musculotendinous junctions of the flexor tendon.

EXAMINATION OF EXTRINSIC FLEXORS

The function of the flexor digitorum profundus can be confined by active flexion of the distal interphalangeal joint. It is the only flexor of this joint.

Since a muscle-tendon unit affects every joint between its origin and insertion, the flexor digitorum profundus may also flex the proximal interphalangeal joint. This makes the diagnosis of superficialis nonfunction more difficult. Each superficialis flexor has its own muscle belly, and each acts independently of the others. The profundus flexors are not as independent, since there is a common muscle for the long, ring, and little finger profundus tendons, and a variable degree of interconnection between these and the index finger profundus. The diagnosis of disruption of flexor digitorum superficialis function is confirmed by check-reining the profundus by holding the other fingers in extension while the patient actively attempts to flex the finger whose superficialis is being tested (Fig. 89–27).

Flexion of the finger at the proximal interphalangeal joint while the distal interphalangeal joint remains loosely extended confirms the functional integrity of the flexor digitorum superficialis.

The thumb, with only two phalanges, has no need for two long flexor tendons. The single flexor pollicis longus bridges all the thumb joints and the wrist joint.

Because the flexor pollicis longus bridges all these joints, it may influence any one by selected fixation of the others. Like the profundus, it may extend its sphere of action beyond that of pure flexion. For example, acute flexion of the interphalangeal joint by the flexor pollicis longus may potentiate an opponens pollicis transfer inserted into the thumb extensor mechanism. It does so by moving the insertion of the opponens transfer distally, thereby increasing its total effectiveness.

The flexor profundi to the third, fourth, and fifth fingers work from a common muscle belly. Acting in unison, they fit the architectural concept of this unit as a stable vise for grasping objects. The independent function of the index profundus frees the index finger for use with the thumb to manipulate an object grasped by the viselike ulnar unit. Independence of action is well developed in the superficialis muscles and the intrinsic muscles.

FINGER INTRINSIC MUSCLES

The interosseous muscles function as ulnar and radial deviators of the fingers as well as

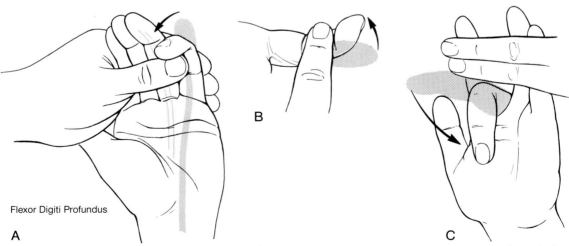

Flexor Digiti Profundus

A **B** **C**

Figure 89–27. Testing for profundus and superficialis function. Note check-reining of the profundus tendon to isolate superficialis function. (Redrawn from Chase, R. A.: Atlas of Hand Surgery. Vol. 2. Philadelphia, W. B. Saunders Company, 1984.)

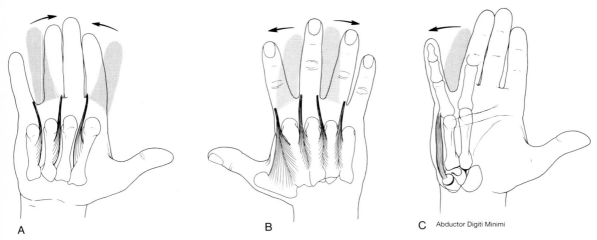

Figure 89–28. *A* to *C,* Function of the palmar interossei to adduct fingers toward the central axis of the hand—the midline of the long finger. Function of the dorsal interossei to abduct the fingers from this line; thus, the second and third dorsal interossei move the long finger radially and ulnarly, respectively. The abductor digiti minimi acts to abduct the little finger acting as a fifth dorsal interosseous muscle. (Redrawn from Chase, R. A.: Atlas of Hand Surgery. Vol. 1. Philadelphia, W. B. Saunders Company, 1973.)

flexors of the metacarpophalangeal joints and extensors of the interphalangeal joints. The dorsal interossei act as abductors from the axis of the hand, which falls in the middle of the long finger. The long finger moves both radially and ulnarly under the influence of the second and third dorsal interossei (Fig. 89–28). The abductor digiti minimi is the dorsal interosseous equivalent of the little fingers.

The palmar interossei adduct the fingers to the hand axis.

The pull of all the interossei palmar to the axis of the metacarpophalangeal joints and dorsal to the interphalangeal joint axis acts to flex the metacarpophalangeal joints and extend the interphalangeal joints. The position assumed is called the "intrinsic plus" posture (Fig. 89–29).

A study of the balance of motors around the digital joints is not only fascinating but most rewarding, since it leads to a better understanding of the changes in adaptability caused by selective paralyses.

The tiny lumbrical muscles harmonize function between the lateral band interphalangeal extensor mechanism and the flexor digitorum profundus. They have a moving site of origin from the profundus tendon and are generally innervated by the same nerve that innervates the corresponding profundus (the ulnar two are innervated by the ulnar nerve and the radial two are innervated by the median nerve, as are the profundi). As

the flexor profundus contracts, the lumbrical origin moves proximally. At the same time the lumbrical insertion moves distally as the extensor is advanced by interphalangeal flex-

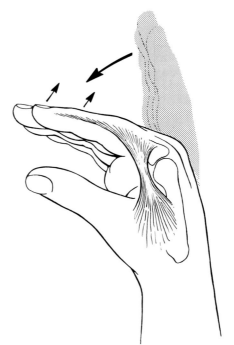

Figure 89–29. All interossei act as prime flexors of the metacarpophalangeal joints since they pass palmar to the joint axis. Extensions into the lateral bands result in extension of the interphalangeal joints. (Redrawn from Chase, R. A.: Atlas of Hand Surgery. Vol. 1. Philadelphia, W. B. Saunders Company, 1973.)

ion. The effective separation of its insertion and origin makes the lumbrical more effective in flexing the metacarpophalangeal joint. Conversely, with a change in balance of power, the lumbrical tends to pull the profundus distally as it shortens the lateral bands. This combination of profundus relaxation and lateral band pull results in extension at the interphalangeal joints.

EXAMINATION OF INTRINSIC MUSCLES

Examination of the hand for finger intrinsic function requires little more than an understanding of the anatomy described above and its related function. Function of the interossei may be assessed by asking the patient to adduct and abduct the fingers from the hand axis in the middle of the long finger. The

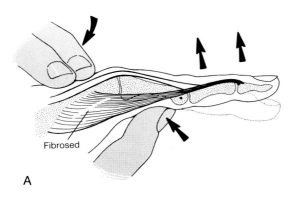

A

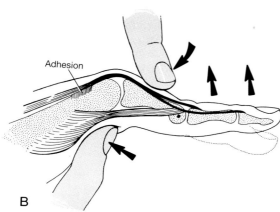

B

Figure 89–30. *A, B,* Testing for tightness or shortening of the interosseous muscles as a cause of passive extension contracture of the interphalangeal joint. The metacarpophalangeal joint is passively extended and the interphalangeal joints passively extend. If the cause of extensor tightness at the interphalangeal joint is a result of long extensor adhesions to the metacarpal, the interphalangeal joints will passively extend on passive flexion of the metacarpophalangeal joint. (Redrawn from Chase, R. A.: Atlas of Hand Surgery. Vol. 2. Philadelphia, W. B. Saunders Company, 1984.)

ability to flex the metacarpophalangeal joints with the interphalangeal joints extended ("intrinsic plus" posture) confirms interosseous function. Paralysis is reflected by clawing of the fingers with hyperextension of the metacarpophalangeal joints and flexion of the interphalangeal joints on attempts actively to extend the fingers ("intrinsic minus").

Lumbrical function is best reflected by having the patient fully flex the finger (extrinsic flexor function), then move the finger smoothly into extension at the interphalangeal joints while holding active flexion at the metacarpophalangeal joint.

Tightness or contracture of the interossei results in inability actively or passively to flex the interphalangeal joints while the metacarpophalangeal joint is extended. Inability to flex the interphalangeal joints may be a result of fixation of the extrinsic extensor tendons proximal to the metacarpophalangeal joint. Testing to differentiate these two possible etiologies is done by passively extending, then passively flexing the metacarpophalangeal joint while assessing the degree of passive extension of the interphalangeal joints. If the interphalangeal joints passively extend when the metacarpophalangeal joint is extended, the interosseous muscle and tendon are short. If by contrast the interphalangeal joints extend when the metacarpophalangeal joint is passively flexed, the extrinsic extensor is adherent proximal to the metacarpophalangeal joint (Fig. 89–30).

THENAR AND HYPOTHENAR MUSCLES

With the hand axis or fixed unit in position the metacarpal arch is adjusted primarily by the thenar and the hypothenar muscle groups. The median nerve generally innervates all the thenar muscles on the radial side of the flexor pollicis longus. These two and one-half muscles (the abductor pollicis brevis, opponens pollicis, and superficial head of the flexor pollicis brevis) are positioning muscles that act to bring the first metacarpal into palmar abduction, thus increasing the concavity of the transverse metacarpal arch. This in turn prepares the thumb for proper pulp to pulp opposition with the fingers.

The thumb is steadied in position by contraction of the antagonist muscles to the abductors and the thumb adductor (Fig. 89–31). Both the adductors and the abductors

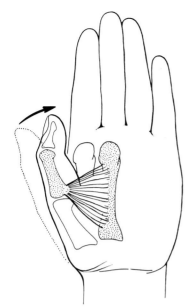

Figure 89–31. The adductor of the thumb originates primarily on the third metacarpal and inserts into the proximal phalanx of the thumb. It functions as an important adductor in pinching. (From Chase, R. A.: Atlas of Hand Surgery. Vol. 1. Philadelphia, W. B. Saunders Company, 1973.)

support flexion of the metacarpophalangeal joint to prevent recurvatum at this joint on pinching, which may occur with paralysis of either or both (Froment's sign) (Fig. 89–32). With graded relaxation of the abductors, the adductor will dominate and pull the thumb against the side of the hand.

The carpometacarpal joint is a saddle joint with a lax capsule. This allows a wide range of circumduction motion and even a small degree of distraction of the joint on traction.

Stability of the thumb root is heavily dependent on the muscles affecting it. The radial-innervated extensor pollicis longus and brevis and abductor pollicis longus secure the metacarpal dorsally. Opposing this to achieve stability are two groups of intrinsic muscles that, together with the extensor and dorsal abductor, triangulate the metacarpal. These two intrinsic groups are the median-innervated palmar abductors (the abductor pollicis brevis, opponens pollicis, and superficial head of the flexor pollicis brevis) and the ulnar-innervated adductors (the adductor pollicis, first dorsal interosseus, and deep head of the flexor pollicis brevis).

When there is paralysis of any of the three major motor nerves, thumb stability is compromised (Fig. 89–33). In median palsy the positioning muscles of the thenar eminence are lost, resulting in inability to oppose the thumb for pulp to pulp opposition with other digits. Ulnar palsy results in adduction weakness and imbalance of the structures influencing the metacarpophalangeal joint. Radial palsy destroys extension and dorsal abduction function, with resultant adduction contracture that becomes fixed after an extended period of unopposed adduction.

The ulnar nerve innervates the hypothenar muscle group, which serves further to develop the concavity of the transverse metacarpal arch. The opponens digiti minimi exemplifies the action of the hypothenar group.

DYNAMICS OF HAND FUNCTION

The central backbone of the hand is positioned in extension by the very important

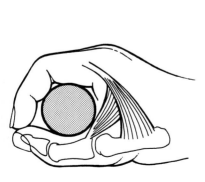

A

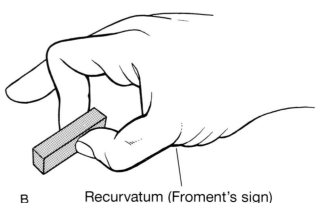

B   Recurvatum (Froment's sign)

Figure 89–32. When paralysis of the thumb adductor, flexor bevis, or abductor pollicis brevis occurs, the loss of primary flexion support at the metacarpophalangeal joint may result in recurvatum collapse of the metacarpophalangeal joint in pulp to pulp pinching. (Froment's sign). (Redrawn from Chase, R. A.: Atlas of Hand Surgery. Vol. 1. Philadelphia, W. B. Saunders Company, 1973.)

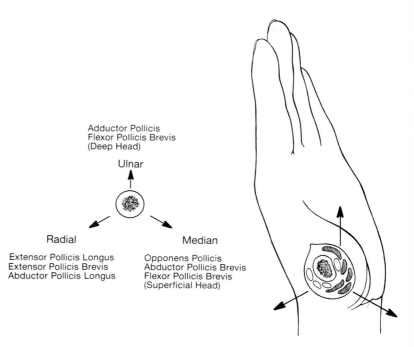

Figure 89–33. The first metacarpal relationship to the fixed carpal bones is dependent on three groups of muscles. Each group receives separate innervation (median, ulnar, and radial). Paralysis of any of these nerves results in imbalance of the forces stabilizing the thumb metacarpal. An abnormal thumb posture and functional deficit result that are classical for each nerve palsy. (From Chase, R. A.: Surgical anatomy of the hand. Surg. Clin. North Am., *44*:1364, 1964.)

extensor carpi radialis brevis and longus. Flexion is effected by the flexor carpi radialis. All three muscles insert on the central two metacarpals (the second and third). These key motors are responsible for positioning the hand axis in preparation for operation of the adaptive hand elements around it.

There are numerous other modifying motors to adjust the hand axis in the exact position desired, such as the flexor carpi ulnaris and extensor carpi ulnaris, which produce ulnar deviation.

The fixed unit of the hand is extended from the radius at the radiocarpal joint. The entire complex is a beam attached to the ulna by the distal radioulnar joint, the interosseous membrane, and the proximal radioulnar articulation. Rotation around the fixed ulna in supination and pronation is largely under the influence of the median-innervated pronator teres and pronator quadratus and the radial-innervated supinator (Fig. 89–34). The biceps and brachioradialis augment supination.

HAND SPACES AND SYNOVIAL SHEATHS

A knowledge of the classical anatomy of the synovial sheaths and potential anatomic spaces in the hand is essential for proper diagnosis and treatment of serious hand infections (Fig. 89–35).

The flexor tendons are shrouded in synovial sheaths, particularly where there is flexion mobility in the longitudinal arch of each ray and at the wrist. The synovial sheath of the flexor pollicis longus generally extends from the flexor insertion to a point proximal to the wrist flexor retinaculum. The same is true of the synovial sheath around the little finger flexors, but as the little finger sheath approaches the proximal palm just distal to the carpal tunnel, it expands to encompass the flexors of the ring, long, and index fingers. At this point it is referred to as the ulnar bursa. Each index, long, and ring finger has a flexor synovial sheath from the point of insertion of the profundus tendon to the level of the distal palmar crease in the palm. The deep space beneath the flexor tendons is divided into two compartments by the heavy vertical septum from the palmar fascia to the third metacarpal. Ulnar to the septum is the midpalmar space, and radial to it lies the thenar space. The thenar space straddles the adductor pollicis muscle like two legs extending between the adductor and deep flexors on the palmar side, and between the adductor and the first dorsal interosseous on the dorsal side.

Infection starting in the digital synovial sheaths may extend to the deep palmar spaces.

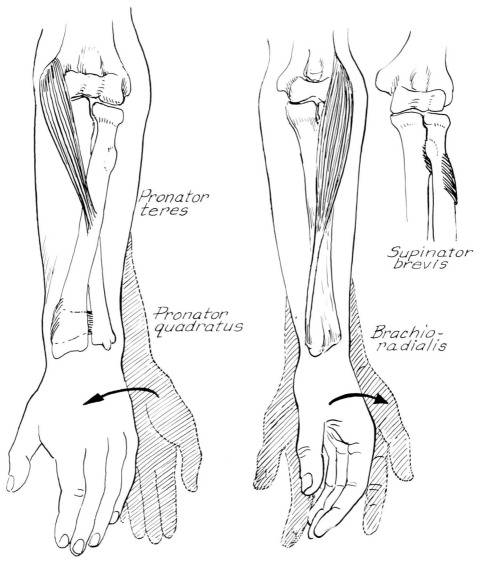

Figure 89–34. The pronator teres and pronator quadratus act to pronate the forearm. The supinator and biceps are supinators. The brachioradialis may augment supination when the arm is extended and already in pronation. (From Chase, R. A.: Atlas of Hand Surgery. Vol. 1. Philadelphia, W. B. Saunders Company, 1973.)

EXAMINATION OF HAND SPACE INFECTIONS

Infections in the digital synovial sheath should be diagnosed when signs of infection occur, such as pain, redness, and fever. The digit is held in a flexed posture. Pain is elicited on passive gentle extension. Such an infection may be obvious if the patient has a paronychia or felon or any other identifiable source of contamination.

BLOOD SUPPLY

The enormous number of variations in arterial and venous patterns of blood supply to the hand are beyond the scope of this chapter. Knowledge of these variations has reached a point of practical importance with the advent of microvascular surgery for revascularization, replantation, and composite tissue transfers. Classic studies for surgeons in need

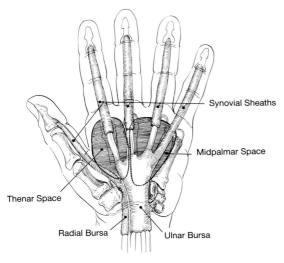

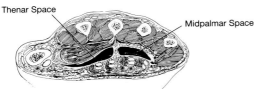

Figure 89–35. The synovial sheaths and major spaces in the hand and fingers. (From Chase, R. A.: Atlas of Hand Surgery. Vol. 1. Philadelphia, W. B. Saunders Company, 1973.)

of detailed knowledge are those by Coleman and Anson (1961) and the detailed studies by Murakami, Takaya, and Outi (1969) and Adachi (1928).

Classical Pattern of Arterial Blood Supply

In general the blood supply of the hand is conveniently divided into palmar vessels, which are subdivided into a superficial and a deep layer and a single dorsal layer. For example, the superficial vascular arch and its branches constitute the superficial group, the deep arch and the palmar metacarpal branches make up the deep layer, and the dorsal arch with its dorsal metacarpal branches forms the dorsal distribution. Although the distribution of blood supply to the thumb is quite different from that to the fingers, it still falls within the same generic groupings by level as those described above.

The ulnar artery emerges from the radial side of the flexor carpi ulnaris at the wrist accompanied by the ulnar nerve. It passes superficially to the flexor retinaculum radial to the pisiform beneath the palmaris brevis

and its fascia. Here it divides into a deep palmar branch and a superficial palmar branch. The superficial branch becomes the dominant contributor to the superficial palmar arch. The superficial arch crosses the palm at the level of the fully abducted thumb. The deep branch contributes to the deep palmar arch.

The radial artery crosses the "anatomic snuffbox" deep to the tendons of the abductor pollicis longus, extensor pollicis brevis, and extensor pollicis longus to plunge through an arcade in the first dorsal interosseous muscle, enter the palm, and form the deep palmar arch. A superficial branch of the radial artery arises at the level of the distal radius before the artery enters the "snuffbox" and courses over or through the abductor pollicis brevis to contribute to the superficial palmar arch. This branch contributes blood supply to the skin over the thenar area and the underlying intrinsic muscles of the thumb.

The superficial palmar arch gives rise to three common digital arteries and multiple branches to intrinsic muscles and skin. The deep vascular arch lies at the proximal ends of the metacarpals deep to all the flexor tendons. It arises chiefly from the radial artery and becomes an arch by anastomosis with the deep branch of the ulnar artery. The deep arch is the major source of blood supply to the thumb and to the radial side of the index finger. This blood supply comes from the first of the four palmar metacarpal arteries. The first metacarpal artery is the prime source of blood supply to the radial and ulnar proper digital arteries of the thumb and the radial proper digital artery of the index finger. These digital arteries generally receive collateral branches from the superficial palmar arch as well. After giving its branch to the index finger, the first metacarpal artery becomes the primary source of blood supply to the thumb and is frequently called the princeps pollicis.

The dorsal arteries originate proximally from the dorsal interosseous artery and a dorsal perforating branch of the volar interosseous artery. These arteries are joined by branches from the radial and ulnar arteries to form a dorsal carpal arch. Dorsal metacarpal arteries arise from this arch and extend distally to the margins of the fingers. These dorsal arteries are joined by a varying number of vessels perforating from the deep palmar metacarpal arteries. In fact, the dominant supply to the dorsal metacarpal arteries may come from these perforators. Dorsal arteries to the thumb come from branches of the radial artery before it plunges through the first dorsal interosseous arcade. Thus, the dorsal arterial blood supply of the thumb is similar to that of the fingers.

EXAMINATION OF VASCULAR SYSTEM

Simple palpation for pulses and arterial mapping using a Doppler are standard examination techniques for quick office examination. Angiography may be necessary if more detailed assessment is required. The most useful gross test for competency of the vascular arches is the simple Allen's test.

Allen's Test. This test (Fig. 89–36) may be used to assess the competence of the major arterial contributors to blood supply in the hand and the functional efficiency of the vas-

cular arches in the hand (Fig. 89–36*A*). Palpate the radial and ulnar pulses at the wrist and prepare to compress these arteries (Fig. 89–36*B*). Have the patient make a very tight fist (Fig. 89–36*C*). Compress the arteries and ask the patient to extend the digits. The hand will be blanched white (Fig. 89–36*D*). Release pressure on one of the arteries and observe the return of a red flush on the hand (Fig. 89–36*E*). Normally, the flush is immediate and progresses across the whole hand without delay. This confirms the patency of the artery and the competence of circulatory collaterals through the vascular arches. The test may be performed to confirm the competence of each of the two major arteries before surgery or to check their competence after repair, thrombectomy, manipulation, or injury.

The Allen's test principle may be used in clinically assessing the competence of the two

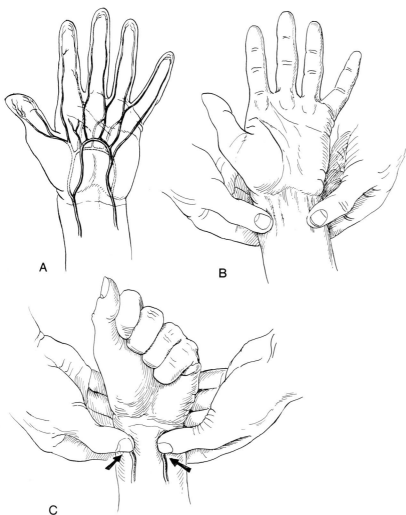

A

B

C

Figure 89–36. *A* to *E,* Allen's test for competency of arterial arches. (Redrawn from Chase, R. A.: Atlas of Hand Surgery. Vol. 1. Philadelphia, W. B. Saunders Company, 1973.)

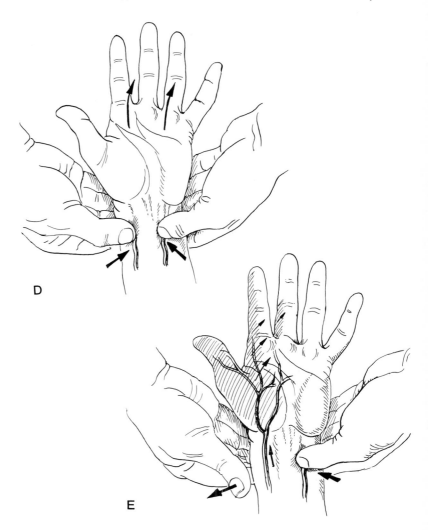

Figure 89–36 *Continued*

proper digital arteries in the fingers. It may be done by observing return of color after compression of both arteries and release of one, or a cutaneous electronic pulsemeter (used by anesthesiologists) may be applied to the digit tip. Compress one artery, then the other, and then both to note the individual proper artery contribution to cutaneous blood supply. The technique may be useful and less trying and dangerous than angiography when one is planning an island pedicle flap from a donor finger whose digital artery may have been damaged by an injury proximal to the finger.

PERIPHERAL NERVES

The peripheral nerves to the upper extremity have anatomic relationships of great im-portance to the surgeon. For example, one needs to know the anatomic availability for nerve block and sites where nerves are subject to compression or injury. Sites of particular susceptibility to injury coincide quite accurately with the sites chosen for anesthesia.

With the advent of fascicular and group fascicular repair of nerves in addition to epineurial repair, it is important for surgeons to understand the generic internal structure of peripheral nerves (Fig. 89–37). The epineurium is the tubular fibrous support structure surrounding the entire nerve; it also courses between the fascicles. Subdivisions consisting of multiple fascicles within the nerve are covered by epineurium. Each fascicle is covered by perineurium. Within each fascicle are separate axons, some myelinated and some unmyelinated. Motor, sensory, and sympa-

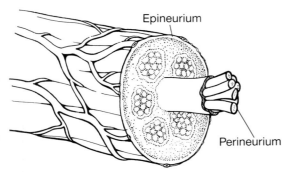

Figure 89-37. Generic structure of peripheral nerves. The epineurium is the tubular external support. Subdivisions within the nerve consisting of multiple fascicles are encased in epineurium as well. Each individual fascicle is covered by perineurium. (Redrawn from Chase, R. A.: Textbook of Hand Surgery. Vol. 2. Philadelphia, W. B. Saunders Company, 1984, p. 79.)

thetic fibers are present within each peripheral nerve. Blood vessels are found on the epineurial surface and in the internal supporting structure of the nerve. The internal topography is plexus-like, as described in detail in the classic monograph by Sir Sidney Sunderland (1978).

The ulnar and median nerves are frequently injured just proximal to the wrist. The nerves are quite superficial and it is a region where injuries to all structures are frequent. Median palsy alone results in anesthesia over the important exploring and manipulating digits (the thumb, index and long fingers, and part of the ring finger) on the palmar surface. The median positioning muscles of the thumb become paralyzed, resulting in an inability to position the thumb for pulp to pulp opposition with other digits. In addition, the two radial lumbricals are paralyzed, but this may be barely perceptible functionally (Fig. 89-38). There is a constant midvolar blood vessel on the median nerve that helps in its identity and in achieving very accurate axial rotation to perfect end to end opposition. The ulnar nerve is far less important from the standpoint of hand sensation but is very important for its motor innervation of all the hypothenar muscles and interossei. In addition, it innervates the thumb adductor, the deep head of the flexor pollicis brevis, and the two ulnar lumbricals (Fig. 89-39). Classically, all the intrinsic muscles on the radial side of the flexor pollicis longus are median nerve innervated (the abductor pollicis brevis, opponens, and superficial head of the flexor pollicis brevis). All other intrinsic muscles in the hand receive their innervation from the ulnar nerve. The tiny two radial lumbricals are the only exceptions to this axiom.

Essentially the flexor pollicis longus divides the hand into a median- and ulnar-innervated part from the motor standpoint. There are often variations from this classical innervation pattern. The pattern of peripheral nerve distributions was studied by Woodhall and Beebe (1956), who pointed out the likely variations based on an analysis of World War II nerve injuries.

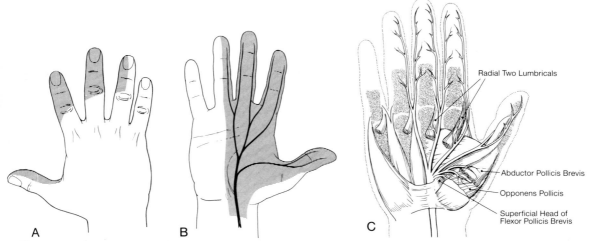

Figure 89-38. *A, B,* The median nerve classically lends sensibility to the palmar aspect and the distal dorsum of the thumb, index, long, and radial half of the ring fingers. Intrinsic muscles radial to the flexor policis longus and the two radial lumbricals receive motor innervation from median nerve. (Redrawn from Chase, R. A.: Atlas of Hand Surgery. Vol. 1. Philadelphia, W. B. Saunders Company, 1973.)

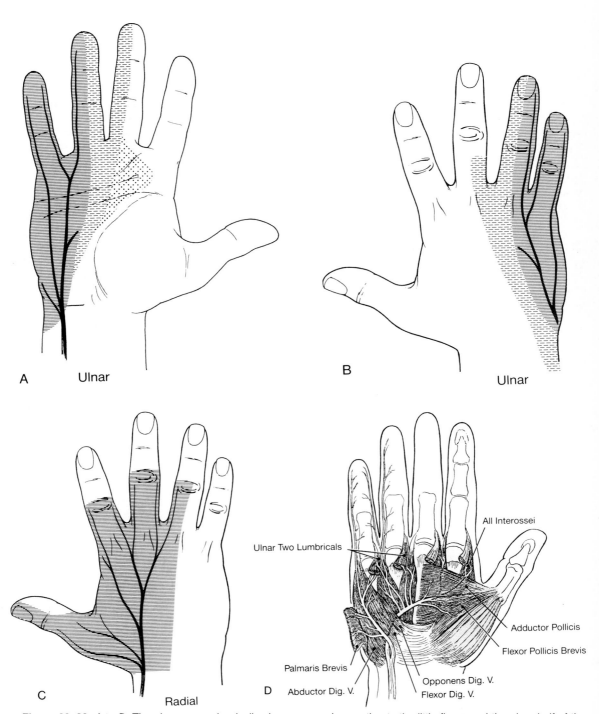

Figure 89–39. *A* to *D,* The ulnar nerve classically gives sensory innervation to the little finger and the ulnar half of the ring finger. All hypothenar muscles, all interossei, the two ulnar lubricals, the adductor pollicis, and the ulnar half of the flexor pollicis brevis are classically innervated by the ulnar nerve. (Redrawn from Chase, R. A.: Atlas of Hand Surgery. Vol. 1. Philadelphia, W. B. Saunders Company, 1973.)

The ulnar nerve divides into a deep motor branch and a superficial sensory branch just beyond the pisiform. Occasionally, stab wounds of the hand result in transection of the motor branch with no sensory loss.

A guide to proper fascicular orientation in the ulnar nerve is the fact that one can identify that portion destined to be the deep or superficial branches well above the wrist. The nerve may be bluntly split and funicular suture done for even greater accuracy.

For detailed studies of the fascicular pattern distribution and the intraneuronal plexuses, the reader is referred to the extensive work of Sunderland and Bedbrook (1949) and Sunderland and Bradley (1949).

Dorsal Branch of Radial and Ulnar Nerves

The dorsal or superficial branch of the radial nerve courses through the forearm in relationship to the brachioradialis muscle on the radial side of the arm (Fig. 89–40).

The nerve crosses the "anatomic snuffbox" between the extensor pollicis brevis and the extensor pollicis longus in the loose subcutaneous tissue. It divides into multiple branches, which give sensibility to the dorsum of the hand over the radial two-thirds, the dorsum of the thumb, and the index, long,

and half of the ring finger proximal to the distal interphalangeal joint.

The dorsal branch of the ulnar nerve courses around the ulnar aspect of the forearm in its distal one-fourth after branching from the main trunk at a variable site in the distal one-third of the forearm. It passes from its position deep to the flexor carpi ulnaris out through the dorsal fascia to become subcutaneous. It branches to innervate the dorsum of the ulnar portion of the dorsum of the hand, the dorsum of the little finger, and at least part of the dorsum of the ring finger (Fig. 89–40).

The deep motor branch of the ulnar nerve passes through the pisohamate and opponens tunnel in company with the deep branch of the ulnar artery. It courses with the deep vascular arch across the depths of the palm, giving off motor branches to the hypothenar muscles, all the interossei, the two ulnar lumbricals, and the thumb intrinsics ulnar to the flexor pollicis longus.

Crowded Areas with Unyielding Boundaries

Flexion and extension motions in the hand occur at two levels, the wrist and the finger joints. Flexion at these joints would surely create volar bowstringing at the long flexor

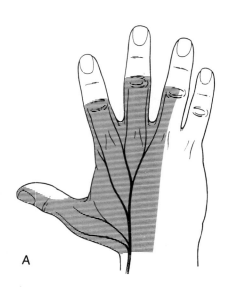

Radial

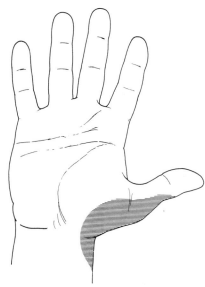

Figure 89–40. *A, B,* The dorsal branch of the radial nerve lends sensibility to the radial dorsal aspect of the hand as shown. (Redrawn from Chase, R. A.: Atlas of Hand Surgery. Vol. 1. Philadelphia, W. B. Saunders Company, 1973.)

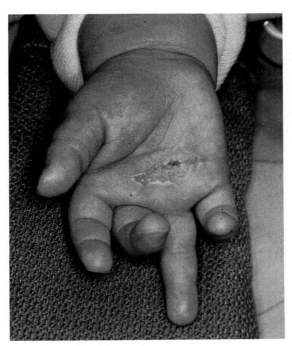

Figure 90–4. Loss of the cascading effect of the fingers in repose indicates tendon laceration.

tained with the wrist in neutral position to evaluate carpal bone alignment.

After the initial evaluation, management is discussed with the patient, or sometimes with a family member. In the case of a child, the management is discussed in depth with the parents. This discussion should include an explanation of the functional units of the hand (see Chap. 89) and agreement on the strategy needed to obtain the best results. Many decisions can be made preoperatively as far as skin, bone, nerve, and tendon injuries are concerned. The radiographs can be reviewed with the parents or another family member. The decision whether treatment should take place in the operating room is made in the emergency room. If the injury is extensive and devascularization is highly probable, transfer of the patient to the operating room is more urgent than when the injury is simple. Only skin lacerations and simple fractures and dislocations are treated definitively in the emergency room.

Replantation Principles

(See also Chap. 93)

With current surgical technology, the only absolute contraindication to replantation (other than the patient's health) is irreversible loss of blood supply. The decision to replant is made by the patient or parents and the surgeon. Many patients who have read glowing newspaper articles demand revascularization or replantation of a part. If the surgeon feels that neither is indicated but the patient still insists on it, another surgeon should be consulted. When the vascular tree is not irreversibly damaged, it is possible to restore circulation in complete amputations at any level in the upper extremity. Principles are established only to provide exceptions.

Factors to consider when making a decision about replantation include the age and general health of the patient and the time and mechanism of amputation. Older patients regain less function. The more distal the level of amputation, the better is the functional result. In the case of replantation above the elbow in an adult, return of elbow function may be expected, but useful function of the hand or wrist is rare. It has been suggested that the only reason for replanting an amputation above the elbow is to provide subsequent fitting with a below-elbow prosthesis. A crushing injury carries a poor prognosis, as does an avulsion injury. The factors necessary for a successful limb replantation include cooling of the severed limb, mastery of the surgical techniques of replantation, and aggressive postoperative management. Many patients prefer replants distal to the proximal interphalangeal (PIP) joint rather than an amputation stump. Replantation of a single digit proximal to the PIP joint has generally yielded unsatisfactory results. The surgeon should tell the patient the degree of functional recovery expected after replantation and then proceed as mutually agreed.

MANAGEMENT IN OPERATING ROOM

Operative Suite Organization

Hand Tables. A variety of tables are available to support the upper extremity during surgery. When magnification is used, it is helpful to have a wide table so that the surgeon's forearms can be supported. An attachment to the table accommodating a catch basin for irrigation is useful. The authors have modified the end of the hand table where it attaches to the operating table: the end that is usually placed beneath the operating table or patient is removed and fitted with a hinge, which fits over the runner on the side of the operating table. This allows the operating table to be raised or lowered to meet the needs of the anesthesiologist without breaking the arm table.

Instrumentation. A wide variety of instruments are required in hand surgery. It is paramount that each surgeon make a list of the instruments needed for each particular operative procedure. A basic pack is prepared and a second pack selected to supplement the basic pack for each procedure. Obviously the instruments used during a wrist fusion differ significantly from those required for a flexor tendon graft or a digital nerve repair. Since tourniquet time is precious, it is important to avoid waiting for instruments to be found or sterilized. Thus, cards are necessary to list the instruments needed for each procedure. This is crucial during replantation surgery, which usually occurs at night. It is advantageous to have the instrument packs in the room and labeled. Even then it is often necessary for one of the replantation team nurses to come in to set up a case. All instruments must be checked by the scrub nurse before the operation begins. It is frustrating to have a drill or saw that does not work properly.

Magnification and Microsurgery. Treatment of neurovascular injuries in the hand requires the specialized skills of the microsurgeon. Precision instruments have been developed for the delicate work needed in microsurgery. Magnification is essential for the adequate treatment of nerve and vascular injuries. A frequently used magnifying device is the surgical loop, usually providing 2 to 6 × magnification. These loops can be worn by the surgeon without fatigue, and are excellent for dissecting; however, many may prefer the operating microscope. Many models are available; the basic features include foot-controlled focus, zoom and X-Y axis mobility, a fiberoptic light source, and binoculars for a first assistant to view the surgical field.

The microscope should be prepared before the operation begins. The nurse must check the light bulbs (keep an extra bulb taped to the microscope), set the eye pieces to accommodate the surgeons, and determine whether the height of the scope has been adjusted to permit focusing on the hand. Some scopes can simply be cranked up or down, while others have to be changed with a hex wrench and a set screw.

Choice of Anesthetics in Hand Surgery (See also Chap. 91)

The surgeon may select local, intravenous regional, regional block, or general anesthesia. Choice of the appropriate anesthetic method is determined by the patient's age and general health, the presence of associated injuries, the anticipated extent of the operative procedure, any history of drug allergies, and recent ingestion of food. If the patient has a significant illness such as coronary artery disease, chronic obstructive airway disease, or compromised hepatic or renal function, local may be safer than general anesthesia. Patients with such conditions may be taking medication that alters the body's ability to respond to the stress of surgery. Every patient who is taking steroids or has a history of having done so within the previous year is given supplemental steroid intraoperatively and immediately postoperatively. The age of the patient is very important. A young child always requires general anesthesia in the author's experience. Under no circumstances should one begin debriding and irrigating a wound before the anesthetic agent has become effective. The author most frequently uses intravenous regional anesthesia (Bier, 1908). The equipment requirements are simple: (1) a double-cuffed tourniquet with color-coded controls to indicate which valve controls which cuff; (2) an Esmarch bandage for exsanguination of the extremity; (3) a Webril roll to pad and protect the skin beneath the tourniquet; (4) the local anesthetic—the author prefers lidocaine without epinephrine; (5) a 23 gauge butterfly needle with a plastic connector for administering the anesthetic; and (6) a saline-filled syringe. The 23 gauge butterfly needle is inserted into a vein on the dorsum of the hand, and 10 ml of saline is infused to ensure that the needle is in the vein. The upper extremity is exsanguinated, using an Esmarch bandage. The proximal tourniquet is inflated and the Esmarch bandage is removed. The needle is irrigated with saline to make sure it has not been dislodged. Forty to 50 ml of 0.5 per cent lidocaine is injected intravenously. The arm assumes a mottled appearance as the anesthetic is instilled. The onset of anesthesia is rapid and complete within 10 to 15 minutes. The needle is removed and pressure is applied to the puncture site to minimize hematoma formation. When the patient begins to complain of discomfort in the upper extremity (usually shoulder pain), the distal tourniquet is inflated and the proximal cuff is deflated. If tourniquet time is less than 30 minutes, the tourniquet is deflated and reinflated within four to five seconds. This is repeated three to four times over a period of five minutes to fractionate the release of the local anesthetic into the circulation, minimizing the risk of a toxic reaction.

Pneumatic Tourniquet

Surgery of the hand would be difficult, if not impossible, without the aid of a bloodless field. The word "tourniquet," which comes from the French *tourner*, to turn, was introduced by Jean Louis Petit (1718). He used a strap which encircled the extremity and a screw device attached to the strap. Tightening the screw compressed the limb until blood flow was interrupted. Lister (1864) used the tourniquet to provide a bloodless field during elective surgery. Esmarch (1873), at the suggestion of von Langenbeck, used a flat rubber bandage to strip blood from the arm and render it ischemic. The pneumatic cuff was introduced by Riva-Rocci (1896) for determining blood pressure. Perthes (1921), a German army surgeon, described a pneumatic device for rendering an extremity ischemic by inflating a tubular piece of rubber around the arm. Cushing's (1904) pneumatic tourniquet, which he inflated with a bicycle pump, was the forerunner of our modern tourniquet, equipped with a gauge for monitoring pressure and a continuing source of pressure supply by compressed air. The tourniquet has undergone many modifications to improve its reliability. Many surgeons have it calibrated with a mercury manometer each day. Some tourniquets have a safety valve installed in the line between the cuff and tank to prevent excessive pressure. The pressure generated by the cuff is greatest at the margins of the cuff. Love (1978) modified the tourniquet to minimize this gradient of pressure at the edges. Many surgeons use padding beneath the cuff in the belief that it may distribute the pressure more evenly and prevent pinching of the skin.

The tourniquet is standardized each day before the operating schedule begins by the operating room head nurse. After the tourniquet has been applied, the times of inflation and deflation are recorded. No standard tourniquet pressure has been agreed upon. It has often been suggested that a tourniquet pressure 100 mm higher than systolic blood pressure is adequate, but the author disagrees and uses 300 mm Hg pressure routinely. If the tourniquet is reinflated, the time between deflation and reinflation is recorded.

Several layers of soft cast padding are placed around the midportion of the arm. The pneumatic cuff is applied snugly and the rubber tubing from the gauge is connected securely to the cuff. A towel is placed around the distal edge of the tourniquet to prevent prep solution from soaking into the padding beneath the tourniquet while the extremity is prepared.

Preparation and Draping

After the patient has been anesthetized, a tourniquet is placed around the arm. If there is bleeding from the wound, the upper extremity is exsanguinated and the cuff is inflated to control bleeding while the wounds are cleansed (Fig. 90–5). If bleeding is minimal, the wound is cleansed and the tourniquet subsequently inflated, thus conserving tourniquet time. The wound must be thoroughly cleansed. The most effective method is by means of a jet lavage. The area around the wound is shaved. Grease in a wound can be removed with tetracycline ointment.

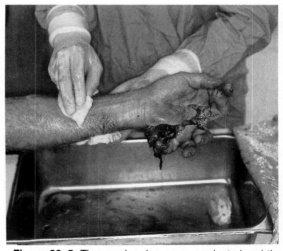

Figure 90–5. The arm has been exsanguinated and the tourniquet inflated to control bleeding because prolonged irrigation of the wound is needed to remove the foreign material (sand in this case).

Wound irrigation and cleansing may require significant operative time, as it must be complete. Foreign body particles, such as grease, sand, or emery dust associated with industrial accidents, evoke an intense inflammatory reaction and fibrosis that compromises subsequent restorative procedures. Occasionally, soft tissues must be removed to eliminate foreign bodies completely (Fig. 90–6). Minimal trimming of the edges of cleanly lacerated wounds is usually necessary.

Hair removal from the operative field is controversial. Some writers consider that shaving is unnecessary and may have an adverse effect on the subsequent sterility of the arm (Seropian and Reynolds, 1971). The author limits the area to be shaved to the immediate surgical field, and this is done in the operating room at the time of surgery, before the skin is prepped. However, the presence of hair on the skin has not been shown to be a significant factor in the development of wound infections (Green, 1982).

The use of high pressure wound irrigation is recommended for most wounds of the upper extremity, especially those resulting from industrial and farm accidents (Fig. 90–7). The irrigation device must be able to deliver fluid under high pressure for irrigation. This not only removes gross contamination but also helps debride nonviable tissue and bone fragments. Normal saline is used as the irrigation fluid, the volume used being dependent on the degree of contamination.

Many techniques of preparing the upper extremity for surgery have been reported. The more common antiseptic solutions used today include pure alcohol (which is an ex-

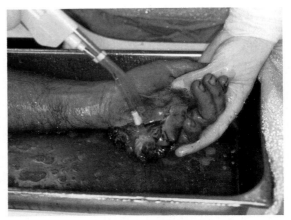

Figure 90–7. A pulsating high pressure jet lavage is required to irrigate contaminated wounds adequately.

cellent skin disinfectant, although its antiseptic properties are short-lived) and hexachlorophene (pHisoHex). Iodine solutions, either iodine in alcohol or the aqueous iodine solutions, are also in regular use. Iodoforms that contain povidone-iodine, such as the aqueous solution Betadine, are undoubtedly the most common skin disinfectants used. Chlorhexidine (Hibiclens) is a 70 per cent alcohol solution that has gained favor. Each of these solutions has advantages and disadvantages. More common disadvantages are skin irritation or allergic reactions from the iodine. In clean, elective upper extremity cases, the author uses an iodine-alcohol solution, which works effectively for skin antisepsis and has a very low rate of skin irritation. Betadine is preferred for contaminated or open wounds.

The skin preparation is designed to eliminate both transient and resident bacteria of the upper extremity. Most transient flora are eliminated by skin preparation, but there may be resident flora around and beneath the fingernails (Hann, 1973), which should be trimmed and cleaned before prepping.

After the extremity has been thoroughly prepared, two sheets are applied over the arm board. The more proximal sheet is folded to provide a cuff just distal to the level of the tourniquet. Two stockinettes are placed over the fingertips and rolled up the arm to the level of the tourniquet. A second sheet is placed over the top of the tourniquet and a clamp is placed on either side of the arm, impaling the upper sheet, the stockinette, and the lower sheet (Fig. 90–8).

The stockinette is rolled up the forearm to

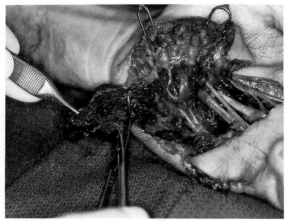

Figure 90–6. Nonviable muscle is debrided, including embedded foreign material.

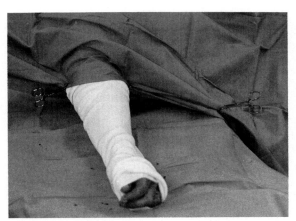

Figure 90–8. Draping as described in the text permits extensive exposure of the upper extremity in any position, and freedom to place the hand on the trunk for flap coverage if needed.

a level above the wound. The incisions for the operative procedure are marked. It is important to dot in any previous lines of laceration or surgical incision to prevent a flap being inadvertently based on a scar. After the incision lines are marked, several 4 × 4 sponges are placed in the palm and the stockinette is unrolled to cover the fingertips. The upper extremity is held suspended by the stockinette while an Esmarch bandage is applied loosely around the level of the hand. The Esmarch is then brought up and tightly wound around the fingers, proceeding proximally by overlapping each turn approximately one-half the width of the bandage. After the arm has been fully exsanguinated, the tourniquet is inflated to 300 mm Hg in adults and 200 mm Hg in children. The time of inflation is recorded. The anesthetist notifies the surgeon after one hour of tourniquet time and then at 30 minute intervals.

How long can a tourniquet be safely used? There is no universal agreement. There is support for using a tourniquet for from 45 minutes to four hours, two hours being the most widely accepted time. Wilgis (1971) obtained venous blood samples in man preoperatively, intraoperatively, and after tourniquet release. After inflation of the tourniquet, he observed a decrease in venous pH from 7.4 to 7.31 after 30 minutes of tourniquet ischemia. Thereafter, a gradual decrease in pH to 7.19 at 60 minutes, 7.04 at 90 minutes, and 6.90 after 120 minutes was observed. There was also noted to be a concomitant fall in the partial pressure of oxygen from a normal

level of 45 mm Hg to 20, 10, and 4 mm Hg after 60, 90, and 120 minutes of ischemia, respectively. After release of the tourniquet, return of these parameters to normal levels required up to 15 minutes when the arm had been ischemic for 90 minutes. At two hours, there was evidence of capillary and cellular damage in striated muscles. Severe acidosis, pH of less than 7.2, has also been associated with hypocoagulability of blood. This may contribute to the profuse oozing that occurs after release of a tourniquet that has been inflated for an extended period.

Other studies have corroborated these findings. After two hours of ischemia, Solonen and Hjelt (1968) reported histologic abnormalities in muscle, but Tountas and Bergmann (1977) noted no irreversible changes after this period. Patterson and Klenerman (1979), using electron microscopic studies, demonstrated that three hours appeared to be the upper limit before significant pathologic changes occurred in muscle.

The following recommendations are made: (1) keep tourniquet time to a minimum; (2) two hours is the upper limit for a single application of the tourniquet; (3) after removal of the tourniquet, do not reapply it until the pH, PCO_2, and PO_2 have returned to normal (keep deflated five minutes for every 30 minutes that the tourniquet was inflated); (4) before attempting to stop oozing after release of the tourniquet, keep direct pressure on the wound and wait until the period of arteriovenous shunting has subsided (usually ten minutes); (5) completely remove the tourniquet cuff and underlying padding after deflating the tourniquet to prevent constriction of the arm (the cuff and padding can act as a venous tourniquet and contribute to further oozing and hematoma formation); and (6) verify tourniquet pressures with a mercury manometer on at least a biweekly basis—a daily basis is preferable.

If an operative procedure will require more than two hours of tourniquet time, it is best to try to plan the procedure so that the tourniquet is released after an hour and a half, and then to wait 20 minutes before exsanguinating the extremity and continuing. During this waiting period much can be accomplished. If there is need for bone, tendon, or nerve grafts, these can be obtained while the tourniquet remains deflated.

When the operative procedure is complete, should the tourniquet be deflated and bleeding controlled, or should dressings be applied and the tourniquet then deflated? There is no standard practice. On all Dupuytren's procedures, the author releases the tourniquet and maintains elevation and compression of the hand for ten minutes by the clock. Any subsequent bleeding is controlled by coagulation. In many other procedures, such as tendon grafts or nerve repairs, the tourniquet remains inflated until the skin wounds have been closed and the dressings applied. In any procedure in which a large dead space will be created or there has been extensive dissection, such as removal of the fibrotic forearm muscles for a Volkmann's ischemic contracture, the tourniquet is released and bleeding is controlled by elevation and compression, with possible insertion of drains.

When the tourniquet is deflated at the conclusion of the procedure, it is completely removed to prevent venous obstruction.

Use of Tourniquet and Local Anesthesia (See also Chap. 91)

Many operative procedures, performed under local anesthesia, require use of a tourniquet to permit the procedure to be carried out swiftly, safely, and carefully. Tourniquet time must be conserved. To do this, the incisions are first outlined, the local anesthetic is injected, and it is necessary to wait until it has taken effect. The extremity then is exsanguinated and the tourniquet is inflated to 200 mm Hg pressure. Patients under local anesthesia tolerate 200 much better than 250 to 300 mm Hg. After about 20 minutes, patients develop discomfort at the tourniquet site, requiring its release. The injection of local anesthetic in the skin beneath the cuff has not been effective in controlling pain; sedation can help but only briefly. Thus, the surgeon must carefully evaluate the extent of surgery required and his technical skills before beginning a case under local anesthesia requiring an arm tourniquet. Skin grafts or fingertip flaps, capsulotomies, and very limited tenolysis can be done readily under local anesthesia.

When surgery is required on a digit, a finger tourniquet can reduce patient discomfort. The author prefers a 1 inch rubber drain lying flat across the proximal phalanx and clamped opposite the operative side. Unfortunately, a finger tourniquet applies an unknown amount of pressure on the underlying structures. Temporary anesthesia can occur postoperatively.

Operative Procedure

Once it has been established that the vasculature is intact, a tissue-oriented evaluation is preferred. A systematic exploration of the wound should be undertaken, and any foreign bodies removed. Skin, bones, joints, nerves, and tendons are evaluated in order. It should first be determined how much, if any, skin is lost. If appropriate, the fracture sites are inspected and loose fragments removed. Joint stability is tested. Continuity of nerves is determined. Tendons are examined as the fingers and thumb are passively flexed and extended. When there is extensive injury, the remnants must be evaluated to determine the potential for functional recovery. It is imperative that the surgeon be able to discern whether or not a part can be of value, and to make this decision he must be aware of the current restorative techniques available for reconstruction. In general, all innervated skin and functional units (e.g., isolated joints) should be preserved. In subsequent operative procedures these units may be used either alone or in combination with others to provide a single functioning unit (Fig. 90–9).

The goals in initial management are the restoration of functional units, the achievement of primary healing with minimal scar formation, and provision of an optimal environment for subsequent surgery. Reconstruction is tissue oriented, beginning with skin and progressing through bone, joint, nerve, and tendon until the restoration of motor unit function can be established by repair, transfer, or grafting of tendons. Such tissue-oriented evaluation allows one to respond to simple questions and proceed as indicated. Is direct wound closure precluded by skin loss?

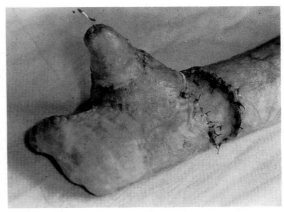

Figure 90–9. A thumb and web space has been constructed using remnants of the index finger.

healing: a disadvantage in the use of power tools. Arch. Surg., *104*:687, 1972.

Kleinert, H. E., and Meares, A.: In quest of the solution to severed flexor tendons. Clin. Orthop., *104*:23, 1974.

Lister, J., Baron: Collected Papers. Vol. I. Oxford, Clarendon Press, 1909, p. 176.

Love, B. R. T.: The tourniquet. Aust. N.Z. J. Surg., *48*:66, 1978.

Mubarak, S. J., Hargens, A. R., Owen, C. A., Akeson, W. H., and Garetto, L. P.: The wick catheter technique for measurement of intramuscular pressure. A new research and clinical tool. J. Bone Joint Surg., *58A*:1016, 1976.

Patterson, S., and Klenerman, L.: The effect of pneumatic tourniquets on the ultrastructure of skeletal muscle. J. Bone Joint Surg., *61B*:178, 1979.

Peacock, E. E., Jr.: Wound Repair. 3rd Ed. Philadelphia, W. B. Saunders Company, 1984, p. 300.

Perthes: Quoted in Boyes, J. H.: On Shoulders of Giants. Philadelphia, J. B. Lippincott Company, 1976, p. 166.

Petit, J. L.: D'un nouvel instrument de chirurgie. Mem. Acad. R. Sci., 1718, p. 254.

Riva-Rocci: Gazz. Med. Torino, *47*:981, 1001, 1896.

Seropian, R., and Reynolds, B. M.: Wound infections after preoperative depilatory versus razor preparation. Am. J. Surg., *121*:251, 1971.

Solonen, K. A., and Hjelt, L.: Morphological changes in striated muscle during ischaemia. Acta Orthop. Scand., *39*:13, 1968.

Tountas, C. P., and Bergman, R. A.: Tourniquet ischemia: ultrastructural and histochemical observations of ischemic human muscle and of monkey muscle and nerve. J. Hand Surg., *2*:31, 1977.

Verth, M.: Zur Frage der Wundausschneidung. Chirurg., *7*:473, 1935.

Weeks, P. M., and Wray, R. C.: Management of Acute Hand Injuries. 2nd Ed. St. Louis, C. V. Mosby Company, 1978, pp. 135–146.

Wilgis, E. F. S.: Observations on the effects of tourniquet ischemia. J. Bone Joint Surg., *53A*:1343, 1971.

91

Nathaniel M. Sims

Upper Extremity Anesthesia

6. Know the principles and limitations of *premedication* and *intraoperative sedation* of patients as an adjunct to regional anesthesia.

7. Have a plan for *monitoring* the patient while surgery is being conducted.

8. Be prepared to manage any and all *complications of regional anesthesia,* including major systemic toxic reactions such as seizures and cardiopulmonary arrest.

In this chapter we cover these issues and discuss specific anesthetic techniques that may be useful for the surgeon when performing regional anesthesia.

EVALUATION OF PATIENT

The goals for anesthetic management of the hand surgical patient include: (1) a safe, comfortable patient; (2) an immobile surgical field, with or without muscle relaxation; (3) satisfactory analgesia intra- and postoperatively; and (4) hemostasis, with or without tourniquet, all with minimal risk of complications. Regional anesthesia is the technique of choice in many instances. The surgeon may wish to perform the block and leave the patient in the hands of a circulating nurse for intermittent monitoring of vital signs. Under other circumstances he may wish to consult the anesthesiologist, for assistance with a specific regional anesthetic technique, for advice with regard to intraoperative monitoring or management of a coexisting medical problem, or for consideration of general anesthesia.

Certain patient groups require special consideration:

1. The *emergency patient* with other pathologic conditions (i.e., a possible head injury

The hand surgeon often finds himself choosing regional anesthesia for the patient, performing the block, and then doing the surgical procedure. Regional anesthesia is well suited for surgery of the hand, being useful in diverse clinical settings where general anesthesia may be impractical. In order to apply regional anesthesia safely, however, the surgeon must:

1. Become expert at *patient selection* for general versus regional anesthesia.

2. Know the possibilities, limitations, and complications of the various *regional anesthetic techniques.*

3. Be familiar with the pharmacology of the *local anesthetic agents,* especially pharmacodynamics, pharmacokinetics, dosage, and toxicity.

4. Understand those aspects of *brachial plexus* and *upper extremity anatomy* that are important to successful regional technique.

5. Choose those blocks that he will routinely *perform himself,* and those for which he will consult the anesthesiologist.

in addition to hand trauma) should be managed during surgery by the anesthesiologist.

2. Any patient with significant *trauma* must be considered to have abnormal gastric and intestinal motility, and therefore must be considered as having a "full stomach." This patient is as much at risk of aspiration as one who has just eaten or who has intra-abdominal hypertension due to pregnancy, ascites, or bowel obstruction. The choice of regional anesthesia, although it apparently avoids the surgeon having to deal with the airway, does not remove the danger of pulmonary aspiration of gastric contents. Regional anesthesia alone does not obtund laryngeal reflexes, but the patient who is secured supine to an operating room table and is then sedated is still at risk. Such a patient may experience nausea or require airway management for treatment of a toxic reaction. An anesthesiologist should be available. Consideration should be given to avoidance of blocks that require near-maximal doses of local anesthetics, and avoidance of excessive intravenous sedation. Under special circumstances the administration of cimetidine, ranitidine, metoclopramide, or a nonparticulate antacid for reduction of gastric acidity may be considered.

3. Similar conditions obtain for the patient with the "difficult airway." Regional anesthesia avoids having to deal with the airway, but a surgeon may be in an extremely difficult position if local anesthesia produces a toxic reaction requiring airway management. Block anesthesia may still be selected and performed by the surgeon, but the anesthesiologist should be available.

4. Elective procedures usually are not performed during *pregnancy.* Emergency surgery involves the potential problem of premature induction of labor and, during the first trimester, of drug-induced fetal effects. Although the available local and general anesthetics do *not* appear to be teratogenic, regional anesthesia may best minimize fetal exposure to drug.

5. In the *pediatric patient,* either regional or general anesthesia may be used. Intravenous regional anesthesia is possible, using dosages listed on page 4309 (Rudzinski and Ampel, 1983). Brachial plexus blocks can be performed, bearing in mind that the patient is unlikely to be able to cooperate or to report paresthesias. Premedication is given before arrival in the operating room, and the anesthesiologist may be able to facilitate performance of a block by giving either a "permissive" (1 to 2 mg/kg) or "anesthetic" (4 to 10 mg/kg) dose of ketamine intramuscularly (Melman, Penuelas, and Marrujo, 1975; Leak and Winchell, 1982; Schulte-Steinberg, 1984). Axillary block can then be performed using either a para-arterial technique or a nerve stimulator (Leak and Winchell, 1982; Schulte-Steinberg, 1984). Winnie (1983) recommends the interscalene technique, using a 25 gauge needle and relying on contact with the transverse process of C6.

6. In the *outpatient,* regional techniques are frequently excellent choices. However, only short or intermediate duration agents should be used in patients who will be discharged after the operation.

7. In patients with significant *medical disease,* a number of issues may need to be worked out in consultation with the anesthesiologist. The presence of significant *pulmonary disease* is a strong relative contraindication to supraclavicular techniques of brachial plexus block, since pneumothorax, sympathetic block, or phrenic or recurrent laryngeal nerve palsy may precipitate respiratory failure. In asthmatics, inadvertent sympathetic block can produce bronchospasm due to unopposed parasympathetic action on the bronchi (Lim, 1979; Thiagarajah and associates, 1984). Patients with emphysema and bullae have increased risk of pneumothorax due to prominence to the lung apices. Patients with excessive pulmonary secretions may not tolerate blockade of the recurrent laryngeal nerve, because this interferes with effective coughing. In patients with *abnormal coagulation,* major brachial plexus block may be relatively contraindicated owing to risk of hematoma formation. In theory, patients with *renal failure* are more susceptible than normals to toxicity from local anesthetics (Bromage, 1972b; Strasser and associates, 1981). Reasons for this include hypoproteinemia and anemia leading to high cardiac output and more rapid systemic absorption of local anesthetic agents, more rapid absorption of epinephrine (if used), and a shortened duration of anesthetic action. Finally, patients with *rheumatoid arthritis* may undergo multiple surgical procedures. They may often require general anesthesia, because of inability to lie supine and immobile during surgery. Airway problems may be significant as a result of kyphoscoliosis, cervical arthritis, cricoarytenoid arthritis, or the presence of an abnormally small glottis. Medications may include

drugs that affect platelet function and cause abnormal coagulation.

8. Patients with a history of *allergy to local anesthetics* or of *malignant hyperthermia* should be seen in consultation well in advance of surgery. "Allergy" most frequently represents reactions to preservative, to inadvertent intravascular injection of epinephrine-containing solutions, or to concurrently administered medications. Almost all true allergies are due to compounds with ester linkage (procaine, chloroprocaine, tetracaine). Only one well-documented case of allergy to an amide (lidocaine, bupivacaine, etidocaine) has been reported (Brown, Beamish, and Wildsmith 1981), and thus it has been accepted practice to proceed with the use of preservative-free amides in patients with a history of allergy to local anesthetics if it is not practical to delay surgery until more extensive evaluation can be performed (Incaudo and colleagues, 1978; Raj, 1985). Regional anesthesia is appropriate in patients with a history of malignant hyperthermia (MH). It has been suggested that amide local anesthetics may cause an MH reaction by releasing calcium from the sarcoplasmic reticulum, but a literature search (Adragna, 1985) has revealed no reports of any MH crises caused solely by the use of amide local anesthetics without epinephrine. In many institutions, lidocaine is used routinely in MH-susceptible patients without problems.

9. Several other surgical situations require close coordination between the surgical and anesthesia teams. These include the patient undergoing *bilateral surgery,* for whom techniques must be chosen so as to reduce or eliminate the risk of bilateral pneumothorax, or bilateral phrenic or recurrent laryngeal nerve block. Bilateral blocks imply large doses of local anesthetic and greater risk of systemic toxic reaction. In patients undergoing *multidigit replantation surgery,* the involvement of the anesthesiologist is advisable for management and sedation. Regional anesthesia may be favored if the operation can be completed within the duration of a single-injection brachial plexus block, or if continuous regional anesthesia can be achieved with a catheter technique. Alternatively, the procedure can be started under axillary block with subsequent transition to general anesthesia. When general anesthesia is chosen, the effects of prolonged exposure to inhaled or intravenous anesthetic agents must be borne in mind (Caplan and Long, 1984; Bird,

1984). In addition, anesthesiologist and surgeon must position the patient meticulously, avoiding pressure on nerves and bony prominences. Cycling inflatable mattresses may help prevent pressure necrosis. In patients with *two surgical sites,* the fact that a donor site for skin, bone, or blood vessel is needed does not preclude regional or infiltration anesthesia. Sada and Kobayashi (1983) reported a case of toe to thumb transfer performed using a combination of spinal anesthesia and continuous axillary block. In patients with *infection* or *tumor* in the operative arm, particularly with lymphangitis or palpable axillary or supraclavicular lymph nodes, regional anesthesia is often considered to be relatively contraindicated, although the author has been unable to find clinical data that justify avoidance of blocks in these patients. Winnie (1983) has recommended that one may proceed with regional anesthesia in the presence of infection or tumor except where technically difficult (e.g., when there is axillary adenopathy), using supraclavicular brachial plexus blocks if the axilla is unsatisfactory. Patients undergoing *nerve repair* or who have a history of *paresthesias* or *neural deficit* pose special problems. The concern has been that the anesthetic technique may be implicated if the disease process worsens or if there is an unsatisfactory surgical result. Others have suggested that it is reasonable to proceed with regional technique provided that a thorough preoperative neurologic evaluation is documented in the patient's record and the risks and benefits are carefully explained to the patient. Finally, patients who *refuse regional anesthesia* need a consultation with an anesthesiologist; in most such cases, general anesthesia is needed.

10. There may be the occasional patient in whom more than the usual amount of effort must be taken to avoid *neural complications* related to surgery or anesthesia. Retrospective studies (Selander, Dhuner, and Lundborg, 1977; Selander, Edshage, and Wolff, 1979; Plevak, Linstromberg, and Danielson, 1983; Sada and Kobayashi, 1983; Winchell and Wolfe, 1985) suggest a 0.36 to 2.2 per cent incidence of neuritis secondary to regional anesthesia or block technique. Vandam, in a review (Woolley and Vandam, 1959) of neurologic sequelae of brachial plexus nerve block, commented: "It may be prudent to avoid the use of brachial plexus nerve block in persons . . . whose fingers and hands are

exceedingly important for the performance of fine work. Musicians, artists, and certain types of technicians may fall into this category." Whatever the occupation, patient care is optimized when the relative risks of general and regional anesthesia are discussed with the patient. There is no one answer that is right for all patients.

In summary, there are very few absolute indications or contraindications for any particular scheme of management of anesthesia in hand surgery.

REGIONAL ANESTHESIA FOR HAND SURGERY

Choosing Right Block for Patient

When regional anesthesia for surgery of the upper extremity is selected for a patient, the surgeon or anesthesiologist must choose a technical approach from the many available. These include intravenous regional block, local infiltration, digital block, wrist block, elbow block, axillary block, or one of the infra- or supraclavicular techniques (see

Fig. 91–1). Continuous regional anesthesia is an option. The choice must be made bearing in mind the answers to three questions:

1. *Which approaches match the duration of analgesia required?* Surgical operations on the hand may usefully be divided into those that can be completed within 50 minutes (the limit of tolerance for a tourniquet without anesthesia) and those that cannot. Well-defined procedures lasting less than 50 minutes can be performed using a combination of upper arm or forearm tourniquets plus local nerve blocks at the elbow, wrist, or fingers, with or without subcutaneous ring anesthesia under the tourniquet (Vatashsky, 1980). Alternatively, tourniquet tolerance can be increased (to approximately 90 minutes) by using intravenous regional anesthesia and a double tourniquet. For longer procedures, blockade of the brachial plexus, either single injection or continuous, or general anesthesia must be used. *Continuous technique* can be achieved with the percutaneous placement of plastic catheters into either the interscalene or the subclavian or axillary perivascular spaces. For *multidigit replantation,* continuous technique performed at the *axillary* level

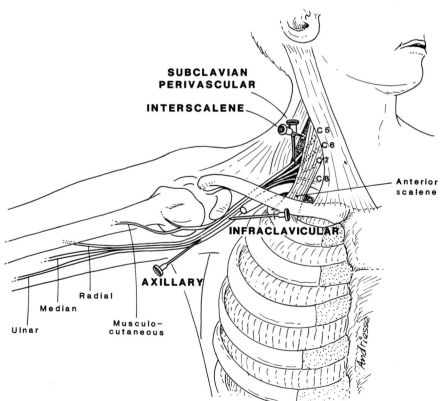

Figure 91–1. Commonly performed brachial plexus blocks.

has been preferred by those reporting large series, because of the appropriate extent of analgesia and the lower incidence of complications seen with this block compared with brachial plexus blocks performed above the clavicle (Matsuda, Kato, and Hosoi, 1982; Sada and Kobayashi, 1983; Neimkin and associates, 1984). Considerations related to the *postoperative course,* such as the need for prolonged sympathetic block and pain relief, or the possibility of reoperation/dressing changes/physical therapy requiring anesthesia, may tip the balance in favor of a continuous technique in certain patients.

2. *Which techniques match the extent of analgesia required?* Such considerations for a hand surgical procedure must take into account the dermatome or sensory nerve distribution of the surgical site, the need for forearm or upper arm analgesia for a tourniquet, and the presence of a second surgical site (if any). The last-named may make general anesthesia mandatory or may simply indicate the necessity of a second regional anesthetic procedure. The need for a tourniquet (1) may be satisfied without anesthesia if its use will be brief, (2) may be satisfied with intravenous regional anesthesia if the time required is less than 90 minutes, or (3) may mandate general anesthesia or brachial plexus blocks, with or without individual blocks of the intercostobrachial or lateral antebrachial cutaneous nerves. Most important, however, the practitioner of regional anesthesia must recognize that the extent of surgical analgesia due to a nerve block is highly dependent on the approach to the nerves to be blocked. For example, not all brachial plexus blocks are equal. Typically, interscalene blocks provide better analgesia in the upper than in the lower cervical nerve distribution, and axillary blocks provide better analgesia in the lower than in the upper cervical nerve distribution. Thus, intravenous regional blocks,

digital or wrist blocks, and axillary blocks are most suitable for hand operations. Blocks near the clavicle are most suitable for upper forearm, elbow, and lower arm analgesia; interscalene techniques are best for surgery on the upper arm and shoulder (Raj, 1985).

Anatomic considerations allow us to predict which portions of the brachial plexus will be difficult to block. With *interscalene* block, anesthesia is most likely to be delayed or absent in the distribution of C_8 and T_1, since those roots are farthest away from the site of anesthetic injection. With blocks near the clavicle, especially in the *subclavian perivascular* technique, the inferior trunk (also C_8 and T_1) may have delayed or absent block because that trunk is farthest from the site of injection, and also because the inferior trunk may reside between the subclavian artery and the upper surface of the first rib, isolating it from the anesthetic agent. With *axillary* block, despite efforts to drive the anesthetic agent centrally, function and sensation may be preserved in the musculocutaneous and axillary nerves, which exit from the axillary sheath at a more proximal level than any of the terminal nerves.

Several clinical studies have been carried out to quantify the frequency with which brachial plexus blocks result in incomplete surgical analgesia (Table 91–1). With *interscalene block,* Lanz, Theiss, and Jankovic (1983), despite using 50 ml of 0.5 per cent bupivacaine, failed to achieve ulnar and medial antebrachial cutaneous anesthesia in about 50 per cent and median nerve anesthesia in about 25 per cent of 50 patients to whom he administered interscalene blocks. Ward (1974) observed lack of analgesia in the ulnar distribution in 11 per cent of 28 patients. Vester-Andersen (1981) failed to achieve analgesia in the medial antebrachial cutaneous nerve in 10 per cent and of the ulnar nerve in 30 per cent of 100 patients,

Table 91–1. Brachial Plexus Blocks: Extent of Analgesia

Block Site	Nerve (% Success)*								
	SC	AX	MC	RA	ME	UL	MA	MB	IC
Interscalene (N = 50)	90	95	98	98	75	50	55	40	25
Subclavian perivascular (N = 56)	40	85	83	85	80	78	78	40	10
Axillary (N = 34)	15	60	60	70	98	95	98	90	10

*Percentage success in blocking each of nine of the nerves of the brachial plexus 20 min after injection of 50 ml 0.5% bupivacaine with vasoconstrictor. SC = supraclavicular; AX = axillary; MC = musculocutaneous; RA = radial; ME = median; UL = ulnar; MA = median antebrachial cutaneous; MB = medial brachial cutaneous; IC = intercostobrachial. Modified from Lanz, E., Theiss, D., and Jankovic, D.: The extent of blockade following various techniques of brachial plexus block. Anesth. Analg., 62:55, 1983.

using 40 ml of agent. With *supraclavicular* and *subclavian perivascular* blocks, Lanz found that all nerves of the brachial plexus, with the exception of the supraclavicular, the medial brachial cutaneous, and the intercostobrachial, were blocked with about the same frequency in 111 patients. Eeckelaert and associates (1984, 100 patients) found similar results. Finally, with regard to *axillary* blocks, Lanz, again using 50 ml of 0.5 per cent bupivacaine, failed to achieve musculocutaneous and axillary nerve sensory block in about 40 per cent of patients. With the *continuous technique,* four large series totaling 836 continuous brachial plexus blocks have been reported, the large majority being axillary blocks. In these studies, catheter technique alone gave adequate surgical analgesia in 77 per cent of 597 patients (Sada and Kobayashi, 1983), 80 per cent of 137 patients (Selander, Dhuner, and Lundberg, 1977), 98 per cent of 52 patients (Ang, Lassale, and Goldfarb, 1984), and 94 per cent of 50 patients (Matsuda, Kats, and Hosoi, 1982). In most instances, supplemental nerve blocks sufficed to permit surgery under regional anesthesia.

In summary, each of the techniques of regional anesthesia may fail to give adequate surgical anesthesia in certain predictable ways, and this should be borne in mind when choosing a particular block for a particular surgical site.

3. *Which techniques offer the smallest chance of complications?* For certain patient groups, even a "minor" complication may lead to significant morbidity. Data on the relative likelihood of complications of particular blocks allow us to distinguish between complications for which there is a known incidence and complications that occur sporadically (Table 91–2). These considerations, as much as any others, may steer us toward or away from a particular block when choosing among approaches that are otherwise equally indicated for a given clinical situation.

Blocks Performed Above Clavicle. There are four complications of blocks performed above the clavicle for which an appropriate incidence can be calculated. Symptomatic *phrenic nerve block* resulting in dyspnea on deep inspiration, or rarely in severe respiratory failure (Hood and Knoblanche, 1979; Schuster, Kafer, and Mandel, 1983), appears to occur with an incidence of 0.4 to 6 per cent (Henderson and Macrae, 1983), but radiographic evidence of unilateral

Table 91–2. Complications of Brachial Plexus Blocks

Interscalene, Supraclavicular, Subclavian, and Subclavian Perivascular Block	
Occasional complications:	Incidence (%)
Phrenic nerve block	30–67
Sympathetic block	50–75
Recurrent laryngeal n. block	1–17
Pneumothorax	0.4–6
Sporadic complications:	
Epidural block	
Total spinal	
Permanent phrenic n. block	
Seizure	
Hemothorax	
Axillary Block	
Occasional complications:	
Toxicity: systemic absorption	0.03–2.8
Sporadic complications:	
Vascular insufficiency	
Intense vasoconstriction	

diaphragmatic paresis was seen in 10 (67 per cent) of 15 patients after single injection subclavian perivascular block in one study (Knoblanche, 1979) and in 0 per cent, 38 per cent, 36 per cent, and 36 per cent of 368 patients having axillary, "classical Kulenkampff, subclavian perivascular, or interscalene blocks, respectively, in another study (Farrar, Scheybani, and Nolte, 1981). Bilateral phrenic nerve block resulting from inadvertent epidural spread of local anesthetic agent, and producing respiratory arrest, is a theoretical possibility and indeed was reported after an interscalene block (Scammell, 1979). Asymptomatic *sympathetic block* resulting in Horner's syndrome (ptosis, miosis, enophthalmos) has been described in 64 per cent of 130 patients (Ramamurthy, cited by Winnie, 1983) and in 52 per cent of 100 patients (Seshadri, cited by Winnie, 1983) following subclavian perivascular block, and in 75 per cent of 100 patients (Vester-Andersen, 1981) following interscalene block. Sympathetic blockade is usually innocuous and transient, but a case of acute bronchospasm concurrent with onset of Horner's syndrome in a known asthmatic was reported by Lim (1979). *Recurrent laryngeal nerve block* causing hoarseness has been reported with a frequency of 1 per cent (Lombard, 1982, 100 patients), 1.5 per cent (Ramamurthy, cited by Winnie, 1983, 134 patients), 6 per cent (Seshadri, cited by Winnie, 1983, 100 patients), and 17 per cent (Vester-Andersen, 1981, 100 patients), and has been innocuous. Bilateral recurrent nerve block has not been reported.

Pneumothorax following brachial plexus blocks above the clavicle has a variable incidence. Symptomatic pneumothorax occurs with a frequency of 0.4 to 6 per cent (Matthes and Denhardt, Schmidt and associates, 1981; Henderson and Macrae 1983; Winnie, 1983) following classical supraclavicular block; following interscalene and subclavian perivascular block the incidence is approximately 1 per cent (Vester-Andersen, 1981, 100 patients; Farrar and associates, 1981, 100 patients).

Other, more severe complications have occurred sporadically following brachial plexus blocks performed above the clavicle. There have been at least ten case reports of *bilateral spread of analgesia via the epidural space* following interscalene block, of which two required intubation and mechanical ventilation for several hours (Kumar and associates, 1971; Cobcroft, 1976; Schoeffler and associates, 1978; Scammell, 1979; McClure and Scott, 1981; Lombard and Couper, 1983; Huang, FitzGerald, and Tsueda, 1986). There are at least five case reports of *total spinal anesthesia* (Ross and Scarborough, 1973; Edde and Deutsch, 1977; Barutell and associates, 1980; Gregoretti, 1980; Winnie, 1983) following interscalene block. *Permanent phrenic nerve paralysis* after interscalene block has been reported several times (Kayerker and Dick, 1983; Bashein, Robertson, and Kennedy, 1985), and has occurred on another occasion known to the author. Several cases of immediate *seizure* following apparent intra-arterial injection (bupivacaine, 15 mg) into the vertebral artery have been reported during performance of interscalene block; Korevar, Burney, and Moore (1979) have calculated that a dose of bupivacaine as small as 7.5 mg injected into the carotid or vertebral artery could result in seizures. *Toxicity from systemic absorption* is discussed elsewhere. *Hemopneumothorax, mediastinal and subcutaneous emphysema* associated with pneumothorax, and a variety of other rare complications have been the subjects of case reports.

Blocks Performed Below Clavicle. There appear to be few complications of infraclavicular or axillary block. There have been sporadic reports of *toxicity from systemic absorption:* Gerstein and associates (1984) reported a series of 11,000 axillary blocks and found three seizures, all in chronic alcoholics, an incidence of 0.03 per cent. Plevak, Linstromberg, and Danielson (1983) reported a 1.5 per cent incidence of seizures in 716 axillary blocks performed with a variety of local anesthetic agents. Sada and Kobayashi (1983) reported systemic toxic reactions (unspecified as to type) in 17 of 597 patients (2.8 per cent) undergoing prolonged hand surgery with continuous axillary block, using up to 600 mg plain lidocaine and mepivacaine as initial doses. Gerstein and associates (1984) also found, during one year of their study, a 0.16 per cent incidence of bradycardia requiring treatment (three of 1922 patients) Several cases of *vascular insufficiency* due to hematoma formation (Sada and Kobayashi, 1983; Restelli and associates, 1984) or *intense vasoconstriction* associated with epinephrine (Merrill, Brodsky, and Hentz, 1981; Matsuda, Kato, and Hosoi, 1982) have been reported. Finally, complications of intravenous regional anesthesia are rare and have involved systemic toxicity resulting from faulty tourniquet technique.

In summary, the choice among regional anesthetic techniques takes many factors into account and must be individualized for each patient. Supraclavicular blocks appear to have much greater potential for morbidity than axillary blocks, and the benefits expected should be worth this added risk.

Local Anesthetic Agents: Basic Pharmacology

Any physician using local anesthetic agents should have a firm understanding of the mechanism of action, structure-function relationships, toxicity, and pharmacodynamics of these drugs. Only then can informed choices be made among the agents and wise decisions made regarding dosage and administration.

Mechanism of Action. The clinically useful local anesthetics produce temporary block of nerve conduction (Strichartz, 1983). They interfere with the function of sodium channels, causing inhibition of sodium conductance, and prevent development of action potentials. They fall into two chemical categories: drugs with an ester link between the aromatic end of the molecule and the intermediate chain, and drugs with an amide link. This difference is reflected biologically in the *site of metabolism* (ester compounds are hydrolyzed in plasma, whereas amide compounds undergo degradation in the liver), and in the *allergic potential,* because a high frequency of sensitizing reactions is observed with the ester derivatives of para-aminobenzoic acid.

sory fibers first, because of the predominance of sensory fibers in the core and greater vascular absorption there.

Patient Management: Consent, Premedication, Sedation

A calm, cooperative patient is important for the performance of regional blocks as well as for surgery itself. If regional anesthesia is contemplated, the doctor and patient must agree in advance that this is the best form of anesthesia. Bearing in mind the sometimes conflicting needs of patient rapport, medical conscience, and legal liability, patients must be made sufficiently aware of risks, alternatives, and benefits in order that "informed consent" may be obtained and appropriately noted in the chart. For elective surgery, the patient should fast for six to eight hours before the procedure.

It is essential to remember that pharmacologic measures are only adjuncts to preoperative counseling. With regard to premedication, *benzodiazepines* (diazepam, lorazepam) as a class are excellent for anxiolysis, reduction of awareness, amnesia, and centrally mediated muscle relaxation. They also decrease the CNS toxic effect of local anesthetics by raising the seizure threshold. They can be potentiated with small intramuscular doses of *droperidol*, which adds an antiemetic effect and produces a calm, cooperative patient who is somewhat indifferent to the surroundings but still capable of responding to instructions. Since some discomfort is inherent in regional anesthesia, the addition of a *narcotic* (morphine, 0.05 to 0.1 mg/kg, or meperidine, 0.5 to 1.0 mg/kg intramuscularly) to the preoperative regimen may be useful. Once in the operating room, these can be supplemented with additional intravenous medications. Winnie (1983) has recommended that for procedures lasting more than 90 minutes, 1.0 to 1.5 mg/kg of *hydroxyzine* be administered intramuscularly into the anesthetized region for long-acting sedation. Others have used *barbiturates* as infusions. *Ketamine,* as discussed earlier, can be used in small intramuscular doses in pediatric patients to permit performance of blocks. *It is essential to bear in mind that all of the above are extremely potent medications capable of causing loss of consciousness, profound respiratory depression, and loss of airway protective reflexes if used inappropriately. General anesthesia may indeed be induced with only*

intravenous diazepam and meperidine or morphine. "Supplementary" medications can never make up for pain from the surgical field due to an inadequate block, and oversedation may be extraordinarily dangerous, especially when the surgeon is acting both as operator and anesthesiologist.

Along with drug therapy, the conscious patient should be afforded other comforts, e.g., pillows, table flexion, warmth, and a quiet operating room or music via headphones.

Block Performance: General Aspects

Before any nerve block is begun, access to resuscitative equipment and medications is mandatory. Appropriate monitoring and resuscitative equipment should include at a minimum (1) a means of administering oxygen by positive pressure (e.g., an anesthesia machine or an anesthetic bag and mask connected to a source of oxygen); (2) airway management equipment including laryngoscope, oropharyngeal airways, cuffed endotracheal tubes, and a suction catheter connected to wall suction; and (3) labeled syringes containing a short-acting barbiturate, diazepam, succinylcholine, and a vasopressor (ephedrine, 5 to 10 mg/ml). An intravenous infusion should be in place, and the patient should be monitored at least with an ECG and a blood pressure cuff. *Record keeping* must be concise but comprehensive, noting at a minimum type of block, supplemental blocks, anesthetic agent and additives, needle type, use of adjunctive equipment (nerve stimulators), paresthesias, puncture of blood vessels, hematomas, tourniquet pressure and time, and unexpected reactions. Postoperative visits and notes should specifically address postanesthetic sequelae.

A variety of devices and logistic arrangements have been advocated to facilitate regional anesthesia. A dedicated anesthesia *block room* has been shown to improve operating room efficiency (Rosenblatt and Shal, 1983). *Nerve stimulators* have improved success in patients who cannot cooperate sufficiently to report paresthesias (Smith, 1976; Yasuda and associates, 1980; Gribomont, 1981; Eeckelaert and associates, 1984; Raj, 1985). Characteristics of useful stimulators include constant current output (0.1 to 5 mA), clear meter reading to 0.1 mA, variable output control, linear output, short pulse width, pulse of 1 Hz, properly marked polarity (allowing the cathode [−] to be attached to the needle), high and low output scale, battery indicator, and high quality alligator-type clips (Ford, Pither, and Raj, 1984; Pither, Raj, and Ford, 1985). Winnie (1983) has popularized the *immobile needle,* consisting of a piece of flexible plastic tubing inserted between the injection needle and the syringe, so that necessary manipulation of the syringe does not cause movement of the needle. In general, *22 or 24 gauge, 1½ inch, 45 degree bevel translucent hub needles* are preferred for nerve block (Winnie, 1983). The clinical advantages of such needles are reduced trauma to nerves (Selander, 1977), easy identification ("fascial click") of tissue planes, and early recognition of intravascular needle placement. *Insulated needles* (Ford, Pither, and Raj, 1984; Bashein, Robertson, and Kennedy 1984) and insulated needles with *pencil points* (Galindo, 1980) offer certain advantages when used with nerve stimulators, but have not gained widespread use. A *modified Seldinger technique* has been recommended (Rosenblatt, Pepitone-Rockwell, and McKillop, 1979; Mehler and Otten, 1983; Ang, Lassale, and Goldfarb, 1984; Postel and Marz, 1984) as a means of advancing a catheter up the axillary sheath for continuous technique. Rarely, *surgical exposure of the axillary sheath* contents (Tonczar and associates, 1983) has been utilized in special situations to permit brachial plexus block.

Specific Blocks

The important regional anesthetic techniques for the upper extremity are brachial plexus blocks at different levels, intravenous regional anesthesia, peripheral nerve blocks at the elbow, and wrist and digital nerve blocks. Numerous techniques have been described, and an excellent historical review with original illustrations has been assembled in a monograph by Winnie (1983). Several important blocks are briefly described below, and the reader is referred to standard anesthesia textbooks for further detail (Cousins and Bridenbaugh, 1980; Winnie, 1983; Raj, 1985).

Interscalene Block (Fig. 91–2). Advantages of the interscalene approach to the brachial plexus include reliable blockade of C3-C4 as well as the remainder of the bra-

chial plexus, making it the only block suitable for shoulder surgery. It is an excellent choice for surgery on the radial aspect of the hand, wrist, or base of thumb "snuff box" where reliable anesthesia requires median, radial, and musculocutaneous blockade. Disadvantages of this block relate to the difficulty of blocking C8-T1, which limits its usefulness for surgery on the ulnar aspect of the wrist, and for elbow surgery. In addition, it is subject to the higher incidence of complications generally seen in brachial plexus blocks performed above the clavicle.

Surface landmarks can best be seen by having the patient lie supine with his head turned away from the side to be blocked. If the patient lifts his head from the table, the sternocleidomastoid muscle becomes taut. The interscalene groove is palpated by rolling the fingers back from the sternocleidomastoid over the anterior scalene and into the groove between the anterior and middle scalene muscles. If the patient takes a deep breath, both scalene muscles contract, confirming correct finger position (Sharrock and Bruce, 1976). The point of needle entry (Fig. 91–2*B*) should be at the level of the transverse process of C6, as determined by the intersection of a line drawn laterally from the cricoid cartilage and the interscalene groove. The external jugular vein usually crosses the scalene muscles near this point. A 1½ inch, 22 or 24 gauge needle is inserted into the interscalene groove perpendicular to the skin in all planes, inward, caudad, and slightly posterior. The needle is advanced until a paresthesia to the fingertips is obtained, at which time the needle is fixed and aspirated for blood or cerebrospinal fluid and 20 to 40 ml of local anesthetic solution is injected. If bone is contacted (usually the transverse process of C6), the needle is repositioned. Digital pressure cephalad to the needle directs the solution toward the lower roots, if analgesia of the hand (C5-T1) is the reason for performing the block. The intercostobrachial and medialbrachial cutaneous nerves should be blocked separately by deposition of a few milliliters of local anesthetic over the axillary artery pulse if a tourniquet is to be used during the procedure, since they arise from C8 and T1, nerve roots that may be incompletely blocked with this technique.

Subclavian Perivascular Block (Fig. 91–3). Subclavian perivascular block is a modification, described by Winnie, of the traditional supraclavicular block of Kulen-

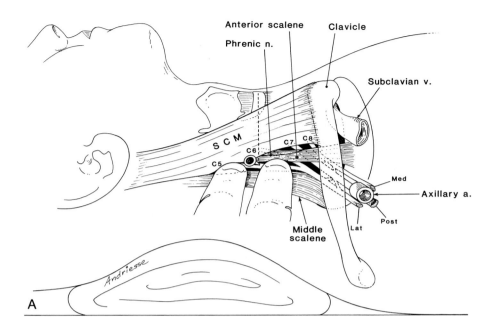

Anterior scalene
Clavicle
Phrenic n.
Subclavian v.
S C M
C6 C7 C8
C5
Med
Axillary a.
Post
Lat
Middle
scalene

Andriesse

A

Carotid a., internal jugular v.,
and vagus n. in carotid sheath

Sternocleidomastoid

Phrenic n.

Anterior scalene

Trachea
Thyroid
Esophagus

Middle scalene

C6

Andriesse

B

Figure 91–2. Interscalene block. *A,* The needle is in the interscalene space, touching the trunks of the brachial plexus. *B,* Cross sectional view.

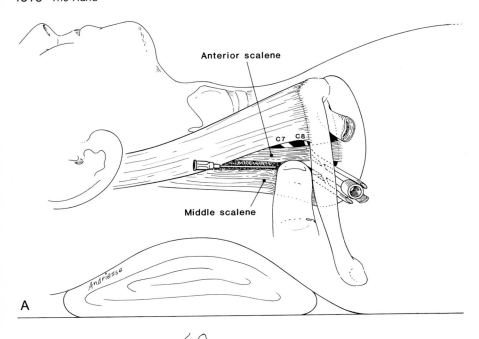

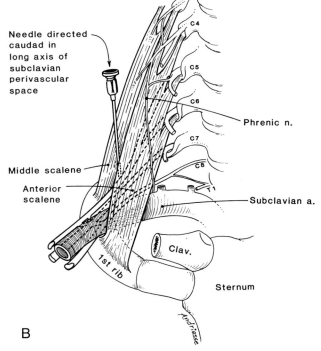

Figure 91–3. *A,* Subclavian perivascular approach to the brachial plexus. The needle is in the interscalene space, directed caudad. *B,* Subclavian perivascular block.

kampff. Its advantages are that it provides reliable blockade of all the roots of the brachial plexus from C5 to T1. It is thus suited for elbow and forearm anesthesia, and for surgery on the radial aspect of the wrist and hand. Disadvantages are that T1-T2 occasionally are not blocked, making the block less suitable for surgery on the ulnar aspect of the hand, and that the block is subject to the higher rate of complications seen with brachial plexus blocks performed above the clavicle.

To carry out the block, the interscalene space is identified as for performance of an interscalene block. The palpating finger is then moved inferiorly along the groove until

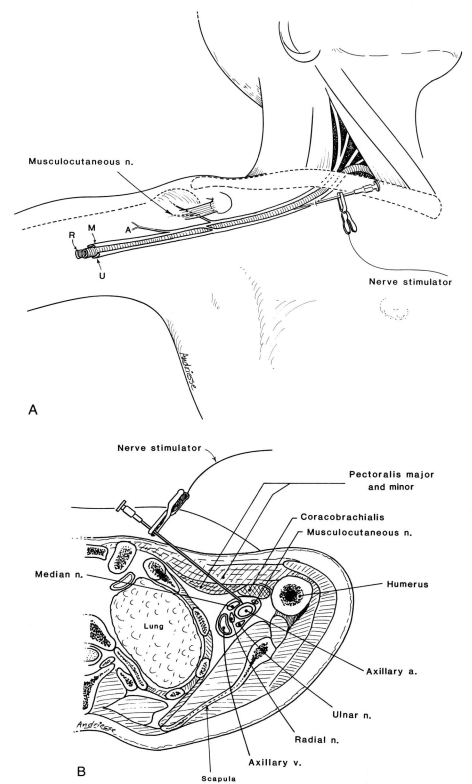

Figure 91–4. *A, B,* Infraclavicular block. The needle enters the skin 1 inch below the midclavicular point. It is directed laterally toward the axillary artery at an angle of 45 degrees to the skin, with the patient's arm abducted to 90 degrees. A nerve stimulator is essential to the technique.

the pulse of the subclavian artery is palpated. A 1½ inch, 21 to 22 gauge needle is inserted just above this point in a direction that is directly caudad (Fig. 91–3A). Since the trunks of the brachial plexus lie closer to the middle scalene muscle than to the anterior, the needle should be inserted into the posterior one-third of the space between the two muscles. The needle is advanced until a paresthesia to below the elbow is obtained, at which time the entire dosage of local anesthetic is injected. The intercostobrachial and medial brachial cutaneous nerves must be blocked separately in the axilla if a tourniquet is to be used.

Infraclavicular Block (Fig. 91–4). An infraclavicular approach to the brachial plexus has been popularized by Raj. The advantage of the technique is that it blocks the cords and branches of the brachial plexus above the level of formation of the musculocutaneous and axillary nerves, thus permitting anesthesia of the entire arm. Its disadvantages are the need for nerve stimulator, and perhaps greater patient discomfort during performance of the block. The technique (Fig. 91–4A) involves use of a 3½ inch 22 gauge spinal needle introduced 1 inch below the inferior border of the clavicle at its midpoint, and aimed laterally toward the brachial artery in the axilla. When proximity to the brachial plexus is confirmed by paresthesias elicited by the nerve stimulator, 40 ml of local anesthetic solution is injected.

Axillary Block (Fig. 91–5). The advantages of axillary block include ease of performance, low incidence of complications, and reliability of analgesia in the C7-C8-T1 distribution. It is thus ideal for surgery on the hand. Many techniques can be used for axillary block. Modification of a perivascular technique described by Winnie, incorporating the prodution of paresthesias, gives a high success rate in adults. The adult patient is positioned with the arm abducted 90 degrees and flexed at the elbow. The axillary artery is then located at its proximal point in the axilla. Once the skin is prepared, a short bevel needle is inserted (Fig. 91–5A), seeking either an ulnar or median nerve paresthesia. Once a paresthesia to the fingers occurs, the needle position is fixed. The anesthetic agent is administered after aspiration tests are negative. Use of large volumes (40 ml) and digital pressure distal to the needle help ensure a block of the musculocutaneous nerve. An alternative technique used in the author's in-

stitution (Kleinert and associates, 1963) involves use of three 12 ml syringes with 25 gauge needles: ulnar, median, and radial paresthesias are sought before injection of the anesthetic. Once an initial injection of local anesthetic has been made, subsequent paresthesias may be harder to elicit. Transfixion of the axillary artery, to facilitate radial nerve block, is routine. In the *pediatric patient* who is uncooperative or unable to report paresthesias, transfixing the artery increases the success rate. In this approach the child is sedated and local anesthetic is injected both above and below the vessel. As with the other major blocks of the plexus, the intercostobrachial and medial antebrachial cutaneous nerves may be blocked separately (Fig. 91–5B), although proximal placement of the local anesthetic agent near the edge of the pectoralis muscle often blocks these nerves.

Intravenous Regional Anesthesia. Intravenous regional anesthesia (IVRA) offers an agreeable combination of ease of administration, safety, and efficacy. The technique is limited in duration on the basis of tourniquet tolerance, and there is no residual analgesia after tourniquet release, unless supplemental nerve blocks have been performed. There is controversy regarding the site of action of IVRA, some investigators favoring sensory nerve endings, some favoring nerve trunks, and others the neuromuscular junction. (Lillie, Glynn, and Fenwick, 1984; Raj, 1985).

The main points regarding IVRA administration are the following. Intravenous access should be available in the contralateral extremity. The cuff inflation apparatus must be reliable. The intravenous cannula is placed distally to avoid high venous pressures near the cuff. The arm must be exsanguinated thoroughly, using elevation and an Esmarch bandage. The proximal cuff must be inflated to at least 100 mm Hg above systolic pressure. Arterial occlusion must be confirmed by a distal pulse check. Injection of local anesthetic must be carried out slowly (over one to two minutes) to avoid leakage, due to high venous pressure, of agent under the cuff. The second (distal) cuff may then be inflated and the proximal cuff deflated to avoid pain from the tourniquet after anesthesia has been established. A "second wrap" technique has been advocated (Landeen, Epstein, and Haas, 1978; Haas and Landeen, 1978) to provide a dry operative field, diminished tourniquet pain, and better anesthesia. A minimum of

levels during continuous interscalene block. Anesthesiology, *62*:65, 1985.

Kleinert, H. E., DeSimone, K., Gaspar, H. E., Arnold, R. E., and Kasdan, M. L.: Regional anesthesia for upper extremity surgery. J. Trauma, *3*:3, 1963.

Knoblanche, G. E.: The incidence and aetiology of phrenic nerve blockade associated with supraclavicular brachial plexus block. Anaesth. Intensive Care, *7*:346, 1979.

Korevar, W. C., Burney, R. G., and Moore, P. A.: Convulsions during stellate ganglion block. Anesth. Analg., *58*:329, 1979.

Kumar, A., Battit, G. E., Froese, A. B., and Long, M. C.: Bilateral cervical and thoracic epidural blockade complicating interscalene brachial plexus block. Anesthesiology, *35*:650, 1971.

Lalka, D., Vicuna, N., Burrow, S. R., Jones, D. J., Ludden, T. M., et al.: Bupivacaine and other amide local anesthetics inhibit the hydrolysis of chloroprocaine by human serum. Anesth. Analg., *57*:534, 1978.

Landeen, F. H., Epstein, L., and Haas, L.: Special regional anesthetic techniques in ambulatory anesthesia. Contemp. Anesth. Pract., *1*:71, 1978.

Lanz, E., and Theiss, D.: Evaluation of brachial plexus block—comparison between supraclavicular and interscalene approach. Regional Anaesthesie, *2*:57, 1979.

Lanz, E., Theiss, D., and Jankovic, D.: The extent of blockade following various techniques of brachial plexus block. Anesth. Analg. *62*:55, 1983.

Lawes, E. G., Johnson, T., Pritchard, P., and Robbins, P.: Venous pressures during simulated Bier's block. Anaesthesia, *39*:147, 1984.

Leak, W. D., and Winchell, S. W.: Regional anesthesia in pediatric patients—review of clinical experience. Regional Anesth., *7*:64, 1982.

Lehman, W. L., and Jones, W. W.: Intravenous lidocaine for anesthesia in the lower extremity. J. Bone Joint Surg., *66a*:1056, 1984.

Lillie, P. E., Glynn, C. J., and Fenwick, D. G.: Site of action of intravenous regional anesthesia. Anesthesiology, *61*:507, 1984.

Lim, E. K.: Interscalene brachial plexus block in the asthmatic patient. Anesthesia, *34*:370, 1979.

Lofstrom, B., Wennberg, A., and Widen, L.: Late disturbances in nerve function after block with local anesthetic agents. Acta Anaesth. Scand., *10*:111, 1966.

Lombard, T. P.: The interscalene approach to block of the brachial plexus. S. A. Med. J., *62*:871, 1982.

Lombard, T. P., and Couper, J. L.: Bilateral spread of analgesia following interscalene brachial plexus block. Anesthesiology, *58*:472, 1983.

Mani, M., Ramamurthy, N., Rao, T. L. K., Winnie, A. P., and Collins, V. J.: An unusual complication of brachial plexus block and heparin therapy. Anesthesiology, *48*:213, 1978.

Matsuda, M., Kato, N., and Hosoi, H.: Continuous brachial plexus block for replantation in the upper extremity. Hand, *14*:129, 1982.

Matthes, H., and Denhardt, B.: Experiences with brachial plexus blocks. Langenbecks Arch. Chir., *345*:505, 1977.

Mazze, R. I., and Dunbar, R. W.: Plasma lidocaine concentrations after caudal, lumbar epidural, axillary block and intravenous regional anesthesia. Anesthesiology, *27*:574, 1966.

McClure, J. H., and Scott, D. B.: Comparison of bupivacaine hydrochloride and carbonated bupivacaine in brachial plexus block by the interscalene technique. Br. J. Anaesth., *53*:523, 1981.

Mehler, D., and Otten, B.: A new set of catheters for continuous axillary plexus block. Regional Anaesthesie, *6*:43, 1983.

Melman, E., Penuelas, J. A., and Marrufo, J.: Regional anesthesia in children. Anesth. Analg., *54*:387, 1975.

Merrill, D. G., Brodsky, J. B., and Hentz, R. V.: Vascular insufficiency following axillary block of the brachial plexus. Anesth. Analg., *60*:162, 1981.

Moore, D. C., Bridenbaugh, L. D., and Bridenbaugh, P. O.: Does compounding of local anesthetic agents increase their toxicity in humans? Anesth. Analg., *51*:579, 1972.

Moore, D. C., Mather, L. E., Lysons, D. F., and Horton, W. G.: Arterial and venous plasma levels of bupivacaine following peripheral nerve blocks. Anesth. Analg., *55*:763, 1976.

Neimkin, R. J., May, J. W., Jr., Roberts, J., and Sunder, N.: Continuous axillary block through an indwelling Teflon catheter. J. Hand Surg., *9A*:830, 1984.

Ogden, P. N.: Failure of intravenous regional analgesia using a double cuff tourniquet. Anaesthesia, *39*:456, 1984.

Pither, C. E., Raj, P. P., and Ford, D. J.: The use of peripheral nerve stimulators for regional anesthesia—a review of experimental characteristics, technique, and clinical applications. Regional Anesth., *10*:49, 1985.

Plevak, D. J., Linstromberg, J. W., and Danielson, D. R.: Paresthesia vs. nonparesthesia—the axillary block. Anesthesiology, *59*:A216, 1983.

Postel, J., and Marz, P.: Electrical nerve localization and catheter technique. Regional Anaesthesie, *7*:104, 1984.

Pratt, J. M.: Analgesics and sedation in plastic surgery. Clin. Plast. Surg., *12*:73, 1985.

Radtke, H., Nolte, H, Fruhstorfer, H., and Zenz, M.: A comparative study between etidocaine and bupivacaine in ulnar nerve block. Acta Anaesth. Scand. Suppl., *60*:17, 1975.

Raj, P. P.: and Jenkins, M. T.: The site of action of intravenous regional anesthesia. Anesth. Analg., *51*:776, 1972.

Raj, P. P.: Ancillary measures to assure success. Regional Anesth., *5*:9, 1980.

Raj, P. P.: Handbook of Regional Anesthesia. New York, Churchill Livingstone, 1985.

Raj, P. P., Katz, R. L., and Carden, E.: Dynamics of local-anesthetic compounds in regional anesthesia. Anesth. Analg., *56*:110, 1977.

Raj, P. P., Montgomery, S. J., and Jenkins, M. T.: Infraclavicular brachial plexus block—a new approach. Anesth. Analg., *52*:897, 1973.

Reiz, S., and Nath, S.: Cardiotoxicity of local anaesthetic agents. Br. J. Anaesth., *58*:736, 1986.

Restelli, L., Pinciroli, D., Conoscente, F., and Cammelli, F.: Insufficient venous drainage following axillary approach to brachial plexus blockade. Br. J. Anaesth., *56*:1051, 1984.

Reynolds, F.: Bupivacaine and intravenous regional anaesthesia. Anaesthesia, *19*:105, 1984.

Rosenberg, P. H., Kalso, E. A., Tuominen, M. K., and Linden, H. B.: Acute bupivacaine toxicity as a result of venous leakage under the tourniquet cuff during a Bier block. Anesthesiology, *58*:95, 1983.

Rosenblatt, R., Pepitone-Rockwell, F., and McKillop, M. J.: Continuous axillary analgesia for traumatic hand injury. Anesthesiology, *51*:565, 1979.

Rosenblatt, R. M., and Shal, R.: The design and function of a regional anesthesia block room. Regional Anesth., *9*:12, 1983.

Ross, S., and Scarborough, C. D.: Total spinal anesthesia following brachial plexus block. Anesthesiology, 39:458, 1973.

Rousso, M., Wexler, M. R., Weinberg, H., Vatashky, E., and Aronson, B.: Subutaneous ring anaesthesia in the prevention of tourniquet pain in hand surgery. Hand, 10:317, 1978.

Rudzinski, J. P., and Ampel, L. L.: Pediatric application of intravenous regional anesthesia. Regional Anesth., 8:69, 1983.

Sada, T., and Kobayashi, T.: Continuous axillary brachial plexus block. Can. Anaesth. Soc. J., 30:201, 1983.

Scammell, S. J.: Inadvertent epidural anaesthesia as a complication of interscalene brachial plexus block. Anaesth. Intensive Care, 7:56, 1979.

Schmidt, E., Racenberg, E., Hilderbrand, G., and Buch, U.: Complications and risks of brachial plexus anaesthesia with special reference to long-term damage. Anasth. Intensivther. Notfallmed., 16:346, 1981.

Schoeffler, P., Haberer, J. P., Concina, D., Mehl, C., and Fornecker, M. L.: Une complication de l'anesthesie par bloc interscalenique du plexus brachial: l'anesthesie peridurale cervico-thoracique. Anesth. Analg. Rean., 35:199, 1978.

Schulte-Steinberg, O.: Regional anaesthesia for children. Ann. Chirurg. Gynaecol., 73:158, 1984.

Schuster, S. B., Kafer, E. R., and Mandel, S.: Phrenic nerve block associated with interscalene brachial plexus block. Regional Anesth., 8:123, 1983.

Schwartz, P. S., Newman, A., and Green, A. L.: Intravenous regional anesthesia. J. Am. Podiatry Assoc., 73:201, 1983.

Scott, D. B.: Toxic effects of local anaesthetic agents on the central nervous system. Br. J. Anaesth., 58:732, 1986.

Selander, D.: Catheter technique in axillary plexus block. Acta Anaesth. Scand., 21:324, 1977.

Selander, D., Dhuner, K. G., and Lundborg, G.: Peripheral nerve injury due to injection needles used for regional anaesthesia. Acta Anaesth. Scand., 21:182, 1977.

Selander, D., Edshage, S., and Wolff, T.: Paresthesiae or no paresthesiae—nerve lesions after axillary blocks. Acta Anaesth. Scand., 23:27, 1979.

Selander, D., Mansson, L. G., Karlsson, L., and Svanvik, J.: Adrenergic vasoconstriction in peripheral nerves of the rabbit. Anesthesiology, 62:6, 1985.

Seltzer, J. L.: Hoarseness and Horner's syndrome after interscalene brachial plexus block. Anesth. Analg., 56:585, 1977.

Shanahan, P. T., and Kleinert, H. E.: Anesthesia management of upper extremity replantation surgery. Anesthesiol. Rev., 10:10, 1982.

Sharrock, N. E., and Bruce, G.: An improved technique for locating the interscalene grove. Anesthesiology, 44:431, 1976.

Sims, J. K.: A modification of landmarks for infraclavicular approach to brachial plexus block. Anesth. Analg., 56:554, 1977.

Smith, B. L.: Efficacy of a nerve stimulator in regional analgesia; experience in a resident training programme. Anaesthesia, 31:778, 1976.

Strasser, K., Abel, J., Breulmann, M., Schumacher, I., Siepmann, H. P., and Trampisch, H. J.: Plasma level of etidocaine within the first two hours after axillary block in healthy adults and patients with renal insufficiency. Regional Anaesthesie, 4:14, 1981.

Strichartz, G. R.: Physiology of nerve transmission (including comments on the mechanisms of local anesthetic action). Semin. Anesth., 2:1, 1983.

Thiagarajah, S., Lear, E., Azar, I., Salzer, J., and Zeiligsohn, E.: Bronchospasm following interscalene brachial plexus block. Anesthesiology, 61:759, 1984.

Thiessen, E., Bergmann, J., and Steinhoff, H.: Prilocaine induced methemoglobinemia after interscalene block. Regional Anaesthesie, 7:94, 1984.

Thompson, G. E., and Rorie, D. K.: Functional anatomy of the brachial plexus sheaths. Anesthesiology, 59:117, 1983.

Tonczar, L, Ilias, W., Mayrhofer, O., Munk, P., and Sandbach, G.: An unusual procedure in performing brachial plexus block. Arch. Orthop. Trauma. Surg., 101:297, 1983.

Tucker, G. T., and Mather, L. E.: Clinical pharmacokinetics of local anesthetics. Clin. Pharmacokinet., 4:241, 1979.

Tuominen, M., Rosenberg, P. H., and Kalso, E.: Blood levels of bupivacaine after single dose, supplementary dose, and during continuous infusion in axillary plexus block. Acta Anaesthesiol. Scand., 27:303, 1983.

Vatashsky, E., Aronson, H. B., Wexler, M. R., and Rousso, M.: Anesthesia in a hand surgery unit. J. Hand Surg., 5:495, 1980.

Vester-Andersen, T., Christiansen, C., Hansen, A., Sørensen, M., and Meisler, C.: Interscalene brachial plexus block: area of analgesia, complications and blood concentrations of local anaesthetics. Acta Anaesth. Scand., 25:81, 1981.

Ward, M. E.: The interscalene approach to the brachial plexus. Anaesthesia, 29:147, 1974.

Wencker, K. H., Fruhstorfer, M., and Nolte, H.: Axillary plexus block with long acting local anaesthetics—a comparative study of etidocaine and bupivacaine. Anaesthetist, 24:521, 1975.

Whiffler, K.: Coracoid block—a safe and easy technique. Br. J. Anaesth., 53:845, 1981.

Wildsmith, J. A. W., Tucker, G. T., Cooper, S., Scott, D. B., and Covino, B. G.: Plasma concentrations of local anaesthetics after interscalene brachial plexus block. Br. J. Anaesth., 49:461, 1977.

Winchell, S. W., and Wolfe, R.: The incidence of neuropathy following upper extremity nerve blocks. Regional Anesth., 10:12, 1985.

Winnie, A. P.: Plexus Anesthesia. Philadelphia, W. B. Saunders Company, 1983.

Winnie, A. P., Tay, C., Patel, K. P., Ramamurthy, S., and Durrani, Z.: Pharmacokinetics of local anesthetics during plexus blocks. Anesth. Analg., 56:852, 1977.

Woolley, E. J., and Vandam, L. D.: Neurological sequelae of brachial plexus nerve block. Ann. Surg., 149:53, 1959.

Yasuda, I., Ojima, T., Ohhira, N., Kaneko, T., and Yammamuro, M.: Supraclavicular brachial plexus block using a nerve stimulator and an insulated needle. Br. J. Anaesth., 52:409, 1980.

92

Nancy H. McKee, M.D.

Amputation Stump Management and Function Preservation

Amputation is defined as the removal of an extremity. When this removal is carried out through a joint, it is described as a disarticulation. Amputation can be congenital, traumatic, or surgical. The goal of surgical amputation is to create a satisfactory stump with maximal function and comfort. The surgeon is responsible for ensuring that the patient is fitted with an adequate prosthesis and educated as to its proper use, as well as for helping the amputee to attain mental and emotional readjustment.

HISTORICAL PERSPECTIVE

Amputations were recorded over 30,000 years ago in the cave paintings of grottos in France and Spain. Many were probably related to frostbite in the Upper Palaeolithic period (Sahly, 1963). Man's ingenuity has been working with the problem of prostheses for centuries. M. Sergius had an iron hand after the Second Punic War (218–202 B.C.) (Rang and Thompson, 1981). Putti (1929) reports fifteenth and sixteenth century prostheses still existing complete with ratchets and pivots to permit grasp and pinch. We also know that detailed arrangements for compensation of loss of fingers were available in the eleventh century (Bertelsen and Capener, 1960). Gillis (1954) provides an interesting historical review of the tools and technique of amputation surgery. The great leaps in technology in the twentieth century should be considered in light of the past.

INDICATIONS

Upper limb amputations present either as emergencies or as elective problems:
1. Trauma. The injuring agent may be mechanical (Arcari, Larsen, and Posch, 1959; Entin, 1964; Swanson, 1963; Grogono, 1973; Ransford and Hughes, 1977; Galway, Hubbard, and Mowbray, 1981); electrical (Solem,

Fischer, and Strate, 1977; Esses and Peters, 1981); thermal; related to frostbite (Page and Robertson, 1983); or chemical (Tooms, 1980).

2. Malignant tumors. Amputations are for cure or for palliation (Carroll, 1957; El-Domeiri and Miller, 1969).

3. Infection. This can be either acute, fulminating, and life threatening or chronic and unresponsive to less ablative procedures.

4. Vascular problems or malformations. Vasculitis, systemic, self-inflicted, or iatrogenic, may lead to amputation (Chase, 1960; Lynch, Key, and White, 1979).

5. Trophic ulceration (Swanson, 1963).

6. A flail useless part may be amputated from a congenital anomaly to improve function. This should not be done if there is any other use for these tissues (Tooms, 1980).

GOALS IN AMPUTATION SURGERY

The goal is first to eradicate any precipitating factor that necessitated the amputation and then to provide maximal function of the residual extremity. A comfortable stump with functional length and useful, painfree sensation is sought. Rapid tissue healing (facilitated by good planning and atraumatic technique) and early rehabilitation help prevent adjacent joint contractures and loss of power and endurance. Early prosthetic fitting enables the patient to achieve the best use of the extremity and an early return to work.

The advantages of early rehabilitation in an amputee center have been extolled by many, including Jones (1977).

COMPLICATIONS

Complications can be classified according to the timing, the specific entity involved, and the level.

Preoperative

Hypovolemic Shock. Fluid losses should be recognized and corrected promptly. A compressive dressing and elevation minimize blood loss from most sites. Direct compression and tourniquet have a role in preventing life-threatening hemorrhagic shock.

Infection. To avoid subsequent infection, it is imperative that dirty, freshly injured extremities be promptly, thoroughly washed. Povidone-iodine (Betadine) solution can be employed as the irrigating fluid before use of copious normal saline solution. A sterile dressing is applied and appropriate intravenous antibiotic started.

Intraoperative. Hemorrhagic shock remains a possible complication until all significant vessels have been securely ligated. Careful hemostasis is the key to prevention of postoperative hematoma. Thorough debridement of all devitalized tissue and foreign material is essential to help prevent infection. Wound cover is thoughtfully planned. Bunnell (1932) illustrates the loss of function from contractures of the hand. Littler (1956)

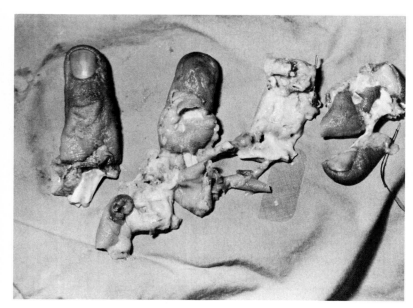

Figure 92–1. Four unreplantable fingers crushed in a punch press making thin aluminum pie plates. Four closed amputation stumps were created on the day of injury.

comments that "more deformity is encountered secondary to skin loss and cicatricial contracture than from any other single factor." In severe crushing injuries, electrolyte imbalances (Entin, 1955) and the complications from myoglobinemia can be fatal.

Postoperative. Early complications include wound hematoma, infection, and necrosis. These are potentially preventable and every effort should be taken to avoid them.

Late complications may be neurologic, musculoskeletal, vascular, skin related, or psychologic.

Neurologic sequelae. Weir Mitchell's book on injuries to the nerves (reprinted in 1965) devotes a chapter to the "neural maladies of stumps." He quotes his patients (injured in the American Civil War) as giving descriptive accounts of phantom limbs ("sensory hallucinations"), altered sensation, stump spasms or chorea, acute neuralgia, and neuromata. Mitchell states that he did not reamputate any of his patients, but was aware of others who had reamputated because of pain and had not been rewarded in their efforts. His treatment included leeches, bandages, hypodermic injections of morphine, large warm poultices, mercurial ointments, and considerable support. Leriche (1939) in his book *The Surgery of Pain* devoted a chapter to "the pain of amputation stumps." With respect to unremitting hyperesthesia of a stump, Leriche describes finding on four occasions a hyperemic arachnoiditis localized to the side of the spinal cord of the amputation. He emphatically states four principles of what *not* to do: (1) "one must not underestimate the complaints of a man who has had an amputation whose stump is painful"; (2) "the patient should not be kept waiting unduly long for the careful examination which alone can determine the method of production of his pains"; (3) "the patient should not be allowed to become a morphine addict"; and (4) "reamputation must be avoided."

Bailey and Moersch (1941) define a phantom limb as "the sensation of feeling in the presence of an extremity following its amputation." It is a common occurrence after amputation, but infrequently leads to incapacitating symptoms. Herrmann and Gibbs (1945) report that the incidence of phantom limb pain was highest after major amputation in an extremity that was severely traumatized. Livingstone (1945) found that a phantom limb began immediately or very soon after amputation and that its pattern did not

change significantly during the healing period. The phantom limb was not a total reproduction of the amputated extremity, but usually had dominance of the more sensory parts, such as fingers, of the extremity. Stimulation of a neuroma did not elicit typical phantom sensations. Feinstein, Luce, and Langton (1968) summarize the schools of thought of peripheral versus central origin of the phenomenon, and conclude that there is no single cause.

Patients undergoing amputations should be informed of phantom limb sensations and reassured about the variations that these sensations can take. After the early postoperative period, many patients cease to be concerned about their phantom.

Neuromas, painful stumps, and Sudeck's are elaborated upon in Chapters 111 and 113. Efforts continue to be made to differentiate between central and peripheral phenomenon. The thalamus (Iselin and Mazars, 1984) is but one central level at which interference in pain pathways has been attempted.

Musculoskeletal Problems

CONTRACTURES. Prevention is of the utmost importance. The patient should be encouraged to keep the extremity mobile to help avoid contractures. Dederich (1963) describes his controversial myoplastic stump correction as capable of creating active muscle movements and relieving pains caused by "cramped and retracted muscles."

FINGER TENDONS. A finger with excess lumbrical pull can result from loss of the insertion of flexor digitorum profundus. Parkes (1970) felt that it most commonly occurred in the middle finger.

Quadriga should be tested for in finger amputations. Owing to the lack of independence of the profundus tendons, the tethering of one (e.g., to an amputation stump) can limit the range of the others (Verdan, 1960). Release of the fixed profundus tendon(s) restores complete gliding to the tendon(s) that had been impaired (Neu, Murray, and McKenzie, 1985).

BONE. Barber (1929) examined 40 postmortem amputation stumps, many of which had formed osteophytes. Aitken and Frantz (1953) reported that spur formation was common in children but did not lead to surgery. In juvenile amputees, the incidence of overgrowth of the humerus exceeds that of the radius and ulna.

Vascular Problems. These are rare, but it is possible to get a symptomatic false aneu-

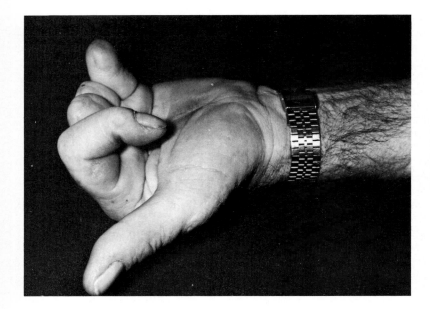

Figure 92–2. The syndrome of Quadriga. The tethering of one or more profundus tendons in the amputation finger stumps limits the excursion of this man's uninjured index finger. (Courtesy of Workers' Compensation Board of Ontario.)

rysm subsequent to an amputation (Hentz, Jackson, and Fogarty, 1978).

Skin Problems. "Daily cleansing of the stump and socket and changing of socks helped to prevent and control the progress of skin lesions" (Nathan and Davidoff, 1965). Folliculitis, furunculosis, sebaceous cysts, miliaria, intertrigo, skin breakdown, and dermatitis medicamentosa can all prevent use of a prosthesis (Slocum, 1949).

Psychologic Problems. Cone and Hueston (1974) concluded that "the final outcome of surgical intervention in hand injuries is determined not only by anatomical reconstruction and tissue repair, but also by the management of the psychological reaction of the patient to the injury." They pointed out the importance of assessing the personality of the patient, the cultural factors, the process of grief and mourning, and the potential primary and secondary gain. Wilkes (1956) found that many workers with hand injuries complained of work-related problems. Miller, Watkins, and Davis (1961) interviewed workers with a disparity between complaints and physical findings, and reported a high incidence of dissatisfaction with some aspect of the job or the administrative handling of their injury. Murray (1982) discussed the nuances of the doctor-patient relationship in dealing with the emotional, personal, and economic problems that may predispose to the injury and influence the rehabilitation. Two non–M.D.s, Clark and Malchow (1984), made some telling comments on the importance of adequate doctor-patient communications in making the decisions to amputate. The doctor has the ultimate challenge and responsibility for "seeing that his disabled patients resume their rightful place in society" (Parry, 1966). There are unfortunately some people who are Sad, Hostile, Anxious, Frustrated, and Tenacious (SHAFT syndrome). Wallace and Fitzmorris (1978) described this syndrome in the upper extremity. Their three patients had a total of 25 operations performed by 11 doctors in five different states. "Mania operativa" is an uncommon, unrecognized cause of limb amputation (Hunter and Kennard, 1982).

Thumb and fingertip injuries are discussed in Chapters 122, 124, 125, and 127 (thumb) and 93 and 99 (fingertip).

PRINCIPLES OF FINGER AMPUTATIONS

The object of a finger amputation "should be to provide a mobile, stable, painless stump with least interference to remaining tendon and joint function" (Thompson, 1963) or in other words a useful stump (Willems, 1936). Milford (1971) reported that amputation revision is still probably the most frequent elective operation in hand surgery. Certainly in primary surgery, efforts can be made to decrease the potential need for revision.

Skin. Viable skin is conserved and utilized to achieve wound cover (Kaplan, 1969). Where possible, the thicker volar skin with good sensibility is utilized in preference to the thinner dorsal skin (Omer, 1982). The skin flaps must cover the bone without tension. The dorsal flap can be cut with the finger in flexion, and the palmar flap designed with the finger in extension to ensure adequate skin cover (Slocum and Pratt, 1944). "Dog ears" in the acute traumatic amputation should often be left, to avoid compromising blood flow to the flaps achieving closure. Most "dog ears" disappear in time; in an elective amputation, they can be trimmed.

The use of split-thickness skin grafts to help achieve wound closure has been controversial throughout the years. Scott (1974) urged the "avoidance, where possible, of skin grafts." Clarkson (1955) referred to the advantage of its being stable cover on most traumatic stumps, but reported the disadvantages that it is poorly sensitized, off-color, and unsightly. Cannon (1958) stressed the value of free skin grafting in achieving wound closure. He considered this especially important when there was a problem with infection. The Toronto Microvascular Team has been using split-thickness skin grafts to help preserve stump length on many of their unreplantable digit stumps for the past 11 years. Most of these skin grafts are still in place. They shrank considerably, bringing normal skin with good sensation over the amputation stump. A few skin grafts have been excised some years after the operation at the request of the patient (Fig. 92–3). This has been possible with minimal bone shortening.

Bone. Crushing of bone is to be avoided. Sharp rongeurs can refine the bone contour. Bulbous tips are undesirable functionally and cosmetically (Chase, 1960). Traumatic or operative bone chips should be removed from the wound by debridement or irrigation (Thompson, 1963). Bone length is not as important as a stump with mobile, nonsensitive cover (Ennis and Huber, 1938; Ratliff, 1969).

Cartilage. Whitaker and associates, 1972 and Graham and associates, 1973a,b explored the experimental and clinical results of finger amputations with preservation of articular cartilage, concluding that it is better to leave the articular cartilage on the end of the stump. To provide a less bulbous stump, the condyles and the anterior protruding aspect of the phalanx can be trimmed. The articular cartilage provides a shock pad for trauma and is less painful during the period of rehabilitation (Omer, 1982).

Nerves. This is probably the most controversial area of amputation surgery. Ideally, neuromas are to be avoided. As this is not yet feasible, the end of the nerve should certainly be in a position away from scar where it will not be exposed to excessive pressure. Thus, the end of a nerve must not be near the wound closure, or at an anticipated point of contact or pressure in pinch and grasp. A frequently applied technique consists of careful isolation of the nerve, dissection proximally, and transection with retraction into soft tissues. Hall and Bechtol (1963) described their disappointment with

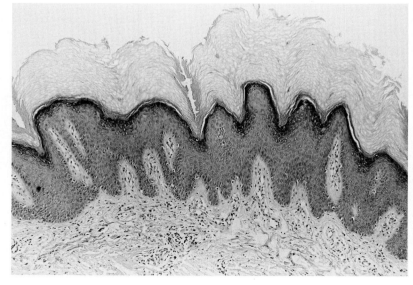

Figure 92–3. Photomicrograph of excised, hyperkeratotic split-thickness skin graft that helped preserve length in the index of a multiple finger amputation. The patient requested that this skin graft be excised five years after the injury. Excision of the graft (1 sq cm) was possible without shortening the bone.

crushing, ligation, injection, coagulation, transection within the perineural sheath, and implantation into bone.

Tendons. Profundus tendons should never be sutured over the end of the finger amputation stump (Slocum, 1959). This could limit the flexion of a normal digit in the syndrome of quadriga (Verdan, 1960). Dirty, retracted tendon ends should be cleaned. Parkes (1970) illustrated how loss of flexor digitorum profundus insertion could precipitate a lumbrical plus finger. Harvey and Harvey (1974) in a review of amputations did not consider this a real problem, and this has been our experience. Preservation of a tendon insertion improves the mobility of an amputation stump. Murray and Harris (1981) described using the superficialis tendons to the index, long, and ring fingers to preserve power and bulk of proximal phalanges amputated proximal to the proximal interphalangeal joint. The suggested attachment is to the thick parts of the tendon pulley system in the appropriate phalanx. Murray also described using excess extensor tendon to place over a raw bony surface of the amputation stump to provide extra padding. Adherence of the profundus tendon to the stump is to be avoided. Care in not pulling a tendon excessively and in avoiding damage to the vincula may help avoid proximal hemorrhage and subsequent adhesions. Early postoperative mobilization of the fingers can minimize unwanted adhesions.

Blood Vessels. Digital arteries should be identified and ligated with fine sutures or by a bipolar cautery. Visible veins can be dealt with in a similar fashion.

LEVELS OF FINGER AMPUTATIONS

Through the Distal Interphalangeal Joint

Kaplan (1965) recommended the preservation of even a few millimeters of the distal phalanx as being very useful. The most difficult part of this level of amputation is thorough removal of the nail bed. If the distal phalanx cannot be saved, an amputation through the distal interphalangeal joint, with appropriately trimmed condyles of the middle phalanx, can provide a good stump. If much dorsal skin is used in the closure, care must be taken to ensure that all the nail bed is removed. If a "lumbrical plus" situation develops, this can be relieved by sectioning the lumbrical tendon (Louis, 1982).

Through the Middle Phalanx

It is desirable to preserve the insertion of the flexor digitorum superficialis, to permit effective participation of this stump in grasping activities. Amputation proximal to the insertion of the superficialis tendon leaves a portion of the middle phalanx that has little or no functional use.

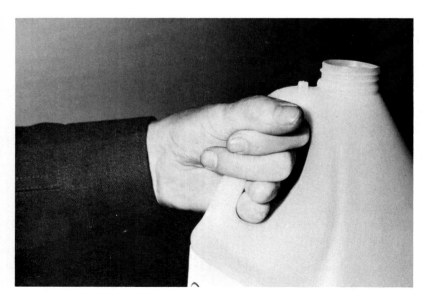

Figure 92–4. The breadth of grip and the control made possible by the length of preserved ring and little finger proximal phalanges are very important to this carpenter.

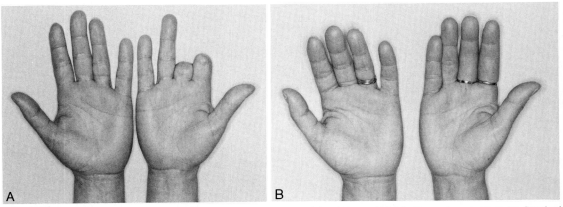

Figure 92–5. *A, B,* This two-finger amputation had the prerequisite 1½ cm distal to the web spaces to be fitted with Pillet prostheses. (Courtesy of Workers' Compensation Board of Ontario.)

Through the Proximal Interphalangeal Joint

The condyles of the head of the proximal phalanx can be trimmed, preserving the terminal articular cartilage. An intact vinculum to the flexor profundus near the base of the proximal phalanx should not be injured. Flexion can be achieved by the interossei muscles (Kaplan, 1965).

AMPUTATIONS OF INDIVIDUAL FINGERS

Index Finger

Although the thumb is the most important digit, the normal index finger is the most important of the other four digits (Mahoney, Phalen, and Frackelton, 1947). The index finger is the primary finger in pinch and is one of the two polar elements responsible for grasping. It is second only to the middle finger in power. When adequate length, sensation, and mobility of an index finger are not maintained, a healthy middle finger is used in preference. When a long finger takes over pinch and most of the fine functions, an index finger stump may hamper general use of the hand.

The level at which an injured index finger becomes a candidate for ray removal has been a controversial subject. Clayton (1963) would consider an amputation proximal to the distal interphalangeal joint if the rest of the fingers are normal. Even in a midproximal phalanx amputation, ray amputation should not be

done primarily (Omer, 1982). In manual workers, the remaining index finger is often found to be highly desirable during its trial period following initial surgery. If the stump is awkward, however, conversion to an index ray amputation is recommended. Chase (1968) emphasized that such an index amputation stump might have important parts for other injuries of either hand. Transfer of an injured digit can be an excellent way to restore thumb function (Dunlop, 1923; Jepson, 1925; Graham and associates, 1947; Peacock, 1960; Harkins and Rafety, 1972).

A review of 21 index transmetacarpal amputations at Toronto General Hospital between 1973 and 1983 revealed that 14 were amputated because of mechanical trauma (all but one late), three were related to scleroderma, one followed an electrical burn, one treated a neglected human bite wound, and one was necessitated by a thrombotic event in conjunction with thrombocytosis. The level of amputation varied from base to beveled head.

The most frequently recommended level of amputation of the index ray is at the base of the metacarpal (Murray, Carman, and MacKenzie, 1977). Farmer (1952) preferred simple disarticulation of the finger at the metacarpal phalangeal joint, with a beveling of the head, thus preserving the transverse metacarpal ligament and the breadth of palm. Harris and Houston (1967), in their series of partial hand amputations, had four patients in whom index metacarpal disarticulations were revised by trimming the metacarpal obliquely through the neck. The new stump was more painful than the old, and all four

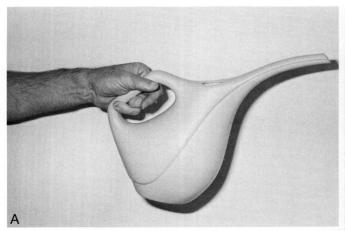

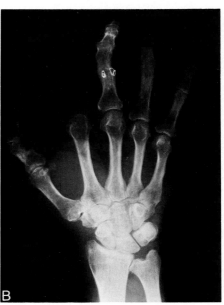

Figure 92–6. *A,* This man has an amputation through the index metacarpophalangeal joint and is shown holding a watering can. He is able to enjoy golf, curling, gardening, and macrophotography. He feels that the breadth of his palm is useful to him. *B,* X-ray demonstrates the bone union of a thumb and index finger on middle finger replantation.

patients felt that the increased space between thumb and middle finger had adversely affected their grasp.

Murray, Carman, and MacKenzie (1977) examined 41 patients with transmetacarpal amputations. Intrinsic transfers had a high incidence of excess intrinsic function and even flexion deformity. One patient had a rotational deformity after an index superficialis tendon was transferred to the base of the long finger (Eversmann, Burkhalter, and Dunn, 1971). In 13 patients definitely lacking an intrinsic transfer, there was no difference in strength from that of the rest of the study population. This suggests that attempts to reinforce abduction of the middle finger are unnecessary. Pronation strength was reduced regardless of the level of the resection of the metacarpal. It was felt that pronation strength was likely to be much better with preservation of even a stump of proximal phalanx. This further supports the advice to permit workmen a trial of use with a short index stump.

There was a 37 per cent incidence of hyperesthesia in the thumb and long finger web, attributable to excessive mobilization of the index finger's radial digital nerve (Murray, Carman, and MacKenzie, 1977). As is true of many other pain situations, a more proximal amputation does not necessarily solve the problem of pain in a more distal stump.

Index ray amputation can provide a visually pleasing hand. Many generations of medical students have often failed to notice the deficient hand demonstrating physical signs in Hamilton Bailey's surgical textbook *Physical Signs in Clinical Surgery* (Brown, 1982).

Long or Ring Finger

The gap created in a hand by a short stump of proximal phalanx of either the middle or ring fingers is significant functionally and cosmetically (Fig. 92–7). The middle finger is the longest finger and normally supports the index in pinch grip (Duparc, Alnot, and May, 1979). Intact middle and ring fingers prevent small objects from falling out of the palm. Deletion of a short ray can improve the function and appearance of the hand (Carroll, 1959; Murray and Harris, 1981). Slocum's 1949 summary of the goals of this surgery includes (1) correcting the rotatory deformity, (2) closing the space between the two adjacent unamputated fingers, and (3) achieving a satisfactory appearance of the hand. Surgically, this has been achieved in a variety of ways:

1. Excision of the metacarpal. The foreshortened ray can be excised, either disarticulated at the carpometacarpal joint or resected close to the base of the metacarpal. Peze and Iselin (1984) included a wedge of the capitate with long finger amputation to help provide a cosmetic hand. Appropriate wedges of skin are excised to help delete the

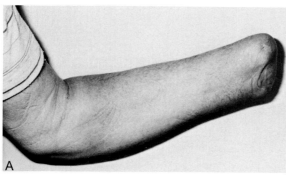 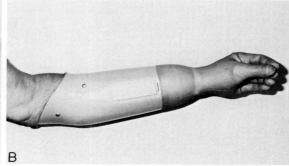

Figure 92–14. *A,* Wrist disarticulation showing the slight distal flare of the radius and ulna. *B,* Myoelectric prosthesis, which has been fitted in a completely below elbow fashion. It has a wrist circumference that exceeds normal shirt cuffs.

Frantz, 1953). With currently available prosthetic design, it is difficult to avoid excessive length of the prosthesis and still have the versatility of interchanging and positioning terminal devices.

BELOW ELBOW AMPUTATION

The recommended maximal length for a below elbow amputation is at least 6 cm above the tip of the ulnar styloid process. This level permits a good wrist unit to be incorporated into the prosthesis as well as the interchange of the various terminal devices. Prosthetic fitting becomes increasingly difficult as proximity to the elbow increases. There is almost no minimal length that can be of some value to the patient.

Bunnell (1956) lengthened a short forearm stump, utilizing bone graft and pedicle flap.

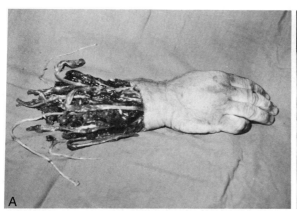 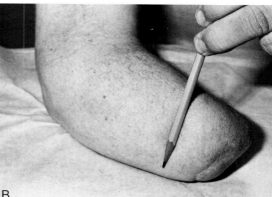

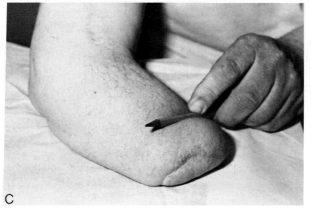

Figure 92–15. Nonreplanted forearm amputation. This farmer caught his dominant hand in a power take-off and avulsed the nerves from the level of his elbow *(A). B, C,* A pencil pressed against the radius and ulna to show the range of pronation and supination. Even with this stump at the junction of the proximal third and distal two-thirds of the forearm, he has at least 70 degrees of pronation and supination.

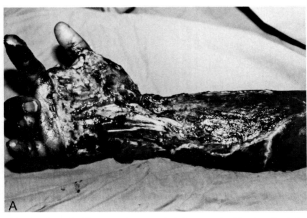 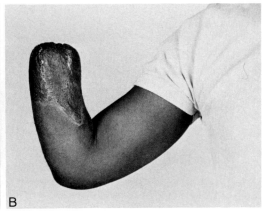

Figure 92–16. Devastating crush injury up to the level of the proximal forearm in the nondominant extremity of an unskilled manual worker *(A).* This man was reluctant to have any other part of his body scarred and he was given time and support to come to the decision of amputation. *B,* A well-healed forearm amputation stump with circumferential mesh skin grafting of the distal 3 inches. The patient was fitted with the temporary prosthesis one month after the amputation and learned to use it well.

With island and free flaps, this is easier in the 1980's than it was in the 1950's. Cutting the biceps tendon can improve the effective length of a short below elbow stump (Blair and Morris, 1946). The brachialis provides adequate flexion.

All possible length below the elbow joint can usefully improve leverage and rotation of the stump. However, rotation is routinely built into the prosthesis.

Surgical Technique. The osteotomies of the radius and ulna are smoothed carefully. Gentle dissection and proximal sectioning of the median, ulnar, and radial nerves is performed (Louis, Hunter, and Keating, 1980). Muscle can be trimmed to prevent a bulbous end of the stump. Skin closure is planned using healthy skin with good sensation where feasible. Skin grafts over adequately padded vascularized tissue can also be serviceable (Fig. 92–16), although rarely needed. Skin wound closure is achieved with primary reliable healing as the goal so that early prosthetic fitting can be feasible.

Yu, He, and Chen (1984) and Yu and He (1985) reported creative use of bone grafting and free vascularized tissue transferred to a forearm amputation stump to achieve functional prehension.

Below Elbow Versus Wrist Disarticulation. Debates about the advantages of a wrist disarticulation as opposed to a below elbow amputation often refer to the improved pronation and supination that can be achieved with a wrist disarticulation. However, if any damage is done to the structures of the radioulnar joint, it is certainly possible

that the pronation and supination of a wrist disarticulation is worse than that of a forearm amputation. Taylor (1968) graphs the natural rotation at different levels in the forearm and the decreasing residual rotation in amputees at progressively shorter forearm lengths. Hunter (1984) was impressed at how little rotation is required by unilateral amputees for adequate function of their prosthesis. The 70 per cent of rotation that is preserved in most long below elbow amputation stumps is more than adequate. Tooms (1972) quoted a survey of surgeons, 60 per cent of whom were in favor of a long forearm amputation in preference to a wrist disarticulation, even when the distal level is feasible. The advantages include ease of fitting, appropriate length of extremity and prosthesis, and avoidance of trouble with the radioulnar joint. Tooms disagreed and considered that, with current prostheses, wrist disarticulation is the more advantageous level. The prosthetic fitting for wrist disarticulation may end up appearing bulkier and longer than the normal arm. For both levels a myoelectric prosthesis can be fitted entirely below the elbow.

KRUKENBERG OPERATION

In 1917, Krukenberg described an ingenious operation that can provide a below elbow amputation with prehensile potential. The operation consists of separating the radius from the ulna and giving each bone an individual muscle and skin covering. The concept of "forcipization" of forearm amputation stumps is attributed to Vanghetti (Henry,

1928). After the operative description by Krukenberg in 1917, the Germans and Russians
mainly worked with this procedure. The operation is simple and can provide prehension
and tactile gnosis. The role that this can play
in rehabilitating a blind bilateral amputee
was appreciated. For the sighted, it has the
advantage of giving effective maneuvering
with sensation in all shoulder positions, even
in the dark. Its main disadvantage is the
unsightly appearance, but a standard prosthesis can be worn over it.

Indications

1. Absolute: Blind bilateral forearm amputees.
2. Relative:
   a. Nonavailability of prosthesis. In under-
      developed countries, this surgery has
      been embarked upon much more freely.
   b. Certain sighted bilateral upper extrem-
      ity amputees. A prosthesis on the non-
      dominant side can be combined with a
      Krukenberg operation on the dominant
      side to provide sensitive grasping. Am-
      putees so equipped find that each ex-
      tremity has different chores at which it
      excels (Tubiana, 1979).
   c. Selected juvenile amputees. Swanson
      (1964), Swanson and Swanson (1980),
      and Chan and associates (1984) re-
      ported excellent results in selected ju-
      venile amputees.

Sung (1957) summarized the salient points
of patient selection:

1. The length of the stump should not be
   shorter than 8 cm from the insertion of
   the biceps, and preferably should be a
   minimum of 9 to 9.5 cm.
2. The forearm tissues should be relatively
   normal, with intact sensation.
3. Patients must accept the operation and its
   appearance and must want their manual
   needs to be met in this way.

Surgical Technique. The areas of refine-
ment and controversy with respect to this
operation have had to do with (1) the amount
of muscle resection; (2) the length of the
separation (Kallio, 1948; Zanoli, 1957); and
(3) the means of achieving skin cover (Colp
and Ransohoff, 1933; Squires, 1937; Purce,
1939; Kallio and Thomson, 1951; Zanoli,
1957; Swanson, 1964; Harrison and Mayou,
1977; Nathan and Trung, 1977; Chan and
associates, 1984). Swanson and Swanson
(1980) concluded that "this procedure should
be extended to more individuals who have
the severe handicap of bilateral hand loss."

ELBOW DISARTICULATION

This operative procedure is thought by
some to be an excellent operation (Tooms,
1972), certainly at an acceptable level (Alldredge and Murphy, 1968; Omer, 1982), and
by others to be less advantageous than above
elbow amputation (McKeever, 1944; Hunter,
1984). The epicondyles of the humerus give
good support and rotatory force transmission
through the prosthesis. The disadvantages lie
within the prosthesis: outside locking hinges
often damage clothing.

ABOVE ELBOW AMPUTATION

The ideal level for above elbow amputation
is at least 8 cm above the lateral epicondyle,
to accommodate the turntable multiple locking unit (Hunter, 1984). A long humeral
stump has good proximal muscular control
and provides a long lever to help maneuver
the prosthesis (McKeever, 1944). Ten cm is
the minimal length of humerus that can be
fitted with a conventional above elbow prosthesis. It is essential to have bone below the
insertion of the pectoralis major.

Operative Technique. The ultimate result is the avoidance of a floppy amputation
stump. In elective cases, anterior and posterior skin flaps are planned to meet over the
end of the stump. The median and ulnar
nerve should be divided at about 4 cm above
the level of bone. Omer (1982) described stag-
gering the skin suture line with that of the
fascial closure. The stability of the prosthesis
can be compromised by excess tissue about
this amputation stump. It is not uncommon
for a flabby amputation stump to need soft
tissue revision (Hunter, 1985). A neoarthrosis
of the shaft of the humerus (Gillis, 1954) and
an angulation osteotomy of the humerus
(Marquardt and Neff, 1974) have both been
created to improve utilization of an above
elbow prosthesis. Few surgeons have seen the
need for either of these modifications.

AMPUTATIONS AROUND THE SHOULDER

An amputation through the humerus above
the level of the humeral insertion of the
pectoralis major has no functional value. The
presence of the humeral head tends to provide
a normally rounded shoulder (Alldredge,

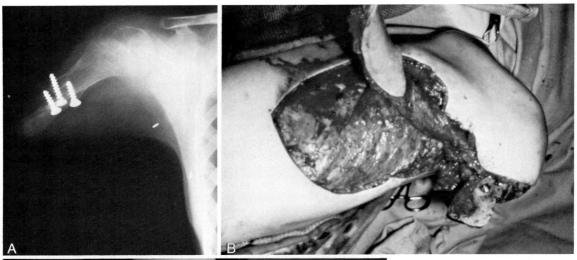

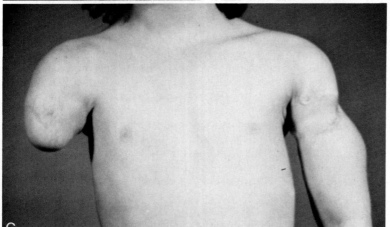

Figure 92–17. Bilateral high level traumatic amputation in a juvenile treated successfully with replantation of the left upper extremity. The short right upper extremity stump was elongated eight months after the amputation with an iliac crest bone graft *(A)*. An ipsilateral latissimus dorsi island myocutaneous flap *(B)* provides cover. The lengthening of the amputation stump has meant that the patient is a good user of an above elbow prosthesis for school activities. Without the prosthesis, this stump is useful in many activities of daily living *(C)*. (Courtesy of Dr. Tsu-Min Tsai and Dr. Kenneth C. Peacock, Louisville, KY.)

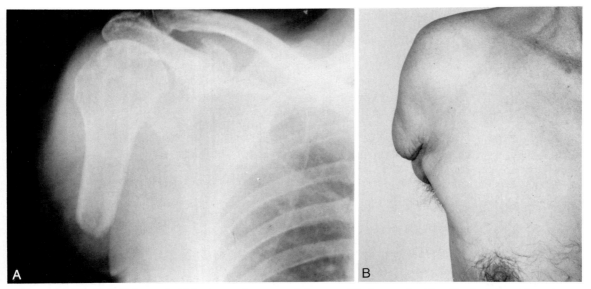

Figure 92–18. *A, B,* This man's high above elbow amputation was fitted as a shoulder disarticulation. There is not enough length of the humerus to control an above elbow prosthesis. (Courtesy of Dr. W. R. Harris and Workers' Compensation Board of Ontario.).

1947). The prosthetic fitting is as for a shoulder disarticulation.

A true shoulder disarticulation has the disadvantage of the prosthesis, also needing to round the shoulder (Louis, 1982). Gillis (1954) gave a step by step description of the surgical procedure of disarticulation at the shoulder using a good deltoid flap. Louis (1982) described utilizing the ends of the latissimus dorsi and pectoralis major to help fill in the hollow defect at the level of the glenoid (Alldredge and Murphy, 1968).

FOREQUARTER AMPUTATION

A forequarter amputation includes the entire upper extremity with its shoulder girdle. Levinthal and Grossman (1939) aptly described this amputation as "being so mutilating and severely shocking that the patient will often not submit to it and the surgeon will hesitate to perform it." The most frequent indications are the presence of malignant tumors (Pack, 1956; El-Domeiri and Miller, 1969), and trauma such as the hay baler injuries described by Hardin (1967) and McKinnon, Robinson, and Masters, (1967). In tumor surgery throughout the years, interscapulothoracic amputation has played an important role in palliation as well as cure of tumors that were not amendable to any lesser degree of surgery (Pack, McNeer, and Coley, 1942).

History. Ralph Cuming in Antigua was credited with the first forequarter amputation in 1808 (Keevil, 1949). In 1836, Dixie Crosby in New Hampshire removed a 25 lb tumor from an emaciated man by performing a forequarter amputation (Crosby, 1875). Berger published a description of an anterior approach to interscapulothoracic amputation in 1887. The operative mortality of Buchanan's series of operations before 1900 was 11 per cent (Pack, McNeer, and Coley, 1942). Littlewood in 1922 published a description of the posterior approach that provided him safe access first to the subclavian artery and then the vein, with a total operative time of 25 minutes. Pack, McNeer, and Coley (1942) found 180 case reports in the medical literature between 1900 and 1942. They comment on the occasionally hazardous anterior approach when only the exposure of resection of the middle third of the clavicle was used. They recommended a more extended anterior approach, credited to Kocher. This approach includes exposure of the axillary vessels before ligation of the subclavian. Pack's own 31 consecutive interscapulothoracic amputations reported in the 1942 paper were performed without an operative death. Patients are relieved to have lost a growth, a fungating mass, or intractable pain. There are also many reports of long-term survivors (Pack, McNeer, and Coley, 1942; Grimes and Bell, 1950; Moseley, 1957; Bailey and Stevens, 1961; Hardin, 1961; El-Domeiri and Miller, 1969).

Surgical Technique. A sound knowledge of anatomy, together with experience in performing a planned operation on a cadaver,

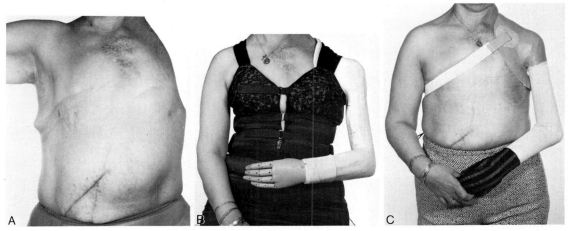

Figure 92–19. *A, B, C,* This woman illustrates the defect of a forequarter amputation. She appreciated a cosmetic prosthesis and chose gloves for the hand to coordinate with dress. (Courtesy of Dr. Peter Fitzpatrick, Princess Margaret Hospital, Toronto.)

will help expedite this surgery. Moseley (1957) illustrated the draping and the dissections.

Posterior Approach. Most surgeons prefer the 1922 posterior technique of Littlewood (Tooms, 1972). The exact skin incisions are probably dictated by the size and position of the tumor or the nature of the trauma. Through the posterior incision the shoulder girdle is freed, permitting the whole extremity to fall away from the trunk and leaving the subclavian vessels and trunks of the brachial plexus stretched and standing out (Haggart, 1940). It is now easy and safe to clamp and ligate the subclavian artery, and then the vein. Care is taken to protect the phrenic and vagus nerves. The trunks of the brachial plexus can be divided. The surgeon can switch sides and create the anterior pectoroaxillary flap. The pectoral muscles are identified and cut. The entire axillary contents can be amputated with the forequarter. The skin, subcutaneous tissue, and deep fascia are sutured over appropriate drains, and the dressing is applied.

Anterior Approach

BERGER. The subclavian artery is ligated through visualization achieved with the middle third of the clavicle removed (Pack, McNeer, and Coley, 1942; Nadler and Phelan, 1966). This limited visualization of the subclavian vessels has been associated with un-desirable hemorrhage (Pack, McNeer, and Coley, 1942).

KOCHER. This is a safer, extended anterior approach whereby the axillary vessels are exposed before ligation of the subclavian artery and vein.

Variations

RADICAL. A thoracotomy combined with the posterior approach provides better visualization of any intrathoracic or inoperable mediastinal involvement before subclavian vessel ligations are carried out (Stafford and Williams, 1958; Wurlitzer, 1973). Thoracic wall resections, with (Wurlitzer, 1973) and without (Stafford and Williams, 1958; El-Domeiri and Miller, 1969) lung and sternum removal have been included with forequarter amputations.

LIMB PRESERVATION. Pack and Baldwin (1955), Pack and Crampton (1961), and O'Brien and associates (1984) reviewed the indications for the Tikhor-Linberg operation in which total or subtotal scapulectomy, partial or complete excision of the clavicle, and resection of the head, neck, and portions of the humerus are removed en bloc. The distal arm, the forearm, the hand and its brachial plexus, and the subclavian artery and vein are preserved. There have been attempts at partial reconstruction with allograft, prosthesis, or vascularized bone grafts (Gross and associates, 1984) (Fig. 92–20).

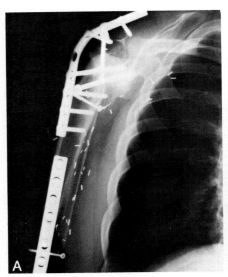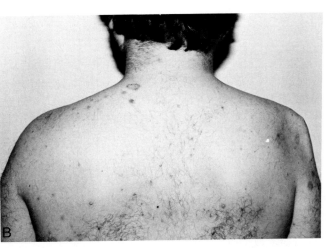

Figure 92–20. *A,* Immediate reconstruction following excision of an intra- and extraosseous chondrosarcoma of the proximal humerus, using allograft and free vascular fibula to fuse the shoulder. The en bloc tumor excision of the proximal humerus included a portion of the glenoid and acromion and the musculature of the shoulder girdle. *B,* He is left with better shoulder contour than the defect of a Tikhor-Linberg operation.

NECK DISSECTION. Combining a neck dissection with an axillary dissection was described by Bowden in 1950 and has been reported along with forequarter amputations (El-Domeiri and Miller, 1969).

TRANSCAPULAR. Levinthal and Grossman (1939) wondered whether preserving part of the scapula would decrease the frequency of scoliosis after interscapulothoracic amputation, but had no experience. De Nancrede (1909) reviewed the literature and his own experience in scapulectomy, concluding that this operation by itself was not a good one for malignant tumors of the scapula.

Sequelae

Persistent phantom limb pain can be a problem (El-Domeiri and Miller, 1969). Levinthal and Grossman (1939) referred to scoliosis as a "frequent sequel to the interscapulothoracic amputation."

CINEPLASTY

Cineplasty is an ingenious attempt to provide direct muscular control of an artificial hand or prosthesis by creating skin-lined tunnels under the same muscle groups that help perform the function of prehension in the normal hand (Kessler, 1944; Alldredge, 1948). The biceps cineplasty appropriately connected to a prosthesis can pull 50 to 80 lb through an excursion of 2 to 2½ inches, and has the potential for some proprioceptive sense in the skin tube, contributing to dexterity (Rank, Wakefield, and Hueston, 1973). There is less harnessing of the shoulder, improved comfort, and an ability to operate the terminal device in any position of the shoulder, including overhead and behind the body (Klopsteg and Wilson, 1968).

The disadvantages include the need for a surgeon who thoroughly understands the operation, the muscle mechanics, and the prosthetic designs. The surgeon must have access to a well-qualified maker of cineplastic limbs. Specific complications have been problems with the tunnels themselves, such as irritations and infections (Mazet, 1958). With improved myoelectric prostheses, the initial goal of the cineplasty to use the local muscles to motor the prosthesis is being achieved without the use of tunnels under muscles.

BILATERAL UPPER EXTREMITY AMPUTATIONS

For bilateral amputations the surgical principles are the same as for unilateral amputations, except that greater effort may be made to save more on at least one limb. As illustrated by Tubiana (1969), the goal is to restore the patient's functional autonomy. Ingenuity in prosthetic fitting and aids for the patient can help restore even high level

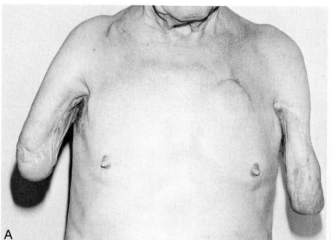 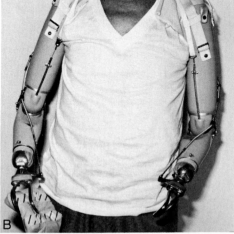

Figure 92–21. *A, B,* This 72 year old man is getting his fourth set of arms for the bilateral above elbow amputations necessitated by a high tension electrical burn injury 18 years earlier. Following the initial prosthetic fitting and rehabilitation at Ontario's Workers' Compensation Rehabilitation Centre, he was able to return to work as an independent meter reader for ten years. He has a wall-mounted device at home that enables him to get the arm prosthesis on and off independently. He is able to cook and eat on his own, but needs help with bathing and dressing. (Courtesy of Workers' Compensation Board of Ontario.)

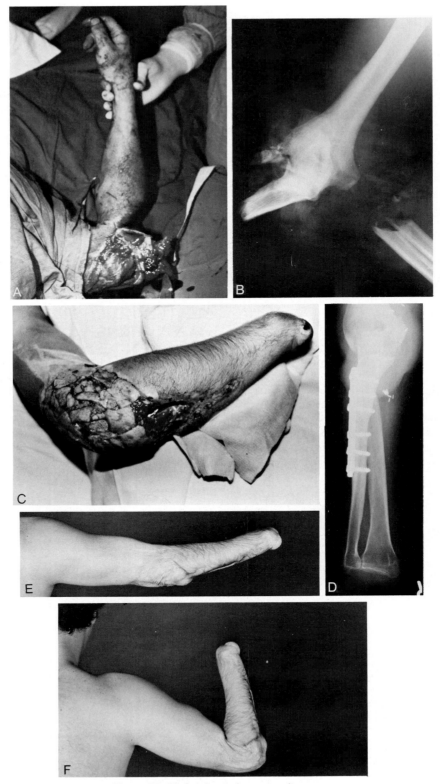

Figure 92–22 *See legend on opposite page*

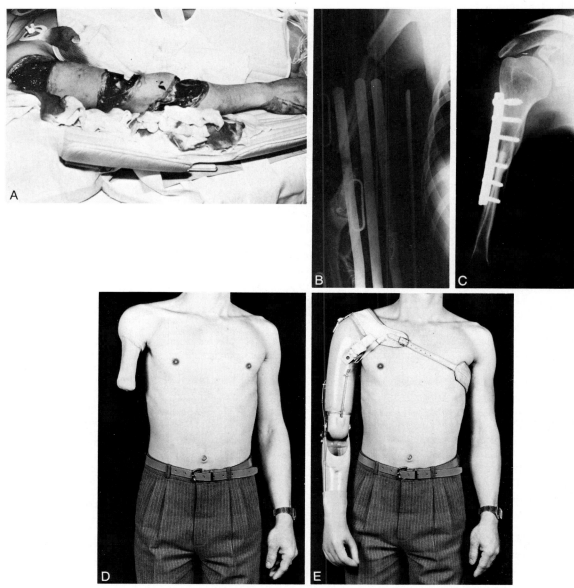

Figure 92–23. *A,* A multilevel incomplete amputation to the dominant right upper extremity of a young punch press worker. *B,* The humerus was shattered. The proximal level of injury would have provided too short an amputation stump for a good upper arm prosthesis. The segment between the wrist and the forearm fractures was replanted to the proximal humerus to increase the length of the stump. *C,* Sensory nerves were repaired to give the stump sensation. *D,* Appearance of the stump three years after the injury. The fitting was more challenging than a normal above elbow fitting because of the flare of the radius. *E,* Once a good fit had been achieved, the patient has more rotational control than do most upper arm amputees.

Figure 92–22. Crushed proximal forearm and elbow. This young man had a 2 ton beam fall on his forearm, pinning him to the ground. *A,* In emergency he could demonstrate good triceps and brachialis function. It was decided to revascularize him to at least preserve the elbow and make what would have been an upper arm amputation into a forearm amputation. The radial head was definitively debrided and the forearm shortened through the ulnar fracture *(B)* before plating this. A wrist disarticulation was completed after the hand was revascularized. The possibility of amputating the hand had been explained to the patient preoperatively. Intraoperatively it was judged that the lack of nerve and muscle would have made it extremely difficult if not impossible to reconstruct a hand that had sensation and mobility. *C,* Two weeks postoperatively with exposed plate on the ulna. Skin grafts have covered the extensor and lateral aspect of the arm. A subsequent further skin grafting and Limberg flap achieved good wound cover of the ulna and its plate. *D,* The fracture united. *E,* Extension and *F,* flexion ranges of the elbow are shown. This man has been a good prosthesis user for several years. His preference is the harness operated hook for work and play. He reserves the myoelectric hand for social occasions.

amputees to relative independence (Kritter, 1972; Friedmann, 1980) (Fig. 92–21).

SALVAGE

Surgeons have long been reluctant to discard amputated tissues. Sir Harold Gillies (1940) suggested burying an amputated digit in an abdominal pocket rather than discarding it. Despite large gaps of soft tissue and bone damage, a useful digit can be salvaged in selected patients by fusing the remaining phalanges (Nemethi, 1955). Chase (1970) emphasized that some parts to be thrown away may be useful for either hand in their total reconstruction. A free flap from an amputated finger can reconstruct and save a severely injured remaining digit (Alpert and Buncke, 1978). May and Gordon (1980) used the palm of an amputated extremity as a free flap to preserve the length of a below elbow amputation. Waterhouse, Moss, and Townsend (1984) salvaged a below knee amputation stump by using a free radial forearm flap from an amputated upper limb. A reluctance to discard tissue, combined with ingenuity as to how to best solve tissue defects, lead to interesting, worthwhile reconstructions.

Elective tissue transfers of the appropriate tissues have saved many an upper extremity (Manktelow, Zuker, and McKee, 1984). Extensive bone defects, whether from trauma, infection, or tumor, have been successfully bridged with free vascularized fibular grafts (Daniel & Weiland, 1982).

Figures 92–22 and 92–23 illustrate attempts to improve an amputation level.

THE CHALLENGE

Two questions to ask when confronted with *an individual* with an amputation are:

1. Can this level be functionally improved?
2. At what level would this replantation cease to be functional?

REFERENCES

History

Bertelsen, A., and Capener, N.: Fingers, compensation and King Canute. J. Bone Joint Surg., *42B*:390, 1960.
Gillis, L.: History of amputations and prostheses. *In* Amputations. London, William Heinemann Medical Books, 1954, Chap. 1.
Putti, V.: Historic artificial limbs, Parts I and II. Am. J. Surg., *6*:111, 246, 1929.
Rang, M., and Thompson, G. H.: History of amputations and prostheses. *In* Kostuik, J. P. (Ed.): Amputation Surgery and Rehabilitation. The Toronto Experience. New York, Churchill Livingstone, 1981.
Sahly, A.: The mutilation of prehistoric hands. J. Bone Joint Surg., *45B*:426, 1963.

Indications

Arcari, F. A., Larsen, R. D., and Posch, J. I.: Injuries to the hand from homemade rockets. Am. J. Surg., *97*:471, 1959.
Carroll, R. E.: Osteogenic sarcoma in the hand. J. Bone Joint Surg., *39A*:325, 1957.
Chase, R. A.: Vascular disorders of the upper extremity. Surg. Clin. North Am., *40*:471, 1960.
Entin, M. A.: Crushing and avulsing injuries of the hand. Surg. Clin. North Am., *44*:1009, 1964.
Esses, S. I., and Peters, W. J.: Electrical burns: pathophysiology and complications. Can. J. Surg., *24*:11, 1981.
Galway, H. R., Hubbard, H., and Mowbray, M.: Traumatic amputations in children. *In* Kostuik, J. P., and Gillespie, R. (Eds.): Amputation Surgery and Rehabilitation. The Toronto Experience. New York, Churchill Livingstone, 1981.
Grogono, B. J.: Auger injuries. Injury, *4*:247, 1973.
Lynch, D. J., Key, J. C., and White, R. R.: Management and prevention of infiltration and extravasation injury. Surg. Clin. North Am., *59*:939, 1979.
Page, R. E., and Robertson, G. A.: Management of the frostbitten hand. Hand, *15*:185, 1983.
Ransford, A. O., and Hughes, S. P. F.: Complete brachial plexus lesions. A ten-year follow-up of twenty cases. J. Bone Joint Surg., *59B*:417, 1977.
Solem, L., Fischer, R. P., and Strate, R. G.: The natural history of electrical injury. J. Trauma, *17*:487, 1977.
Swanson, A. B.: Restoration of hand function by the use of partial or total prosthetic replacement. Part II: Amputation and prosthetic fitting for treatment of the functionless asensory hand. J. Bone Joint Surg., *45A*:284, 1963.
Tooms, R. E.: Amputations. *In* Edmonson, A. S. (Ed.): Campbell's Operative Orthopaedics. 6th Ed. Vol. I. St. Louis, MO, C. V. Mosby Company, 1980, Chap. 8.

Complications

Aitken, G. T., and Frantz, C. H.: The juvenile amputee. J. Bone Joint Surg., *35A*:659, 1953.
Bailey, A. A., and Moersch, F. P.: Phantom limb. Can. Med. Assoc. J., *45*:37, 1941.
Barber, C. G.: Immediate and eventual features of healing in amputated bones. Ann. Surg., *90*:985, 1929.
Bunnell, S.: Contractures of the hand from infections and injuries. J. Bone Joint Surg., *14A*:27, 1932.
Clark, J. D., and Malchow, D.: How to avoid errors in limb salvage decisions. Orthop. Rev., *13*:47, 1984.
Cone, J., and Hueston, J. T.: Psychological aspects of hand injury. Med. J. Aust., *61*:104, 1974.
Dederich, R.: Plastic treatment of the muscles and bone in amputation surgery. J. Bone Joint Surg., *45B*:60, 1963.
Entin, M. A.: Roller and wringer injuries. Plast. Reconstr. Surg., *15*:290, 1955.
Feinstein, B., Luce, J. C., and Langton, J. N. K.: The influence of phantom limbs. *In* Klopsteg, P. E., and

Wilson, P. D. (Eds.): Human Limbs and Their Substitutes. New York, Hafner, 1968, p. 79.

Hentz, V., Jackson, I., and Fogarty, D.: Case report: false aneurysm of the hand secondary to digital amputation. J. Hand Surg., 3:199, 1978.

Herrmann, L. G., and Gibbs, E. W.: Phantom limb pain: its relation to the treatment of large nerves at time of amputation. Am. J. Surg., 67:24, 1945.

Hunter, G. A., and Kennard, A. B.: Mania operativa: an uncommon, unrecognized cause of limb amputation. Can. J. Surg., 25:92, 1982.

Iselin, F., and Mazars, G.: Painful digital amputation stumps. Ann. Chir. Main, 3:156, 1984.

Leriche, R.: The pain of amputations stumps. *In* Young, A. (Ed.): The Surgery of Pain. London, Bailliere, Tindall & Cox, 1939, Chap. 8.

Littler, J. W.: Principles of reconstructive surgery of the hand. Am. J. Surg., 92:88, 1956.

Livingstone, K. E.: The phantom limb syndrome. A discussion of the role of major peripheral nerve neuromas. J. Neurosurg., 2:251, 1945.

Miller, M. F., Watkins, K. C., and Davis, C. L.: Some attitudes commonly found in patients injured on the job. Industr. Med. Surg., 30:135, 1961.

Mitchell, S. W.: Neural maladies of stumps. *In* Injuries of Nerves and Their Consequences. New York, Dover Publications, 1965, Chap. 14.

Murray, J. F.: The patient with the injured hand. J. Hand Surg., 7:543, 1982.

Nathan, L., and Davidoff, R. B.: A multidisciplinary study of long-term adjustment to amputation. Surg. Gynecol. Obstet., 120:1278, 1965.

Neu, B., Murray, J. F., and McKenzie, J. K.: Profundus tendon blockage: Quadriga in finger amputations. J. Hand Surg., 10A:878, 1985.

Parkes, A.: The "lumbrical plus" finger. Hand, 2:164, 1970.

Parry, C. B. W.: Rehabilitation of the Hand. 2nd Ed. London, Butterworths, 1966.

Slocum, D. B.: Complications of the final amputation stump. *In* An Atlas of Amputations. St. Louis, MO, C. V. Mosby Company, 1949, Chap. 8.

Verdan, C.: Syndrome of the quadriga. Surg. Clin. North Am., 40:425, 1960.

Wallace, P. F., and Fitzmorris, C. S.: The S-H-A-F-T syndrome in the upper extremity. J. Hand Surg., 3:492, 1978.

Wilkes, R.: A social and occupational study of injured hands. Br. J. Industr. Med., 13:119, 1956.

Finger Amputations: General

Brown, P. W.: Less than ten—surgeons with amputated fingers. J. Hand Surg., 7:31, 1982.

Cannon, B.: In discussion of McCormack, R. M., and Craft, J. W.: Primary reparative and reconstructive procedures in the severely injured hand. J. Bone Joint Surg., 40A:949, 1958.

Chase, R. A.: Functional levels of amputation in the hand. Surg. Clin. North Am., 40:415, 1960.

Clarkson, P.: The care of open injuries of the hand and fingers with special reference to the treatment of traumatic amputations. J. Bone Joint Surg., 37A:521, 1955.

Duparc, J., Alnot, J-Y., and May, P.: Single digit amputations. *In* Campbell Reid, D. A., and Gosset, J. (Eds.): Mutilating Injuries of the Hand. Edinburgh, Churchill Livingstone, 1979.

Ennis, W. M., and Huber, H. S.: Traumatic amputations of the fingers. Surg. Clin. North Am., 18:305, 1938.

Graham, W. P., Kilgore, E. S., and Whitaker, L. A.: Transarticular digital joint amputations: preservation of the articular cartilage. Hand, 5:58, 1973a.

Graham, W. P., Pataky, P. E., Whitaker, L. A., Kilgore, E. S., Riser, W. A., et al.: Transarticular joint amputations: the value of preserving articular cartilage. J. Surg. Res., 14:524, 1973b.

Harris, W. R., and Houston, J. K.: Partial amputations of the hand: a follow-up study. Can. J. Surg., 10:431, 1967.

Harvey, F. J., and Harvey, P. M.: A critical review of the results of primary finger and thumb amputations. Hand, 6:157, 1974.

Kaplan, E. B.: Amputations and reconstruction operations. *In* Functional and Surgical Anatomy of the Hand. 2nd Ed. Philadelphia, J. B. Lippincott Company, 1965, p. 308.

Kaplan, I.: Functional levels of amputation of fingers. S.A. Med. J., 43:1113, 1969.

Milford, L.: *In* Crenshaw, A. H. (Ed.): Campbell's Operative Orthopaedics. Vol. 1. St. Louis, MO, C. V. Mosby Company, 1971.

Murray, J. F., and Harris, W. R.: Amputations in the hand. *In* Kostuik, J. P., and Gillespie, R. (Eds.): Amputation Surgery and Rehabilitation. The Toronto Experience. New York, Churchill Livingstone, 1981.

Ratliff, A. H. C.: Amputation of the fingers and thumb. Hand, 1:137, 1969.

Scott, J. E.: Amputation of the finger. Br. J. Surg., 61:574, 1974.

Slocum, D. B.: Amputations of the fingers and the hand. Clin. Orthop., 15:35, 1959.

Slocum, D. B., and Pratt, D. R.: The principles of amputations of the fingers and hand. J. Bone Joint Surg., 26:535, 1944.

Swanson, A. B.: Levels of amputation of fingers and hand—considerations for treatment. Surg. Clin. North Am., 44:1115, 1964.

Thompson, R. V.: Essential details in the technique of finger amputation. Med. J. Aust., 50:14, 1963.

Whitaker, L. A., Graham, W. P., Riser, W. H., and Kilgore, E.: Retaining the articular cartilage in finger joint amputations. Plast. Reconstr. Surg., 49:542, 1972.

Willems, J. D.: Amputation of the fingers. Surg. Gynecol. Obstet., 62:892, 1936.

Finger Amputations: Specific

Carroll, R. E.: The level of amputation in the third finger. Am. J. Surg., 97:477, 1959.

Chase, R. A.: The damaged index digit: a source of components to restore the crippled hand. J. Bone Joint Surg., 50A:1152, 1968.

Clayton, M. L.: Index ray amputation. Surg. Clin. North Am., 43:367, 1963.

Eversmann, W. W., Burkhalter, W. E., and Dunn, C.: Transfer of the long flexor tendon of the index finger to the proximal phalanx of the long finger during index-ray amputation. J. Bone Joint Surg., 53A:769, 1971.

Mahoney, J. H., Phalen, G. S., and Frackelton, W. H.: Amputation of the index ray. Surgery, 21:911, 1947.

Murray, J. F., Carman, W., and MacKenzie, J. K.: Transmetacarpal amputation of the index finger: a clinical assessment of hand strength and complications. J. Hand Surg., 2:471, 1977.

Peze, W., and Iselin, F.: Cosmetic amputation of the long finger with carpal osteotomy. Ann. Chir. Main., 3:232, 1984.

Metacarpal Transfers

Carroll, R. E.: Transposition of the index finger to replace the middle finger. Clin. Orthop., *15*:27, 1959.

Chase, R. A.: Metacarpal transfer. *In* Atlas of Hand Surgery. Chap. 40, Philadelphia, W. B. Saunders Company, 1973, Chap. 40.

Colen, L., Bunkis, J., Gordon, L., and Walton, R.: Functional assessment of ray transfer for central digital loss. J. Hand Surg., *10A*:232, 1985.

Dunlop, J.: The use of the index finger for the thumb: some interesting points in hand surgery. J. Bone Joint Surg., *5*:99, 1923.

Graham, W. C., Brown, J. B., Cannon, B., and Riordan, D. C.: Transposition of fingers in severe injuries of the hand. J. Bone Joint Surg., *29*:998, 1947.

Harkins, P. D., and Rafety, J. E.: Digital transposition in the injured hand. J. Bone Joint Surg., *54A*:1064, 1972.

Hyroop, G. L.: Transfer of a metacarpal with or without its digit, for improving the function of the crippled hand. Plast. Reconstr. Surg., *4*:45, 1949.

Jepson, P. N.: Transformation of the middle finger into a thumb. Minn. Med., *8*:552, 1925.

Kaplan, E. B.: Replacement of an amputated middle metacarpal and finger by transposition of the index finger. Bull. Hosp. Joint Dis. Orthop. Inst., *27*:103, 1966.

Peacock, E. E.: Reconstruction of the hand by the local transfer of composite tissue island flaps. Plast. Reconstr. Surg., *25*:298, 1960.

Peacock, E. E.: Metacarpal transfer following amputation of a central digit. Plast. Reconstr. Surg., *29*:345, 1962.

Posner, M. A.: Ray transposition for central digital loss. J. Hand Surg., *4*:242, 1979.

Razemon, J-P.: Digital transfers after amputation of fingers. *In* Campbell Reid, D. A., and Gosset, J. (Eds.): Mutilating Injuries of the Hand. Edinburgh, Churchill Livingstone, 1979, Chap. 12.

Metacarpal Hand

Esser, J. F. S., and Ranschburg, P.: Reconstruction of a hand and four fingers by transplantation of the middle part of the foot and four toes. Ann. Surg., *111*:655, 1940.

Gottlieb, O.: Metacarpal amputation: the problem of the four-finger hand. Acta Chir. Scand. Suppl. *343*:143, 1965.

Kessler, I.: Transposition lengthening of a digital ray after multiple amputations of fingers. Hand, *8*:176, 1976.

Krylov, V. S., Milanov, N. O., Borovikov, A. M., Trofimov, E. I., and Shiriaev, A. A.: Functional reconstruction of both hands by free transfer of combined second and third toes from both feet. Plast. Reconstr. Surg., *75*:584, 1985.

Manktelow, R. T., and Wainwright, D. J.: A technique of distraction osteosyntheses in the hand. J. Hand Surg., *9A*:858, 1984.

Michon, J., and Dolich, B. H.: The metacarpal hand. Hand, *6*:285, 1974.

Morrison, W. A., O'Brien, B. McC., and MacLeod, A. M.: Ring finger transfer in reconstruction of transmetacarpal amputations. J. Hand Surg., *9A*:4, 1984.

Paneva-Holevich, E., and Yankov, E.: A distraction method for lengthening the finger metacarpals: a preliminary report. J. Hand Surg., *5*:160, 1980.

Tsai, T. M., Jupiter, J. B., Wolff, T. W., and Atasoy, E.: Reconstruction of severe transmetacarpal mutilating hand injuries by combined second and third toe transfer. J. Hand Surg., *6*:319, 1981.

Tubiana, R., and Roux, J-P.: Phalangization of the first and fifth metacarpals. J. Bone Joint Surg., *56A*:447, 1974.

Mutilating Hand Injuries

Brown, H. C., Williams, H. B., and Woolhouse, F. M.: Principles of salvage in mutilating hand injuries. J. Trauma, *8*:319, 1968.

Bunnell, S.: The management of the nonfunctional hand—reconstruction vs. prosthesis. Artif. Limbs, *4*:76, 1957.

Campbell Reid, D. A.: The severely mutilated hand. *In* Campbell Reid, D. A., and Gosset, J. (Eds.): Mutilating Injuries of the Hand. Edinburgh, Churchill Livingstone, 1979.

Farmer, A.: Treatment of avulsed skin flaps. Ann. Surg., *110*:951, 1939.

Findlay, R. T.: Conservative treatment vs. immediate amputation in severe crushing injuries of the hand and forearm. Surg. Clin. North Am., *18*:297, 1938.

Fry, R. M.: The importance of skin cover in the injured hand. J. Fla. Med. Assoc., *50*:142, 1963.

Harris, W. R., and Houston, J. K.: Partial amputations of the hand: a follow-up study. Can. J. Surg., *10*:431, 1967.

Kleinman, W. B., and Dustman, J. A.: Preservation of function following complete degloving injuries to the hand: use of simultaneous groin flap, random abdominal flap, and partial-thickness skin graft. J. Hand Surg., *6*:82, 1981.

Lewin, M. L.: Severe compression injuries of the hand in industry. J. Bone Joint Surg., *41A*:71, 1959.

Lilly, D.: Rehabilitation of patients with partial amputation of the hand. Can. J. Occup. Ther., *41*:72, 1974.

London, P. S.: Simplicity of approach to treatment of the injured hand. J. Bone Joint Surg., *43B*:454, 1961.

Midgley, R. A., and Entin, M. A.: Management of mutilating injuries of the hand. Clin. Plast. Surg., *3*:99, 1976.

Robinson, D. W., and Masters, F. W.: Severe avulsion injuries of the extremities including the degloving type. Surg. Clin. North Am., *47*:379, 1967.

Sanguinetti, M. V.: Reconstructive surgery of roller injuries of the hand. J. Hand Surg., *2*:134, 1977.

Swanson, A. B.: Restoration of hand function by the use of partial or total prosthetic replacement. Part I: The use of partial prostheses. J. Bone Joint Surg., *45A*:276, 1963.

Tubiana, R.: Planning of surgical treatment. Hand, *7*:223, 1975.

Tubiana, R., Stack, H. G., and Hakstian, R. W.: Restoration of prehension after severe mutilations of the hand. J. Bone Joint Surg., *48B*:455, 1966.

Vilain, R., and Mitz, V.: Vascular flaps in secondary surgery after hand trauma. Hand, *7*:56, 1975.

Upper Extremity: Inclusive

Louis, D. S.: Amputations. *In* Green, D. P. (Ed.): Operative Hand Surgery. New York, Churchill Livingstone, 1982, Chap. 3.

Omer, G. E.: Upper Extremity Amputations. *In* Flynn, J. E. (Ed.): Hand Surgery. 3rd Ed. Baltimore, Williams & Wilkins Company, 1982, Chap. 11.

Slocum, D. B.: An Atlas of Amputations. St. Louis, MO, C. V. Mosby Company, 1949.

multiple finger replantation procedures (Teal, personal communication).

It is important for a replantation team that the equipment be available in a standard place and in good condition. Obviously, replantation procedures are not elective, and therefore the equipment must be mobilized quickly, sometimes at short notice. A unified team of technicians, nurses, and doctors can facilitate this goal.

Medical centers that do not have a replantation team or skilled hand surgeon capable of replantation can readily refer their patients for care. Since with proper cooling of the amputated part the replantation procedure can be initiated up to 24 hours after the injury, there are few injuries outside the reach of a replantation center.

Regardless of the number of surgeons involved in the replantation attempt, they must be trained in both hand surgery and microsurgery (Strauch and Terzis, 1978). Experience in hand surgery is esssential in evaluating the patient before replantation, in order to try to determine the potential for regaining a functional part; except for the microvascular anastomosis, the basic problem is one of complex upper extremity reconstruction. Moreover, the excellence of repair of all structures, such as tendons, nerves, and bones, will greatly affect the ultimate function, and this work must be performed by someone who understands both acute and reconstructive hand surgery.

The replantation surgeon must obviously be well practiced in microsurgery. As with any other technical skill, significant efforts are required to learn the techniques, and continual application is necessary to maintain skill. Because microvascular anastomotic patency is so important and because the techniques of microvascular surgery are so demanding, it is important that the replantation surgeon have access to a microvascular laboratory where his skills can be honed on experimental animals. The surgeon who is seeing a particularly large volume of patients for microsurgery may not need constant practice in a laboratory, but those treating a smaller number of patients do.

PATIENT CARE

Initial Care

All patients who have an amputated or partially amputated part should be regarded as candidates for an attempt at replantation: not all will be selected or are appropriate for replantation, but all deserve careful consideration. As more emergency medical personnel become aware of the opportunities for replantation, more patients will be referred for this surgery. The appropriateness of attempting a replantation procedure is best determined after the patient is seen by the replantation team. Except in extreme circumstances, it will require their combined expertise to determine whether the patient and the amputated part are suitable for replantation. However, before transfer to the replantation center, the patient's major life-threatening problems must be cared for. With proper cold ischemia, parts may be replanted more than 24 hours after amputation (Hayhurst and colleagues, 1974; Leung, 1981b; May, Hergrueter, and Hansen, 1986). If the amputated part is properly cooled, the patient may be stabilized before transfer or surgery.

The amputated part should be cooled from the time it is retrieved (Fig. 93–2). The part should be wrapped in moist saline gauze,

EARLY CARE OF AMPUTATED PART

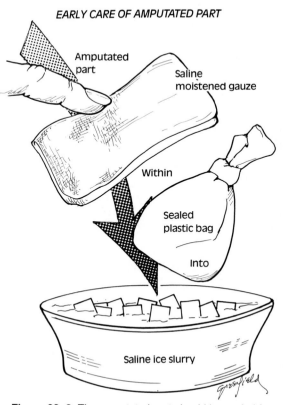

Figure 93–2. The amputated part should be cooled from the time it is retrieved by wrapping it in moist saline gauze, placing it in a sealed plastic bag, and immersing it in an iced saline container.

placed in a sealed plastic bag, and immersed in an iced saline container. It should not be allowed to become waterlogged or frost-bitten. At the primary emergency room the amputated part and the stump should be carefully examined and x-rayed, so that accurate referral to the replantation center can be made. At this time any bleeding should be controlled by direct compression and not by hemostats, ligation, or proximal tourniquets.

It is better that an inappropriate patient and part be referred for the possibility of replantation than that appropriate patients and parts should not be referred.

Initial Emergency Room Care

When the patient arrives at the replantation center, full attention should be given to major life-threatening problems, as for major trauma care. Since the replantation procedure is quite prolonged, other major problems must be diagnosed and cared for before initiation of the replantation surgery. The higher the level of amputation, the greater is the chance that significant injuries may have occurred to other systems (Chen and associates, 1981). Major limb amputations may also have resulted in considerable blood loss. Tetanus prophylaxis should not be overlooked. Intravenous antibiotics and rectal aspirin to initiate the impairment of platelet function are administered in the emergency room. Self-inflicted amputating injuries require immediate consultation with a psychiatrist; postoperative assistance of a psychiatrist may be warranted not only in these patients, but in the majority of patients in whom adaptation to the injury may be difficult (Stewart and Lowrey, 1980; Schweitzer and Rosenbaum, 1982; Strain and DeMuth, 1983).

GOALS OF REPLANTATION AND REVASCULARIZATION

The first goal of replantation surgery is a viable extremity. However, the prime indication for attempting replantation, the second goal, is the surgeon's estimation that a functioning extremity, which will be better than a prosthesis, can be returned to the patient. Furthermore, function must be seen in the larger sense of not just measurable joint motion and sensibility, but value in the normal activities of life. The indications for attempting replantation or revascularization surgery are influenced by both of these goals. If viability cannot be attained, such as when the part is badly crushed or injured at multiple levels, amputation revision is the only possible therapy. If the part has been injured so severely that functional motion and sensibility are unlikely, revascularization or replantation may be contraindicated. Patients rarely allow a replaced part to be reamputated later, even though function might be better with a prosthesis. Therefore, the indications for replantation and revascularization must be considered very carefully in the short, busy time between injury and surgery.

INDICATIONS FOR REPLANTATION

Several authors have developed lists of indications and contraindications for replantation surgery based on up to 30 years' experience analyzing patients' results (O'Brien, 1974; Buncke and Zide, 1979; May and Gallico, 1980a; Chen and associates, 1981; Gallico and Stirrat, 1983). The amputated parts that are generally recommended for replantation are summarized in Tables 93–1 and 93–2. However, it is important to emphasize that each patient must be evaluated individually and should not be included or excluded on the basis of those lists alone. The extenuating circumstances discussed below must be taken into account in determining whether part replacement is warranted. The goal of the operation must be kept in mind: the reattachment of an optimally functioning hand or limb that will be preferable to amputation with or without a prosthesis.

Age of Patient

The age of the patient is an important consideration. The younger the patient, the

Table 93–1. Amputations to Replant

The thumb
Zone I amputations
Multiple digits
Bilateral amputations
Hemi-hand amputations
Hand amputations, wrist to upper forearm
Pediatric amputations

Certain amputated parts almost always deserve careful consideration for replantation.

Table 93–2. Discretionary Replantations

Single finger
Zone II amputations
Severe crush or avulsion injuries
Geriatric amputations
Major limb amputations

Some amputated parts should be considered for replantation surgery only in particular circumstances.

better are the functional results (Jaeger, Tsai, and Kleinert, 1981; Black, 1982). Joint stiffness and limited nerve regeneration in older patients limit functional return. Although the ages of patients who have undergone replantation surgery range from less than 1 year to 83 years, the young patients are a technical challenge, and the old patients a functional failure (Sekiguchi and Ohmori, 1979; Leung, 1979a). Some replantation centers have suggested a cut-off age of 50 to 55 years beyond which replantation will not be performed (Kleinert, Jablon, and Tsai, 1980). However, well-motivated older patients may show good results, and careful preoperative discussion is necessary. Although extremes of age are not a barrier to attempting replantation, most patients who will be seen for replantation or revascularization are in the third and fourth decades because of the higher incidence of such injuries in this age group.

Patient's Motivation

The patient's desire for replantation and an estimate of his motivation are also important in judging the appropriateness of replantation. Although these factors may be difficult to assess in the emergency room in the midst of trauma, and although it may be difficult for patients to understand fully the advantages or disadvantages of a replantation procedure, it is important to inform them as fully as possible of the potential outcome of the replantation procedure. They must help in the decision whether to replace the limb or not. However, even though patients may ardently desire replantation of the part, this expressed interest should not encourage the replantation of potentially useless or limiting parts. Patients' occupations may also be important, since a limb with limited function may be acceptable to a desk worker but not to an industrial worker.

Ischemic Time

The warm ischemic time sustained by the amputated part will influence the chance of revascularizing the part and the ultimate function. Muscle necrosis can be seen after two to three hours of tourniquet ischemia (Harman, 1947; Williams, 1966; Strock and Majno, 1969; Miller and colleagues, 1979). Anoxia leads to progressive cellular damage, resulting in "no-reflow" to the ischemic tissues, and necrosis (May and associates, 1978). The more proximal an amputation, the more likely will the part be susceptible to ischemic damage. The permissible warm ischemic time for a proximal limb amputation, which contains a large amount of muscle, is six hours; the permissible warm ischemic time for more distal amputations is eight to 12 hours. Replantation may be partly successful with a longer warm ischemic time, but partial necrosis and impaired function will surely follow (Chiu and Chen, 1984). Cold ischemia can be sustained by the amputated part for a longer time than warm ischemia (Hayhurst and associates, 1974; May, Hergrueter, and Hansen, 1986). Cooling should be maintained by the technique outlined above or by constant perfusion or immersion (Caffee and Hankins, 1982; Nakayama and Soeda, 1985). A finger or hemi-hand amputation may be maintained in a cold ischemic state for more than 24 hours, whereas a proximal arm or forearm amputation may only be replantable for up to 12 hours after amputation despite proper storage (Leung, 1981b).

Perfusion of Parts

Previous attempts at perfusion with various solutions in order to store amputated parts, as is done in organ transplantation, have not been successful (Chait and colleagues, 1978). However, more recent experimental studies indicate that solutions can be determined that will prolong the ischemic time of various tissues (Rosen and associates, 1985, 1987). Such solutions have been used in clinical replantation surgery with partial success (Smith and colleagues, 1985). However, until the laboratory evidence regarding perfusion preservation has been corroborated in patients, simple cooling of the part is sufficient.

Mechanism of Injury

The mechanism of injury, as one might expect, is an important predictor of the chance of immediate vascular success and the eventual functional outcome (Fig. 93–3). Mechanisms are frequently categorized as guillotine, avulsion, or crush. Each of these mechanisms of injury produces a zone of injury within the amputated part and the stump. The extent of the zone of injury in the vascular supply determines the ease of revascularization. The extent of the zone within the nerves determines the excellence of nerve regeneration and the final sensibility of the part. Tendons and muscles that have been avulsed from their proximal origins may have lost the routes for potential vascular and nerve supply, and because of subsequent fibrosis will certainly contract and glide very poorly. Avulsing and crushing injuries produce a zone of injury proximally and distally to the amputation site that requires more debridement and increases the risk of infection. The greatest immediate failure rate and

the least good long-term functional results are seen in avulsing or diffusely crushing injuries (Hamilton and associates, 1982). Guillotine or clean-cut injuries are the least common, but have the best chance of viability and good ultimate function.

Level of Amputation

The ease of replantation, the duration of acceptable ischemia, and the ultimate function of a replanted part correlate with the level of amputation. Distal amputations do better than more proximal ones. Proximal amputations require a great force of injury to have occurred and frequently have a significant avulsion or crush component in their mechanism. Moreover, the large distal muscle bulk and the length of nerve regeneration required compromise the functional result. Avulsing shoulder amputations are particularly poor candidates for replantation. A considerable amount of force is necessary to cause an amputation at the shoulder level,

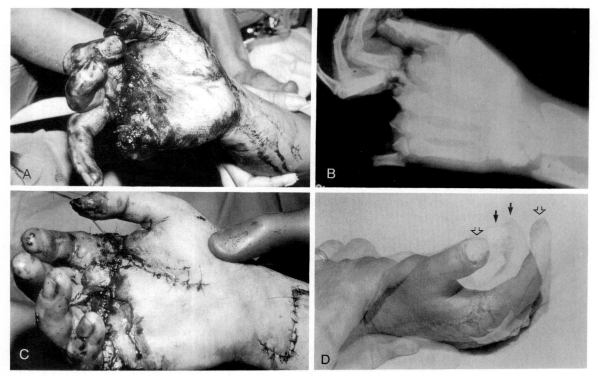

Figure 93–3. Severe crush injury. *A,* One finger has been amputated and three fingers devascularized by crushing in a railroad car coupling. *B,* Because of proximity to the metocarpophalangeal joints, interosseous wires were used for bone fixation. *C,* All structures were repaired. *D,* The extent of the zone of crushing injury leads to significant scar, which hampers the final flexion *(closed arrows)* and extension *(open arrows)* of the fingers shown in double exposure.

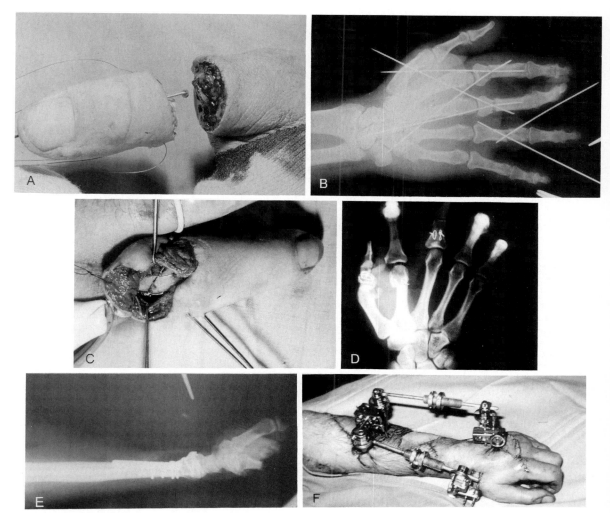

Figure 93–7. Bone fixation techniques. *A,* An axial K-wire is the simplest fixation for distal amputations. *B,* Crossed K-wires are commonly employed, but there is a risk of injuring structures to be anastomosed. *C,* Interosseous wires require elevation of considerable periosteum, but allow anatomic fracture reduction. *D,* Interosseous wires are particularly useful adjacent to joints. *E,* Compression plates are usually employed in amputations proximal to the wrist. *F,* In rare situations, external fixation is required to hold comminuted fractures.

can be seen in the long term (Guerra and colleagues, 1984). Sympathetic nerve impairment may also lead to bone resorption and articular change.

Tendon Repairs

The flexor and extensor tendons should be shortened by a similar amount to the bone to maintain normal resting muscle tension. The tendons are shortened by different amounts on the proximal and distal ends so that the junction of the tendon and the bone union do not directly overlie each other. The ultimate

mobility of the replanted part is dictated by scar-inhibiting tendon motion. Repair of tendons should be performed according to the standard technique (see Fig. 93–9).

Extensor Tendons

The extensor tendons are repaired before the dorsal venous anastomosis is performed (Fig. 93–8). The tendon shortening should be commensurate with bone shortening. The ends are approximated with interrupted 4–0 nylon figure-of-eight or horizontal mattress sutures. The lateral bands should be specifi-

DORSAL RECONSTRUCTION

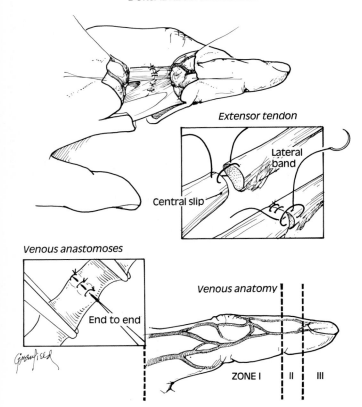

Extensor tendon

Lateral band

Central slip

Venous anastomoses

End to end

Venous anatomy

ZONE I   II   III

Figure 93–8. Dorsal reconstruction. The extensor tendons are approximated in the standard fashion. Vein anastomosis follows extensor tendon repair. A familiarity with the anatomy of the dorsal veins on the fingers will save hours of surgery. Two or three end to end venous anastomoses are safest.

cally repaired to restore flexor-extensor balance as much as possible.

Flexor Tendons

Flexor tendon repair should be performed with the same care as if these tendons alone were divided (Fig. 93–9). Future mobility of the replanted part is dictated to a large extent by the scarring surrounding the flexor tendon. Although the replanted digit will have more scar than the one with flexor division alone, the future gliding of these tendons will be improved by the tenets of Kleinert (Kleinert, Kutz, and Atasoy, 1973) and Verdan (Verdan and Michon, 1961). Both profundus and superficialis tendons should be repaired in Zone II if possible (Lister and colleagues, 1977). In this double repair, the tendons should be shortened either proximally or distally so that the repairs do not overlie each other. A Mason-Allen-Kessler-Kleinert suture technique provides a smooth tendon

junction with minimal interference of the internal blood supply to the healing tendon ends. Although in the case of replantation and revascularization surgery early mobilization of the digit is not usually performed, the aforementioned suture allows early passive motion. A lateral grasping suture described by Becker and associates (1978, 1979) may cause less damage to the internal blood supply of the tendon and have sufficient early strength that active motion can be employed. However, because of the vascular and nerve anastomoses, the digits are not usually moved for the first ten days. The annular pulleys are retained or reconstructed (Lister and colleagues, 1977; Delattre and associates, 1983). Some authors have advocated free grafts of extensor synovial sheath from the foot to replace the lost synovial sheath in the zone of injury (Eiken and Rank, 1977). The immediate placement of Hunter Silastic rod spacers has been advocated when tendon injury has been severe, but may lead to increased risk of infection (Marshall, Wolfort, and Edlich, 1978).

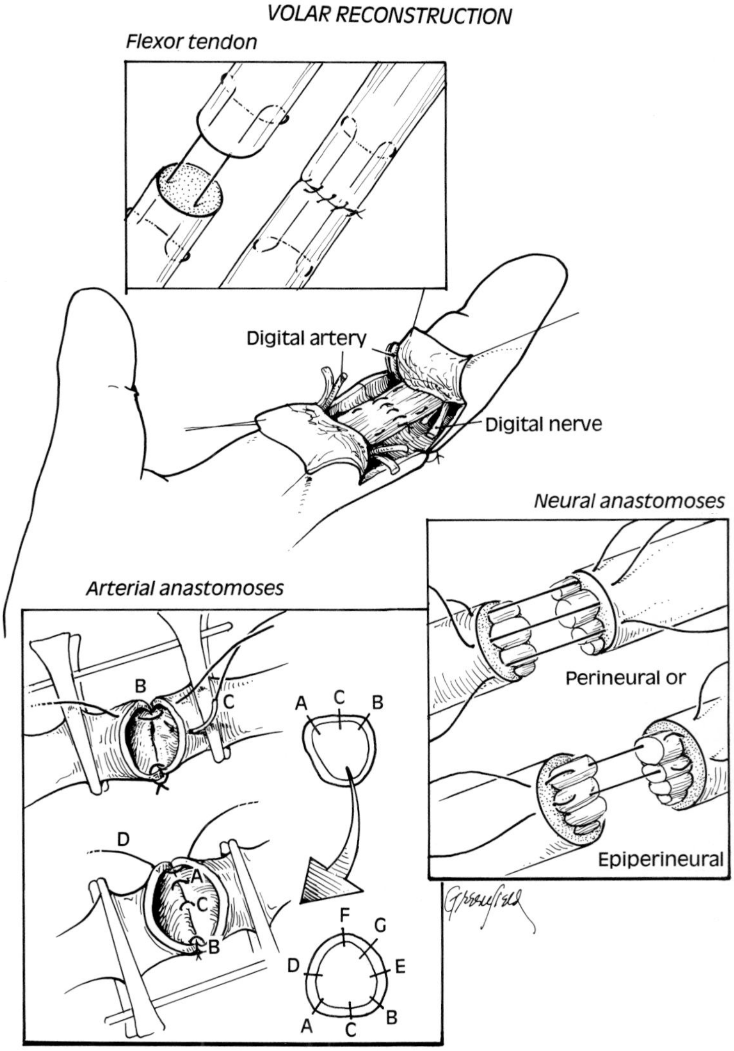

VOLAR RECONSTRUCTION

Flexor tendon

Digital artery

Digital nerve

Neural anastomoses

Arterial anastomoses

Perineural or

Epiperineural

Figure 93–9. Volar reconstruction. The flexor tendons are repaired at all levels, using standard suture techniques, depending on the level of tendon division. One or two arteries are anastomosed with interrupted nylon sutures under the microscope. The nerves are repaired just before skin closure, but must receive careful attention because of the importance of sensibility to ultimate function.

TECHNIQUES OF MICROVASCULAR SURGERY

Zone of Vascular Injury

Successful replantation requires the apposition of healthy, clean, well-vascularized tissues. Depending on the nature of the injury, debridement of each of the individual tissues from the proximal and distal cut ends is necessary. The bone is shortened, both to debride the nonviable cut or crushed surfaces and to allow the apposition of soft tissues. Even though the amputated part does not have a blood supply, the surgeon can usually estimate from the mechanism of injury and the appearance of the tissues which distal parts cannot be salvaged. At this time the structures are dissected out and carefully labeled. It is extremely important to identify draining veins carefully, as they may be difficult to identify later (see Fig. 93–8). The arteries are debrided proximally back to a level at which there is an excellent spurt of blood from the cut end. Distal debridement is performed under microscopic control until the arterial wall shows no signs of crush or avulsion injury.

Patency of the vascular repairs relies on careful assessment of the length of the injured vessel. Within the zone of injury, and sometimes even for a distance on either side of it, the veins and particularly arteries have sustained injuries to the vessel walls that will

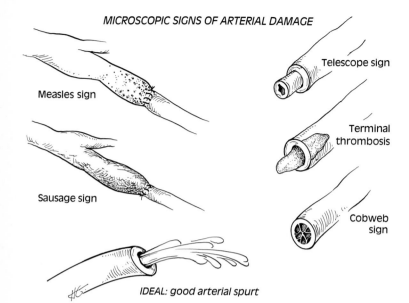

MICROSCOPIC SIGNS OF ARTERIAL DAMAGE

Measles sign

Sausage sign

Telescope sign

Terminal thrombosis

Cobweb sign

IDEAL: good arterial spurt

Figure 93–10. Microscopic signs of arterial damage. The arteries must be debrided back to an uninjured level to provide a good proximal inflow and maintain a patent anastomosis. The telescope sign, terminal thrombosis, and the cobweb sign indicate damage to the intima and media and must be excised. The petechiae of the measles sign and the ballooning of the sausage sign after anastomosis indicate that insufficient debridement was performed.

lead to thrombosis unless debrided. Knowledge of the mechanism of injury combined with clinical signs of vessel damage (May and Gallico, 1980a; Acland, 1972; VanBeek, Kutz, and Zook, 1978) will aid the surgeon in determining how much of the vessel needs debridement before anastomosis (Fig. 93–10). If there is only meager flow from the cut end of the proximal artery, there is remaining vessel damage leading to platelet aggregation or spasm. The zone of injury should be expected, if anything, to be greater than that which is visible (Mitchell and associates, 1985).

Vascular Anastomosis

The vessels are usually repaired after either the extensor or the flexor tendon repairs have been completed. At this stage in the operation, the operating microscope will aid in examination and debridement of the vessels at 6 to 9 power magnification. Lidocaine (Xylocaine) can be used on the proximal artery as a temporary plegic agent, but unless there is continued excellent inflow from the proximal vessel, no sutured anastomosis will remain patent. Vascular anastomotic failure is avoided by thorough vessel debridement even if the debridement results in a need for a vein graft.

The suture anastomosis is the "gold standard" of microvascular surgery (see Fig. 93–9). Most replantation surgery involves the standard end to end anastomosis. An end to side anastomosis has been described, but is not commonly required or indicated in replantation surgery (Godina, 1979). Arteries and veins are anastomosed with interrupted nylon sutures under the operating microscope at magnifications from 6 to 18 times. Vessels as small as 0.5 mm in diameter can be successfully repaired by these techniques. No. 11–0 nylon sutures are used for veins and arteries at the fingertips; 10–0 sutures from the fingertips through the midpalm; and 9–0 sutures at the wrist through forearm levels. Although the vascular repairs can be performed with loupes, the operating microscope is preferred at all levels.

By the time of arterial repair, the finger may need to remain in a flexed position to protect the flexor tendon anastomoses as well as to approximate the arterial ends. The standard laboratory technique of anastomosis is not applicable, and some contortions of the microscope head and the surgeon's hands may be required. An arterial anastomosis that proceeds from 6 o'clock alternately around to 12 o'clock may be an important technique to know in these circumstances, since the vessel does not have to be turned over and the repair can be done with the vessel in an almost vertical position.

Techniques for anastomosis of microvascular vessels using laser beams to weld the open end together have been described, but lead to an unacceptably high incidence of delayed pseudoaneurysm formation (Vale and colleagues, 1986). A biodegradable microvas-

C.: The mechanical role of the digital fibrous sheath: application to reconstructive surgery of the flexor tendons. Anat. Clin., 5:187, 1983.

Dell, P. C., Seaber, A. V., and Urbaniak, J. R.: The effect of systemic acidosis on perfusion of replanted parts. J. Hand Surg., 5:433, 1980.

Douglas, B.: Successful replacement of completely avulsed portions of fingers as composite grafts. Plast. Reconstr. Surg., 23:213, 1959.

Doi, K.: Replantation of an avulsed thumb, with application of a neurovascular pedicle. Hand, 8:258, 1976.

Doi, K.: Replantation of amputated distal phalangeal parts of fingers without vascular anastomoses, using subcutaneous pockets [letter]. Plast. Reconstr. Surg., 64:626, 1979.

Earley, M. J., and Watson, J. S.: Twenty four thumb replantations. J. Hand Surg. (Br.), 9:98, 1984.

Eiken, O., and Rank, F.: Experimental restoration of the digital synovial sheath. Scand. J. Plast. Reconstr. Surg., 11:213, 1977.

Elsahy, N. I.: Replantation of a completely amputated distal segment of a thumb: case report. Plast. Reconstr. Surg., 59:579, 1977a.

Elsahy, N. I.: When to replant a fingertip after its complete amputation. Plast. Reconstr. Surg., 60:14, 1977b.

Emerson, D. J., and Page, R. E.: Immediate excision and skin graft of a friction burn in a replanted thumb with a note on its usefulness and indications. Br. J. Plast. Surg., 37:624, 1984.

Eriksson, E., Anderson, W. A., and Replogle, R. L.: Effects of prolonged ischemia on muscle microcirculation in the cat. Surg. Forum, 25:254, 1974.

Faibisoff, B., and Daniel, R. K.: Management of severe forearm injuries. Surg. Clin. North Am., 61:287, 1981.

Finseth, F. F., May, J. W., and Smith, R. J.: Composite groin flap with iliac bone for primary thumb reconstruction. J. Bone Joint Surg., 58A:130, 1976.

Flagg, S. V., Finseth, F. J., and Krizek, T. J.: Ring avulsion injury. Plast. Reconstr. Surg., 59:241, 1977.

Fossati, E., and Irigaray, A.: Successful revascularization of an incompletely amputated finger with serious venous congestion—a case report. J. Hand Surg. (Am.), 8:356, 1983.

Furnas, D. W., Salibian, A. H., and Achauer, B. M.: Genesis of a replantation program. Am. J. Surg., 136:21, 1978.

Gallico, G. G., III, and Stirrat, C. R.: Extremity replantation. Surg. Annu., 15:229, 1983.

Gelberman, R. H., Urbaniak, J. R., Bright, D. S., and Levin, L. S.: Digital sensibility following replantation. J. Hand Surg., 3:313, 1978.

Gillies, H. D.: Autograft of amputated digit. Lancet, 1:1002, 1940.

Gingrass, R. P., Fehring, B., and Matloub, H.: Intraosseous wiring of complex hand fractures. Plast. Reconstr. Surg., 66:466, 1980.

Glas, K., Biemer, E., Duspiva, K. P., Werber, K., Stock, W., and Herndl, E.: Long-term follow-up results of 97 finger replantations. Arch. Orthop. Trauma Surg., 100:95, 1982.

Glosovac, S. V., Bitz, D. M., and Whiteside, L. A.: Hydrogen washout technique in monitoring vascular status after replantation surgery. J. Hand Surg. (Am.), 7:601, 1982.

Glubo, S. M., Lenet, M., and Sherman, M.: Lawnmower foot: the surgical reconstruction of the traumatically injured forefoot. J. Foot Surg., 16:78, 1977.

Godina, M.: Preferential use of arterial end-to-side an-

astomoses in free-flap transfers. Plast. Reconstr. Surg., 64:673, 1979.

Goldwyn, R. M., and Murray, J. E.: Letter: function of replanted fingers. N. Engl. J. Med., 291:1088, 1974.

Gordon, L., Leitner, D. W., Buncke, H. J., and Alpert, B. S.: Partial nail plate removal after digital replantation as an alternative method of venous drainage. J. Hand Surg. (Am.), 10:360, 1985.

Gordon, S.: Autograft of amputated thumb. Lancet, 2:823, 1944.

Gould, J. S., Gould, S. H., and Caudill-Babkes, E. L.: Interpositional microvascular vein grafting. Hand, 11:332, 1979.

Graham, B., Laulus, D. A., and Caffee, H. H.: Pulse oximetry for vascular monitoring in upper extremity replantation surgery. J. Hand Surg. (Am.), 11:687, 1986.

Graham, B. H., Gordon, L., Alpert, B. S., Walton, R., Buncke, H. J., and Leitner, D. W.: Serial quantitative skin surface fluorescence: a new method for postoperative monitoring of vascular perfusion in revascularized digits. J. Hand Surg. (Am.), 10:226, 1985.

Guerra, J., Jr., Resnick, D., Gelberman, R. H., Reznek, R., and Cone, R. O., III: Replantation of digits or hands followed by destructive joint disease. Radiology, 152:591, 1984.

Hales, P., and Pullen, D.: Hypotension and bleeding diathesis following attempted arm replantation. Anesth. Intensive Care, 10:359, 1982.

Hall, R. H.: Whole upper extremity transplant for human beings: general plans of procedure and operative technique. Ann. Surg., 120:12, 1944.

Halmagyi, A. F., Baker, C. B., Campbell, H. H., Evans, J. G., and Mahoney, L. J.: Replantation of a completely severed arm followed by reamputation because of failure of innervation. Can. J. Surg., 12:222, 1969.

Halsted, W. S., Reichert, F. L., and Reid, M. R.: Replantation of entire limbs without suture of vessels. Trans. Am. Surg., Assoc., 140:160, 1922.

Hamilton, R. B., O'Brien, B. M., Morrison, W. A., and MacLeod, A. M.: Replantation and revascularization of digits. Surg. Gynecol. Obstet., 151:508, 1980.

Hamilton, R. B., O'Brien, B. M., Morrison, W. A., and MacLeod, A. M.: Survival factors in replantation and revascularization of the amputated thumb—10 years' experience. Scand. J. Plast. Reconstr. Surg., 19:55, 1982.

Harashina, T., and Buncke, H. J.: Study of washout solutions for microvascular replantation and transplantation. J. Plast. Reconstr. Surg., 56:542, 1975.

Harman, J. W.: Histological study of skeletal muscle in acute ischemia. Am. J. Pathol., 23:551, 1947.

Harris, G. D., Finseth, F., and Buncke, H. J.: The hazard of cigarette smoking following digital replantation. J. Microsurg., 1:403, 1980.

Harris, W. H., and Malt, R. A.: Late results of human limb replantation: eleven year and six year follow-up of two cases with description of a new tendon transfer. J. Trauma, 14:44, 1974.

Harrison, D. H., and Watson, J. S.: Use of the polypropylene pegs for immediate stabilization in digital replantation. J. Hand Surg. (Am.), 5:203, 1980.

Hayhurst, J. W., O'Brien, B. M., Ishida, H., and Baxter, T. J.: Experimental digital replantation after prolonged cooling. Hand, 6:134, 1974.

Heden, P. G., Hamilton, R., Arnander, C., and Jurell, G.: Laser Doppler surveillance of the circulation of free flaps and replanted digits. Microsurgery, 6:11, 1985.

Honda, T., Nomura, S., Yamauchi, S., Shimamura, K.,

and Yoshimura, M.: The possible applications of a composite skin and subcutaneous vein graft in the replantation of amputated digits. Br. J. Plast. Surg., 37:607, 1984.

Höpfner, E.: Über Gefässnaht, Gafässtransplantationen und Reimplantation von amputierten Extremitäten. Arch. Klin. Chir., 70:417, 1903.

Ikuta, Y.: Method of bone fixation in reattachment of amputations in the upper extremities. Clin. Orthop., 133:169, 1978.

Ikuta, Y., and Tsuge, K.: Micro-bolts and micro-screws for fixation of small bones in the hand. Hand, 6:261, 1974.

Irigaray, A.: New fixing screw for completely amputated fingers. J. Hand Surg., 5:381, 1980.

Jacobson, J. H.: Microsurgical technique in repair of the traumatized extremity. Clin. Orthop., 19:132, 1963.

Jacobson, J. H., and Suzrez, E. L.: Microsurgery in the anastomosis of small vessels. Surg. Forum, 9:243, 1960.

Jaeger, S. H., Tsai, T. M., and Kleinert, H. E.: Upper extremity replantation in children. Orthop. Clin. North Am., 12:897, 1981.

Johansen, K., Bandyk, D., Thiele, B., and Hansen, S. T., Jr.: Temporary intraluminal shunts: resolution of a management dilemma in complex vascular injuries. J. Trauma, 22:395, 1982.

Jones, J. M., Schenck, R. R., and Chesney, R. B.: Digital replantation and amputation—comparison of function. J. Hand Surg. (Am.), 7:183, 1982.

Kader, P. B.: Therapist's management of the replanted hand. Hand Clin., 2:179, 1986.

Kattapuram, S. V., and Phillips, W. C.: Severed body parts: radiologic evaluation following replantation. Radiology, 149:59, 1983.

Kay, S.: Venous occlusion plethysmography in patients with cold related symptoms after digital salvage procedures. J. Hand Surg. (Br.), 10:151, 1985.

Keiter, J. E.: Immediate pollicization of an amputated index finger. J. Hand Surg. (Am.), 5:584, 1980.

Keller, H. P., and Lanz, U.: Objective control of replanted fingers by transcutaneous partial O_2 (PO_2) measurement. Microsurgery, 5:85, 1984.

Kleinert, H. E.: Techniques of axillary block. J. Trauma, 3:3, 1963.

Kleinert, H. E., Jablon, M., and Tsai, T. M.: An overview of replantation and results of 347 replants in 245 patients. J. Trauma, 20:390, 1980.

Kleinert, H. E., and Kasdan, M. L.: Restoration of blood flow in upper extremity injuries. J. Trauma, 3:461, 1963a.

Kleinert, H. E., and Kasdan, M. L.: Salvage of devascularized upper extremities including studies on small vessel anastomosis. Clin. Orthop., 29:29, 1963b.

Kleinert, H. E., and Kasdan, M. L.: Anastomosis of digital vessels. J. Ky. Med. Assoc., 63:106, 1965.

Kleinert, H. E., Kasdan, M. L., and Romero, J. L.: Small blood vessel anastomosis for salvage of the severely injured upper extremity. J. Bone Joint Surg., 45A:788, 1963.

Kleinert, H. E., Kutz, J. E., and Atasoy, E.: Primary repair of flexor tendons. Orthop. Clin. North Am., 4:865, 1973.

Kleinman, W. B., and Dustman, J. A.: Preservation of function following complete degloving injuries to the hand: use of simultaneous groin, random abdominal flap, and partial thickness skin graft. J. Hand Surg., 6:82, 1981.

Komatsu, S., and Tamai, S.: Successful replantation of a completely cut off thumb: case report. Plast. Reconstr. Surg., 42:374, 1968.

Kotani, H., Kawai, S., Doi, K., and Kuwata, N.: Automatic milking apparatus for the insufficient venous drainage of the replanted digit. Microsurgery, 5:90, 1984.

Kubo, T., Ikita, Y., Watari, S., Okuhira, N., and Tsuge, K.: The smallest digital replant yet? Br. J. Plast. Surg., 29:313, 1976.

Kutz, J. E., Sinclair, S. W., Rao, V., and Carlier, A.: Cross-and replantation—preliminary case report. J. Microsurg., 3:251, 1982.

Lapchinsky, A. G.: Recent results of experimental transplantation of preserved limbs and kidneys and possible use of this technique in clinical practice. Ann. N.Y. Acad. Sci., 87:539, 1960.

Lauritzen, C.: A new and easier way to anastomose microvessels: an experimental study in rats. Scand. J. Plast. Reconstr. Surg., 12:291, 1978.

Layton, T. R., Villella, E. R., and Marrangoni, A. G.: Traumatic forequarter amputation. J. Trauma, 21:411, 1981.

Lee, S.: Microvascular surgical teaching rounds using rat organ transplantation model with twelve year biography. J. Res. Inst. Med. Sci. (Korea), 5:215, 1973.

Leung, P. C.: Hand replantation in an 83 year old woman—the oldest replantation? Plast. Reconstr. Surg., 64:416, 1979a.

Leung, P. C.: The "throbbing sign"—an indication of early venous congestion in replantation surgery. J. Hand Surg. (Am.), 4:409, 1979b.

Leung, P. C.: Use of an intramedullary bone peg in digital replantations, revascularization, and toe-transfers. J. Hand Surg., 6:281, 1981a.

Leung, P. C.: Prolonged refrigeration in toe to hand transfer—case report. J. Hand Surg. (Am.), 6:152, 1981b.

Leung, P. C.: Analysis of complications in digital replantations. Hand, 14:25, 1982.

Lister, G.: Intraosseous wiring of the digital skeleton. J. Hand Surg., 3:427, 1978.

Lister, G. D., Kleinert, H. E., Kutz, J. E., and Atasoy, E.: Primary flexor tendon repair followed by immediate controlled mobilization. J. Hand Surg., 2:441, 1977.

Lobay, G. W., and Moysa, G. L.: Primary neurovascular bundle transfer in the management of avulsed thumbs. J. Hand Surg., 5:584, 1981.

Lu, S. Y., Chiu, H. Y., Lin, T. W., and Chen, M. T.: Evaluation of survival in digital replantation with thermometric monitoring. J. Hand Surg. (Am.), 9:805, 1984.

Malt, R. A., and Harris, W. H.: Long term results in replanted arm. Br. J. Surg., 56:705, 1969.

Malt, R. A., and McKhann, C. F.: Replantation of severed arms. J.A.M.A., 189:716, 1964.

Malt, R. A., Remensnyder, J. P., and Harris, W. H.: Long-term utility of replanted arms. Ann. Surg., 176:334, 1972.

Manke, D. A., Sumner, D. S., Van Beek, A. L., and Lambeth, A.: Hemodynamic studies of digital and extremity replants and revascularizations. Surgery, 88:445, 1980.

Marshall, K. A., Edgerton, M. T., Rodeheaver, G. T., Magee, C. M., and Edlich, R. F.: Quantitative microbiology: its application to hand injuries. Am. J. Surg., 131:730, 1976.

Marshall, K. A., Wolfort, F. G., and Edlich, R. F.: Immediate insertion of silicone rubber rods in fingers with cut flexor tendons. Plast. Reconstr. Surg., *61*:77, 1978.

Matsen, F. A., Bach, A. W., and Wyss, C. R., and Simmons, C. W.: Transcutaneous PO₂: a potential monitor of the status of replanted limb parts. Plast. Reconstr. Surg., *61*:77, 1978.

Matsuda, M., Kato, N., and Hosoi, M.: The problems in replantation of limbs amputated through the upper arm region. J. Trauma, *21*:403, 1981.

Matsuda, M., Kato, N., and Hosoi, M.: Continuous brachial plexus block for replantation in the upper extremity. Hand, *14*:129, 1982.

May, J. W., Jr.: Successful digital replantation after 28 hours of cold ischemia. Plast. Reconstr. Surg., *67*:566, 1981.

May, J. W., Jr., and Bartlett, S.: Staged groin flap in reconstruction of the pediatric hand. J. Hand Surg., *6*:163, 1981.

May, J. W., Jr., Chait, L. A., O'Brien, B. M., and Hurley, J. V.: The no-reflow phenomenon in experimental free flaps. Plast. Reconstr. Surg., *61*:256, 1978.

May, J. W., Jr., and Gallico, G. G., III: Upper extremity replantation. Curr. Probl. Surg., *17*:12, 1980a.

May, J. W., Jr., and Gallico, G. G., III: Simultaneous structure repair in replantation surgery: ideas and innovations. Plast. Reconstr. Surg., *66*:466, 1980b.

May, J. W., Jr., and Gordon, L.: Palm of hand free flap for forearm length preservation in non-replantable amputations: case report. J. Hand Surg., *5*:377, 1980.

May, J. W., Jr., Hergrueter, C. A., and Hansen, R. H.: Seven-digit replantation: digit survival after 39 hours of cold ischemia. Plast. Reconstr. Surg., *78*:522, 1986.

May, J. W., Jr., Toth, B. A., and Gardner, M.: Digital replantation distal to the proximal interphalangeal joint. J. Hand Surg., *7*:161, 1982.

McDonald, H. D., Buncke, H. J., and Goodstein, W. A.: Split thickness skin grafts in microvascular surgery. Plast. Reconstr. Surg., *68*:731, 1981.

Mehrotra, O. N.: Hand reconstruction using a damaged index finger. N.Z. Med. J., *86*:137, 1977.

Meuli, H. C., Meyer, V., and Segmuller, G.: Stabilization of bone in replantation surgery of the upper limb. Clin. Orthop., *133*:179, 1978.

Miller, S. H., Price, G., Buck, D., Neeley, J., Kennedy, T. J., et al.: Effects of tourniquet ischemia and post-ischemic edema on muscle metabolism. J. Hand Surg., *4*:547, 1979.

Mitchell, G. M., Morrison, W. A., Papadopoulos, A., and O'Brien, B. M.: A study of the extent and pathology of experimental avulsion injury in rabbit arteries and veins. Br. J. Plast. Surg., *38*:278, 1985.

Mitz, V., Staub, S., and Morel-Fatio, D.: Advantages of interpositional long venous grafts in microvascular surgery. Ann. Plast. Surg., *2*:16, 1979.

Moneim, M. S., and Chacon, N. E.: Salvage of replanted parts of the upper extremity. J. Bone Joint Surg., *67A*:880, 1985.

Morrison, W. A., O'Brien, B. M., and MacLeod, A. M.: A long term review of digital replantation. Aust. N.Z. J. Surg., *47*:767, 1977a.

Morrison, W. A., O'Brien, B. M., and MacLeod, A. M.: Evaluation of digital replantation—a review of 100 cases. Orthop. Clin. North Am., *8*:295, 1977b.

Morrison, W. A., O'Brien, B. M., and MacLeod, A. M.: Results of digital replantation and revascularization. Hand, *10*:125, 1978.

Morrison, W. A., O'Brien, B. M., and MacLeod, A. M.:

Experience with thumb reconstruction. J. Hand Surg., *9*:223, 1984.

Moss, S. H., Schwartz, K. S., vonDrasen-Ascher, G., Ogden, L. L., II, Wheeler, C. S., and Lister, G. D.: Digital venous anatomy. J. Hand Surg. (Am.), *10*:473, 1985.

Murphy, A. L., Conlay, L., Ryan, J. F., and Roberts, J. T.: Malignant hyperthermia during a prolonged anesthetic for reattachment of a limb. Anesthesiology, *60*:149, 1984.

Nakayama, Y., and Soeda, S.: A simple method for cooling fingers during replantation surgery. Plast. Reconstr. Surg., *75*:750, 1985.

Neimkin, R. J., May, J. W., Jr., Roberts, J., and Sunder, N.: Continuous axillary block through an indwelling Teflon catheter. J. Hand Surg. (Am.), *9*:830, 1984.

Nichter, L. S., Haines, P. C., and Edgerton, M. T.: Successful replantation in the face of absent venous drainage: an experimental study. Plast. Reconstr. Surg., *75*:686, 1985.

Nissenbaum, M.: A surgical approach for replantation of complete digital amputations. J. Hand Surg. (Am.), *5*:58, 1980.

Nissenbaum, M.: Class IIA ring avulsion injuries: an absolute indication for microvascular repair. J. Hand Surg. (Am.), *9*:810, 1984.

Nunley, J. A., Coman, L. A., and Urbaniak, J. R.: Arterial shunting as an adjunct to major limb revascularization. Ann. Surg., *193*:271, 1981.

Nylander, G., Vilkki, S., and Ostrup, L.: The need for replantation surgery after traumatic amputations of the upper extremity—an estimate based upon the epidemiology of Sweden. J. Hand Surg. (Br.), *9*:257, 1984.

O'Brien, B. M.: Replantation surgery. Clin. Plast. Surg., *1*:405, 1974.

O'Brien, B. M., Franklin, J. D., Morrison, W. A., and MacLeod, A. M.: Replantation and revascularization surgery in children. Hand, *12*:12, 1980.

Peck, J. J., Fitzgibbons, T. J., and Gaspar, M. R.: Devastating distal arterial trauma and continuous intraarterial infusion of tolazoline. Am. J. Surg., *145*:562, 1983.

Phelps, D. B.: Should a torn off little finger ever be replanted? Plast. Reconstr. Surg., *61*:592, 1978.

Phelps, D. B., Rutherford, R. B., and Boswick, J. A.: Control of vasospasm following trauma and microvascular surgery. J. Hand Surg., *4*:109, 1979.

Pho, R. W.: Vessels and nerve transfer in reconstructive microsurgery. Ann. Acad. Med. Singapore, *8*:385, 1979.

Pho, R. W., Chacha, P. B., and Yeo, K. Q.: Rerouting vessels and nerves from other digits in replanting an avulsed and degloved thumb. Plast. Reconstr. Surg., *64*:330, 1979.

Pho, R. W., Chacha, P. B., Yeo, K. Q., and Caruwalla, J. S.: Replantation of digits using microvascular technique. Ann. Acad. Med. Singapore, *8*:398, 1979.

Pho, R. W., and Satkunanantham, K.: Problems of a double level amputation—a case report. Ann. Acad. Med. Singapore, *11*:273, 1982.

Pitzler, D., and Buck-Gramcko, D.: Secondary operations after replantation. Ann. Chir. Gynaecol., *71*:19, 1982.

Poletti, L. S.: Subcutaneous flap as an alternative to venous anastomosis in replantation surgery. Plast. Reconstr. Surg., *68*:233, 1981.

Poole, M. D., and Bowen, J. E.: Two unusual bleedings during anticoagulation following digital replantation. Br. J. Plast. Surg., *30*:267, 1977.

Rapoport, S., Glickman, M. G., Solomon, J. C., and Cuono, C. B.: Aggressive postoperative pharmacotherapy for vascular compromise of replanted digits. A. J. R., *144*:1065, 1985.

Reichert, F. L.: The importance of circulatory balance in the survival of replanted limbs. Bull. Johns Hopkins Hosp., *49*:86, 1931.

Rich, R. H., Knight, P. J., Erickson, E. L., Broadhurst, K., and Leonard, A. S.: Replantation of the upper extremity in children. J. Pediatr. Surg., *12*:1027, 1977.

Rose, E. H., and Buncke, H. J.: Selective finger transposition and primary metacarpal ray resection in multidigit amputations of the hand. J. Hand Surg. (Am.), *8*:178, 1983.

Rose, E. H., and Hendel, P.: Primary toe-to-thumb transfer in the acutely avulsed thumb. Plast. Reconstr. Surg., *67*:214, 1981.

Rosen, H. M., Slivjak, M. J., and McBrearty, F. X.: Preischemic flap washout and its effect on the noreflow phenomenon. Plast. Reconstr. Surg., *76*:737, 1985.

Rosen, H. M., Slivjak, M. J., and McBrearty, F. X.: Delayed microcirculatory hyperpermeability following perfusion washout. Plast. Reconstr. Surg., *79*:102, 1987.

Russell, R. C., O'Brien, B. M., Morrison, W. A., Pamamull, G., and MacLeod, A.: The late functional results of upper limb revascularization and replantation. J. Hand Surg. (Am.), *9*:623, 1984.

Sadahiro, T., and Endoh, H.: Continuous blood letting for congestion in replantation of the amputated finger. J. Hand Surg. (Br.), *9*:83, 1984.

Schlenker, J. D.: Single K-wire in thumb replantation (letter). Ann. Plast. Surg., *3*:387, 1979.

Schlenker, J. D., Kleinert, H. E., and Tsai, T. M.: Methods and results of replantation following traumatic amputation of the thumb in sixty-four patients. J. Hand Surg., *5*:63, 1980.

Schweitzer, I., and Rosenbaum, M. B.: Psychiatric aspects of replantation surgery. Gen. Hosp. Psychiatry, *4*:271, 1982.

Scott, F. A., Howar, J. W., and Boswick, J. A.: Recovery of function following replantation and revascularization of amputated hand parts. J. Trauma, *21*:204, 1981.

Sekiguchi, J., and Ohmori, K.: Youngest replantation with microsurgical anastomoses: a successful replantation of a finger on an infant—aged 12 months and 15 days—by microsurgical repair is reported. Hand, *11*:64, 1979.

Serafin, D., Kutz, J. E., and Kleinert, H. E.: Replantation of a completely amputated distal thumb without venous anastomosis. Plast. Reconstr. Surg., *52*:579, 1973.

Shafiroff, B. B., and Palmer, A. K.: Simplified technique for replantation of the thumb. J. Hand Surg., *6*:623, 1981.

Sixth People's Hospital, Shanghai: Reattachment of traumatic amputations: a summing up of experience. Chin. Med. J., *1*:392, 1967.

Sixth People's Hospital, Shanghai: Replantation of severed limbs and fingers. Chin. Med. J., *1*:3, 1973.

Sixth People's Hospital, Shanghai: Replantation of severed fingers: clinical experience in 217 cases involving 373 severed fingers. Chin. Med. J., *1*:184, 1975.

Sloan, G. M., and Sasaki, G. H.: Noninvasive monitoring of tissue viability. Clin. Plast. Surg., *12*:185, 1985.

Smith, A. R., Sonneveld, G. J., Kort, W. J., and van der Meulen, J. C.: Clinical application of transcutaneous oxygen measurements in replantation surgery and free tissue transfer. J. Hand Surg. (Am.), *8*:139, 1983.

Smith, A. R., Sonneveld, G. J., and van der Meulen, J. C.: AV anastomosis as a solution for absent venous drainage in replantation surgery. Plast. Reconstr. Surg., *71*:525, 1983.

Smith, A. R., Van Alphen, B., Faithful, N. S., and Fennema, M.: Limb preservation in replantation surgery. Plast. Reconstr. Surg., *75*:227, 1985.

Snelling, C. F., and Hendel, P. M.: Avascular necrosis of bone following revascularization of the thumb. Ann. Plast. Surg., *3*:77, 1979.

Sudahiro, T., and Endoh, H.: Continuous blood letting for congestion in replantation of amputated fingers. J. Hand Surg. *9B*:83, 1984.

Snyder, C. C., Knowles, R. P., Mayer, P. W., and Hobbs, J. C.: Extremity replantation. Plast. Reconstr. Surg., *26*:251, 1960.

Stewart, D. E., and Lowrey, M. R.: Replantation surgery following self-inflicted amputation. Can. J. Psychiatry, *25*:143, 1980.

Stirrat, C., Seaber, A. V., Urbaniak, J. R., and Bright, D. S.: Temperature monitoring in digital replantation. J. Hand Surg., *3*:342, 1978.

Strain, J. J., and DeMuth, G. W.: Care of the psychotic self-amputee undergoing replantation. Ann. Surg., *197*:210, 1983.

Strock, P. E., and Majno, G.: Vascular responses to experimental tourniquet ischemia. Surg. Gynecol. Obstet., *129*:309, 1969.

Strauch, B., and Terzis, J. K.: Replantation of digits. Clin. Orthop., *133*:35, 1978.

Suadge, H., Kutz, J. A., Kleinert, H. E., Lister, G. D., Wolff, T. W., and Atasoy, E.: Perichondrial resurfacing arthroplasty in the hand. J. Hand Surg., *9*:880, 1984.

Tamai, S.: Digit replantation: analysis of 163 replantations in an 11 year period. Clin. Plast. Surg., *5*:105, 1979.

Tamai, S.: Twenty years' experience of limb replantation—review of 293 upper extremity replants. J. Hand Surg. (Am.), *7*:549, 1982.

Tamai, S., Hori, Y., Fukui, A., and Shimizu, T.: Finger replantation. Int. Surg., *66*:9, 1981.

Tamai, S., Hori, Y., Tatsumi, Y., et al.: Microvascular anastomosis and its application on the replantation of amputated digits and hands. Clin. Orthop., *133*:106, 1978.

Tamai, S., Tatsumi, Y., Shimizu, T., et al.: Traumatic amputation of digits: the fate of remaining blood. J. Hand Surg., *2*:13, 1977.

Tsai, T.: A complex reimplantation of digits: a case report. J. Hand Surg., *4*:145, 1979.

Tsai, T. M., Manstein, C., DuBou, R., Wolff, T. W., Kutz, J. E., and Kleinert, H. E.: Primary microsurgical repair of ring avulsion amputation injuries. J. Hand Surg., *9A*:68, 1984.

Tsai, T. M., Singer, R., Elliot, E., and Klein, H.: Immediate free vascularized joint transfer from second toe to index finger proximal interphalangeal joint: a case report. J. Hand Surg. (Br.), *10*:85, 1985.

Tsui, D. Y., Shih, Y. F., Tang, C. Y., and Wang, W. H.: Successful restoration of a completely amputated arm. Chin. Med. J., *85*:536, 1966.

Tupper, J. W.: Techniques of bone fixation and clinical experience in replanted extremities. Clin. Orthop., *133*:165, 1978.

Urbaniak, J. R., Evans, J. P., and Bright, D. S.: Microvascular management of ring avulsion injuries. J. Hand Surg., *6*:25, 1981.

Urbaniak, J. R., Hayes, M. G., and Bright, D. S.: Management of bone in digital replantations: free vascularized and composite bone grafts. Clin. Orthop., *133*:184, 1978.

Urbaniak, J. R., Roth, J. H., Nunley, J. A., Goldner, R. D., and Koman, L. A.: The results of replantation after amputation of a single finger. J. Bone Joint Surg. (Am.), *67*:611, 1985.

Usui, M., Sakata, H., and Ishii, S.: Effect of fluorocarbon perfusion upon the preservation of amputated limbs. An experimental study. J. Bone Joint Surg., *67B*:473, 1985.

Vale, B. H., Frenkel, A., Trenka-Benthin, S., and Matlaga, B. F.: Microsurgical anastomosis of rat carotid arteries with the CO_2 laser. Plast. Reconstr. Surg., *77*:759, 1986.

VanBeek, A. L., Kutz, J. E., and Zook, E. G.: Importance of the ribbon sign, indicating unsuitability of the vessel, in replanting a finger. Plast. Reconstr. Surg., *61*:32, 1978.

VanBeek, A. L., Wavak, P. W., and Zook, E. G.: Microvascular surgery in young children. Plast. Reconstr. Surg., *63*:457, 1979.

Verdan, V., and Michon, J.: Le traitement des plaies des tendons fléchisseurs de doigts. Rev. Chir. Orthop., *47*:285, 1961.

Vilkki, S. K.: Postoperative skin temperature dynamics and the nature of vascular complications after replantation. Scand. J. Plast. Reconstr. Surg., *16*:151, 1982.

Wang, S. H., Young, K. F., and Wei, J. N.: Replantation of severed limbs—clinical analysis of 91 cases. J. Hand Surg. (Am.), *6*:311, 1981.

Webster, M. H. C., and Patterson, J.: The photoelectric plethysmograph as a monitor of microvascular anastomoses. Br. J. Plast. Surg., *29*:182, 1976.

Weeks, P. M., and Young, V. L.: Revascularization of the skin envelope of a denuded finger. Plast. Reconstr. Surg., *69*:527, 1982.

Wei, F. C., Chaung, C. C., Chen, H. C., Tsai, Y. C., and Noordhoff, M. S.: Ten digit replantation. Plast. Reconstr. Surg., *74*:826, 1984.

Weiland, A. J., Robinson, H., and Futrell, J.: External stabilization of a replanted upper extremity. J. Trauma, *16*:239, 1976.

Weiland, A. J., Villarreal-Rios, A., Kleinert, H. E., Kutz, J., Atasoy, E., and Lister, G.: Replantation of digits and hands: analysis of surgical techniques and functional results in 71 patients with 86 replantations. J. Trauma, *2*:1, 1977.

Weiland, A. J., Villarreal-Rios, A., Kleinert, H. E., Kutz, J., Atasoy, E., and Lister, G.: Replantation of digits and hands: analysis of surgical techniques and func-

tional results in 71 patients with 86 replantations. Clin. Orthop., *133*:195, 1978.

Wild, J. J., Jr., Hanson, G. W., Bennett, J. B., and Tullow, H. S.: External fixation use in the management of massive upper extremity trauma. Clin. Orthop., *164*:172, 1982.

Williams, G. R.: Replantation of amputated extremities. Monogr. Surg. Sci., *3*:53, 1966.

Wilson, C. S., Alpert, B. S., Buncke, H. J., and Gordon, L.: Replantation of the upper extremity. Clin. Plast. Surg., *10*:85, 1983.

Wilson, G. R., and Jones, B. M.: The damaging effect of smoking on digital revascularization: two further case reports. Br. J. Plast. Surg., *37*:613, 1984.

Wood, M. B., and Cooney, W. P.: Above elbow limb replantation; functional results. J. Hand Surg. (Am.), *11*:682, 1986.

Wray, R. C., Young, V. L., and Weeks, P. M.: Flexible implant arthroplasty and finger replantation. Plast. Reconstr. Surg., *74*:97, 1984.

Yamano, Y.: Replantation of the amputated distal part of the fingers. J. Hand Surg. (Am.), *10*:211, 1985.

Yamano, Y., Matsuda, H., Nakashima, K., and Shimazu, A.: Some methods for bone fixation for digital replantation. Hand, *14*:135, 1982.

Yamano, Y., Namba, Y., Hino, Y., Hasegawa, T., Ugawa, A., and Ise, M.: Digital nerve grafts in replanted digits. Hand, *14*:255, 1982.

Yamauchi, S., Nomura, S., Yoshimura, M., Veno, T., Iwai, Y., and Shimamura, K.: Recovery of sensation in replanted digits—time of recovery and degree of two point discrimination. J. Microsurg., *3*:206, 1982.

Yamauchi, S., Nomura, S., Yoshimura, M., Veno, T., Iwai, Y., and Shimamura, K.: A clinical study of the order and speed of sensory recovery after digital replantation. J. Hand Surg., *8*:545, 1983.

Yoshimura, M., Nomura, S., Ueno, T., Yamauchi, S., and Shimamura, K.: Clinical replantation of digits and its problem. Ann. Acad. Med. Singapore, *11*:218, 1982a.

Yoshimura, M., Nomura, S., Ueno, T., Yamauchi, S., Iwai, Y., and Shimamura, K.: Evaluation of digital replantation. Acta Chir. Belg., *82*:161, 1982b.

Yoshizu, T., Katsumi, M., and Tajima, T.: Replantation of untidily amputated fingers, hands, and arms: experience of 99 replantations in 66 cases. J. Trauma, *18*:194, 1978.

Zdeblick, T. A., Shaffer, J. W., and Field, G. A.: An ischemia-induced model of revascularization failure of replanted limbs. J. Hand Surg. (Am.), *10*:125, 1985.

Robert W. Beasley

Upper Limb Prostheses

Despite impressive advances in reparative surgery of the hand, management of amputees remains an important area of responsibility. The generally negative aura that surrounds amputations negates due concern. It favors quick dispositions, whereas amputation should be given the same concern as any reconstructive procedure. The parts should be left in the most pain-free and useful condition and the operation undertaken with the same thoughtful planning and skills as any other hand procedure. Early surgical decisions and treatments often are irreversible. The surgeon bears prime responsibility for management and he determines to a great extent the ultimate degree of physical, social, and vocational reintegration a patient achieves. Thoughtful and realistic consideration must

be given to both the physical impairment and the psychologic impact of the loss for each individual.

Brown (1981) emphasized that logical conclusions can be made only after comparison of all alternatives. The surgeon dealing with amputations, therefore, must be thoroughly knowledgeable not only of the possible reconstructive procedures available for an amputee but also of the prosthetic potentials and requirements for the fitting. No longer is it acceptable for the surgeon to "go as far as he can" and then refer the patient for prosthetic fitting in the hope that he may be helped. The two disciplines must be integrated in the interest of optimal care. The surgeon is charged with recommending the best route to the best recovery in the least time. A realistic and definitive plan made at an early stage is best and for many amputees this will include prosthetic fitting. If this is not appreciated from the beginning, the surgeon may perform well-intended but ill-advised procedures that seriously delay or compromise the amputee's ultimate degree of recovery (Fig. 94–1). Contrary to this, with a thorough knowledge of prosthetics, the surgeon will include them when appropriate in his master plan and leave the parts in good condition for prompt fitting.

Time is important. Mistakes and unrealistic undertakings are costly, they submit the patient to needless risks and discomforts, and they have a profoundly adverse effect on the prognosis. It is a constant observation with all hand injuries that there is an inverse relation between the duration of treatment and the ultimate degree of recovery achieved (Beasley, 1981). Therefore, the early determination of the best definitive plan is of great importance. It is a responsibility the surgeon

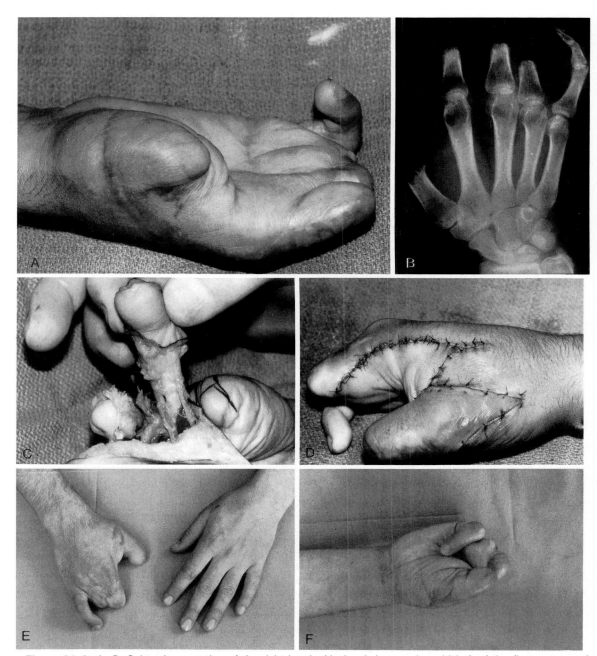

Figure 94–6. *A, B,* Subtotal amputation of the right hand with thumb loss at the midshaft of the first metacarpal illustrates optimal improvement resulting from a plan that combined realistic surgical reconstruction with prosthetic fitting. *C,* Isolation of the useful proximal phalanx of the index finger on intact neurovascular pedicles. *D,* Thumb lengthened to a very functional level by transfer of the remnant of index finger to the first metacarpal midshaft by one-stage neurovascular pedicle technique. *E, F,* The almost useless multilate hand has recovered excellent capability, even enabling the patient to remain right dominant.

Illustration continued on following page

Active prostheses have various moving mechanical parts incorporated in them, whereas passive prostheses intentionally do not. The prime purpose of the active prosthesis is to improve prehensile capability, yet there is no active mechanical device that can begin to compete with the improvement in prehension that will result from fitting a partially amputated hand with an appropriate passive prosthesis (Fig. 94–7). Thus, the common

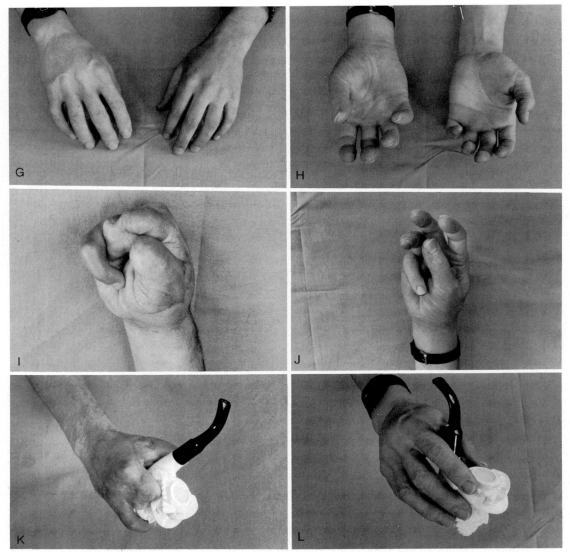

Figure 94–6 *Continued G, H,* Custom partial hand prosthesis alongside the uninjured left hand. *I, J,* Demonstration that none of the hand capabilities resulting from the reconstruction are impaired by the prosthesis. *K, L,* Hand capability demonstrated with and without the prosthesis. *L* illustrates the great esthetic edge that the prosthesis holds over even this excellent reconstruction.

practice of using the term "functional" interchangeably with "active" in describing prostheses is incorrect. It wrongly implies that only active prostheses are functional and all other prostheses are nonfunctional. All types of prostheses are functional if they prove to fulfill some definite need (none fill all needs). Some patients may even benefit from more than one type of prosthesis to meet different requirements at different times, such as one for their work and another for socialization.

Prostheses meet rather specific and limited objectives. None begin to replace the incredible scope of capabilities of a hand. Therefore, just as the term "functional" should be dropped from use, so should the term "artificial hand" also be discarded. There is substantial overlapping, but in general the active devices are principally directed toward trying to improve mechanical prehension. Passive prostheses give high priority to restoring appearance but they also improve capability for many amputees, especially with digital and

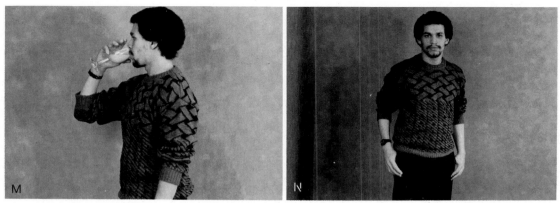

Figure 94–6 *Continued* *M,* The patient comfortably takes drink from a wine glass in the expected manner. *N,* Normal presentation. (Courtesy of American Hand Prosthetics, Inc., New York, NY.)

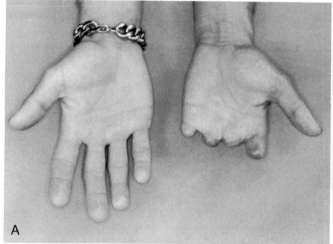

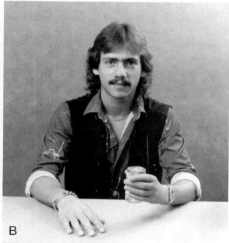

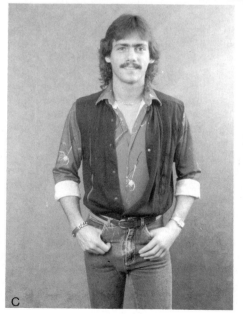

Figure 94–7. *A,* Subtotal left hand amputation. *B,* A passive partial hand prosthesis restores excellent prehension, far better than any active prosthesis. It is incorrect to speak of only active prostheses as "functional." *C,* In addition to greatly improving prehension, the partial hand prosthesis restores normal social presentation. (Courtesy of American Hand Prosthetics, Inc., New York, NY.)

partial hand losses. The relative importance of each of these objectives to the individual patient must be accurately determined by the physician in deciding which type of prosthesis should be fitted, if indeed any.

Active Upper Limb Prostheses

An active prosthesis is a mechanical device designed to improve simple prehension for very specific tasks. It is no more than a vise. It is capable of closing to hold objects put into it, but without the sensibility necessary for automatic control, there is absolutely no potential for precision manipulations. The active prosthesis is a tool that extends the remaining part for specific and limited jobs. It is like a hammer extending the normal hand for the task of driving in a nail. A person would never think of doing this with the butt of the hand; instead he extends the hand with a wooden stick on the end of which there is a heavy steel piece whose characteristics have been worked out to be best for effective nail driving. Such is the basic nature of active or carrier-tool prostheses.

Obviously, the more distal the amputation, the more natural parts remain and the better will be the results of prosthetic fitting. There is a tremendous difference between the benefits of fitting a patient who has a below elbow loss and the results for one who has an upper arm amputation. Few unilateral upper arm amputees today continue trying to use an active prosthesis for which control of an elbow hinge is required in addition to the terminal vise. It is just too complicated and laborious. Most jobs are done by the normal hand automatically before they can get even the first step of the complex prosthetic system into action.

Active prostheses should be divided into two basic categories according to the motive power used to move the articulating parts of the vise mechanism: (1) body powered and (2) externally powered.

BODY POWERED ACTIVE PROSTHESES

There are several possibilities for using body or arm muscles to provide power for operation of an active prosthetic device: (1) the pull of thoracic and shoulder movements transmitted through a cable attachment to the prosthesis, (2) active wrist movements powering the prosthesis like tenodesis mech-

anisms, and (3) cineplastic attachment directly to a muscle.

An important advantage of body powered prosthetic systems is that they provide some sensory feedback, an essential for any degree of automatic control. Simpson (1971) coined the term "extended physiologic proprioception" and attributed much importance to it. He observed that a person quickly develops good control over the trajectories of such items as a golf club or hammer extending the normal hand. He concluded that after loss of a hand the extension of the remaining natural parts with a securely fitting device allows use of this same ability and thus gives useful sensory feedback to aid nonvisual control for prosthetic positioning. This is in fact observed to occur with body powered prostheses. However, such crude position sense is limited to spatial relations and there is little or no information about the performance of the terminal device after it is positioned. No externally powered system has any degree of this indirect positioning sense of body powered units, which Baumgartner (1981) also emphasized to be very important.

Shoulder Cable Powered Active Prostheses. By far the most commonly encountered active, body powered upper limb prosthesis is that powered through a cable attached to a harness arrangement across to the opposite shoulder. The harness is basically the same today as when first introduced in the early part of the nineteenth century. It consists of two essential components: (1) a harness for secure suspension of the prosthesis and (2) the attachment of a cable in such a manner that when the shoulders are shrugged apart, the cable is pulled. There is active pull in only one direction.

As with tendon transfer operations, a basic design concept is that effective transfer of mechanical power to a terminal location requires that every joint across which the power is transmitted must be controlled: otherwise, the system simply buckles and the power is dissipated. Thus, with an arm prosthesis powered by a cable with pull from the opposite shoulder, control of the elbow joint (or hinge) across which the cable passes is essential. When elbow control has to be provided because of above elbow amputation, the complexity of the system is greatly increased. With a single source of power, power is available for only one function at a time. This can be either the elbow or the prehensile terminal device. There has to be a locking mechanism at the elbow level that can be engaged at various angles to stabilize it and free the cable power for the terminal vise unit. Another control problem arises if the patient is grasping when he wishes to change the elbow angle. To do this with the single power source, it is necessary to release the grasping with the terminal device in order to make available the cable power to release the elbow locking mechanism. For many unilateral above elbow amputees the benefit does not justify the trouble and work involved. Below elbow amputees, who do not require an elbow mechanism, benefit much more.

Primarily active systems often incorporate one or more passive units. The most common example is a friction stabilized wrist rotation joint that allows the terminal device to be pre-positioned advantageously before it is used. This again illustrates how incorrect it is to assign the term "functional" only to active prosthetic devices.

The enormous variety of prosthetic terminal devices available further attests to the fact that active prostheses must be looked on simply as tools for rather specific tasks and in no sense comparable with a hand. The list of terminal devices is almost limitless, each relatively effective for very specific jobs and none effective for all. Thus far there has been little success in developing relatively effective active terminal devices whose appearance approaches social acceptability for most people.

The terminal devices of basically split-hook design have proved the most useful in general, especially for heavy work (Fig. 94–8). Their slender configuration facilitates positioning, which has to be guided by the eye, even about small objects. The simple design makes them reliable and resistant to wear and tear. They are inexpensive and silent in operation.

Controversy continues over whether a voluntary opening or a voluntary closing terminal device is best. Both are available and obviously the answer lies in which each patient finds to be most useful for his individual needs. At a glance one would expect the voluntary closing prosthesis to be more normal and useful, since a person does not relax his muscles to grasp as with a voluntary opening prosthesis. This is physiologically incorrect, but most users find that it serves them best. They open the split hook with a shrug of the opposite shoulder, pulling against elastic bands holding the prosthesis closed. As they release the shoulder tension, the hook is closed by the elastic bands that have been stretched in opening it. Thus, sustained grasping with the "vise" is maintained without continuous muscle contractions, energy being required only briefly for the opening and controlled closing of the hook. Experience has shown that relatively small elastic-band closing power is needed. For the unilateral amputee the elastic bands are usually built up to give a closing force of only about 3 or 4 lbs. Complex clutch and locking mechanisms have been tried with voluntary closing systems, giving them sustained grasping without continuous muscle contraction. Their apparently only small benefit for most patients does not seem to justify the cost and complexity and has prevented their widespread use. The vast majority of unilateral upper limb amputees using a split-hook, body powered prosthesis prefer the mechanically simple voluntary opening system.

Wrist Powered Active Prostheses. For the infrequently encountered patient who has a distal carpal or proximal transmetacarpal amputation with preservation of a normal wrist, a custom active prosthesis can be developed that uses wrist movements to open and close prosthetic digits. The device is essentially like the common tenodesis splint used by patients with high spinal cord injuries. According to Law (1981), most patients prefer to have the fingers close with wrist flexion, again a nonphysiologic action that one would not anticipate. The reason is that positioning is easier for table surface pickups than if the fingers close with wrist dorsiflexion.

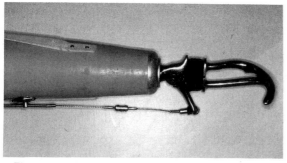

Figure 94–8. A split-hook active prosthesis is designed for heavy work and is body powered by a cable attached to a shoulder harness. This gives it a crude spatial position sense that is an advantage over all externally powered prostheses. Also, the split-hook terminal device is easiest to position by visual guidance. (Courtesy of American Hand Prosthetics, Inc., New York, NY.)

Common to all active prostheses in the form of a hand is the question of which is the most useful prehensile pattern (if only one can be provided, as is the usual case). Again, the specific needs of each patient must be considered, for they are often different even though physical losses are similar. However, it should be remembered that the prosthesis is never more than a minor assisting device to the other normal hand. Thus, a pulp to pulp flat contact between thumb and the index–middle finger unit is usually best. This provides stable grip for papers and moderately small objects as well as palmar grasp around cylindric objects of considerable diameter.

Cineplastic Powered Active Prostheses. Just after World War I, Sauerbruch in Germany introduced the direct attachment of an active prosthesis to the biceps muscle to power it. He detached the biceps tendon distally, rammed a tunnel through the big muscle, and passed a medially based, tubed skin flap through this. Only the biceps had enough amplitude to survive this damage with adequate power and amplitude remaining, and efforts to use smaller forearm muscles failed. An ivory peg was passed through the skin-lined tunnel through the muscle, and a cable was attached to transmit power to the prosthesis. This attractive idea was used for only a short time, primarily because of problems with the dennervated skin tubes through the muscle.

EXTERNALLY POWERED UPPER LIMB PROSTHESES

There are a number of considerations in selecting a power system for prostheses. One is the amount of energy available, and equally important is the rate at which the energy can be delivered. It must be readily available, and as a practical matter there must be a high ratio of energy available to the weight and volume of the storage containers. Two systems for externally powered prostheses have been used, electric and gas.

Gas systems are attractive as they can deliver energy at a very high rate if gases of a low critical temperature which do not liquefy under pressure are used. Another desirable feature is the light weight and versatility of the pneumatic motors, with easily variable rates of action resulting in more normal motions, in contrast to electric motors. The problem with gas systems lies in the storage of high energy "permanent" gases required for these advantages. Safe containers for this hazardous material are too heavy to be portable. If condensable gases that are liquid under pressure are used, the rate of energy delivery is low, varying greatly with temperature, so they cannot be used directly from a container but must be run through a regulator, sustaining a great energy loss. Also, energy lost in exhausts is not easily recaptured. Practical solutions to these problems do not exist so there are today almost no pneumatic powered prostheses.

The development of extremely efficient electric storage cells and the ready availability of electricity for recharging the cells has led to the use of electric motors as the power system for almost all externally powered upper limb prostheses. As indicated, the chief problem with electric motors is the very low rate at which they can deliver energy.

Some efforts have been made to develop a hybrid system using electric power to drive a hydraulic pump, the mechanism of which forces fluid, in turn compressing a gas from which it is separated by a rubber diaphragm, the liquid thus acting as an energy reservoir. The energy can be added over a long period at the motor's slow rate, but drawn off at the high rate characterizing the pneumatic systems. Although attractive, the systems are little used because of their complexity, the dangers of the fluids under such high pressures, and the fact that leaks develop as the prosthesis is used.

Control Problem of Externally Powered Prostheses. The factor limiting the development of truly effective active prostheses is the problem of control. All are "blind" in that they do not have any sensory feedback, which is essential to automatic control. Even an apparently simple task such as taking a sip of water from a glass is an extremely complex operation. Our brain sends out commands to muscles that through experience it has observed perform the desired action. As the muscle or functional muscle group comes into action, there is normally an instantaneous feedback of information, indicating the degree of the desired action that has been accomplished. In turn, the brain processes this information in relation to its desired accomplishment, and issues further commands to each muscle or group involved to continue its action, accelerate it, retard it, and so forth. With even the simplest activity many muscle groups are involved simultaneously in this complex trial and er-

surgically corrected. The use of glue or efforts to suspend the prosthesis from rings on adjacent fingers is not satisfactory. In the case of multiple finger amputations, it is better to fit each finger with its own prosthesis to maintain maximal independent motion. However, if even one of the finger amputations is too short for independent fitting, the much less desirable glove over the hand will be required for fixation (Fig. 94–15).

The finger to be fitted should be nicely tapered, with good soft tissue coverage but no skin redundancy. Ideally it should be smaller than the corresponding finger on the other hand, which is the case if one or both of the flexor tendons are missing. If the finger to be fitted is the same size as that of the other hand, the prosthesis covering it will have to be slightly larger than the normal one. It must have minimal neuroma symptoms and must be well healed. Before the fitting it must be free of edema and have reached a constant size; wrapping with elastic tape facilitates this.

The exception to the recommendation that condyles be tapered is when a distal interphalangeal disarticulation is being fitted with a "mini" digital prosthesis. The "mini" prosthesis has its proximal limit immediately distal to the proximal interphalangeal joint, so there is absolutely no restriction of this joint which contributes greatly to the digital flexion arc. If the flare of the condyles at the distal end of the middle phalanx is reduced greatly, secure fixation of the short prosthesis may not be possible.

It is not possible to have a finger of good appearance without a fingernail, a loss for which a satisfactory surgical solution does not exist. A "sub-mini" prosthesis, so short as to cover only the distal phalanx for fixation but with a perfectly duplicated fingernail, can be useful for some patients.

The thumb is a special digit, obviously of greater importance than any finger. From a prosthetic point of view, it differs from the fingers chiefly in requiring especially secure fixation and in the difficulty of making the proximal limit of the prosthesis inconspicuous. It is difficult to generalize on the exact length of the thumb that can be fitted with an independent prosthesis, as it depends on the soft tissues of the area, the shape of the remaining part of the proximal phalanx, the opposing forces to which it will be subjected, and many subtle but critical factors. The color difference in a finger from the constantly changing color of the normal skin can in most instances be disguised by wearing a ring, especially for females. This advantage is lost for the thumb, as with the index and middle fingers of males. For these the proximal end of the prosthesis is made thin and is not pigmented. With good motion and free use of the part, the color differences are not noticed in casual contacts, but a common Band-Aid or strip of skin-toned surgical tape can be worn across the juncture if desired.

When thumb amputation is through the middle of the proximal phalanx, prosthetic fitting is very secure. When the loss is proximal to this level, independent digital pros-

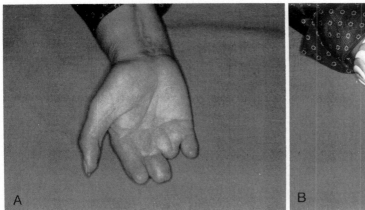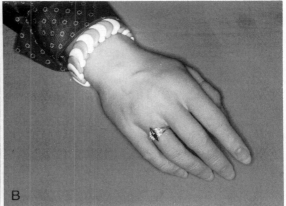

Figure 94–15. *A,* With multiple finger amputations it is best to fit each with a prosthesis for maximal independence. However, if even one of the fingers is too short for fitting, a glove over the hand must be used for fixation. *B,* Fingers of the passive prosthesis provide opposing parts for the thumb, but the glove is required because the one short finger imposes some restriction on movements. (Courtesy of American Hand Prosthetics, Inc., New York, NY.)

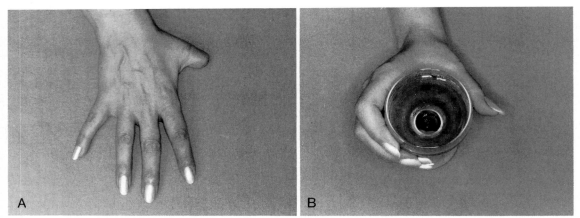

Figure 94–16. *A,* Thumb amputation through the middle of its proximal phalanx permits very satisfactory prosthetic fitting. *B,* The thumb prosthesis contributes to the normal handling of objects. (Courtesy of American Hand Prosthetics, Inc., New York, NY.)

thetic fitting is increasingly difficult or impossible (Fig. 94–16). In some cases a glove on the hand may be used for fixation, but this is less than satisfactory (Fig. 94–17). For such situations, surgical lengthening of the thumb, with or without a planned conjunction with a prosthetic fitting, should be considered. The exact method obviously depends on many individual considerations, but the requirements for prosthetic fitting should be included in the planning. Use of a great toe precludes this option, which the patient may desire after seeing the surgical results. For lengthening by toe transfer, the second toe is pre-

ferred. Osteoplastic thumb lengthening with a prosthetic fitting or the wrap-around toe flap offers the best solution for many patients.

PARTIAL HAND PROSTHESES

Again, only a passive prosthesis can be fitted for the partial hand amputation, with the exception of the rare proximal transmetacarpal amputation for which a complex, wrist driven active device might be considered for special needs. Strictly speaking, this term should include even single digit amputations, but it is generally used to indicate

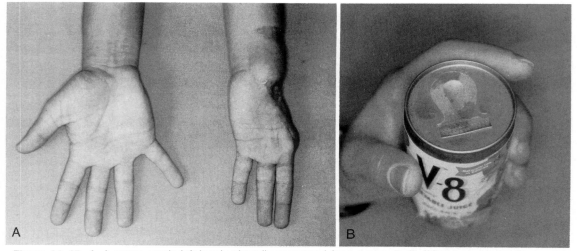

Figure 94–17. *A,* A young man's left hand subtotally amputated for a tumor. *B,* The thumb and index finger of the prosthesis are made with passively adjustable armatures. The normal middle, ring, and small fingers are brought through the prosthesis so that their normal movements and skin sensibility are not impaired. (Courtesy of American Hand Prosthetics, Inc., New York, NY.)

major losses requiring a hand glove, as individual finger fitting is not possible. The amputations can be basically *transverse* (the thumb may be spared or included), *central* (the marginal digits may be spared), or *oblique* in either direction. Obviously the possible combinations are almost unlimited.

The objective of the partial hand prosthesis is to provide prosthetically the missing parts against which remaining natural parts can work while avoiding any restriction of the capabilities of the latter in the process. With finger amputations in which part of the palm has been lost, there may be sufficient room in the prosthesis for anchorage of adjustable armatures extending into the fingers of the prosthesis to improve further physical capabilities. Fitting partial hand amputations constitutes the most difficult of all prosthetic challenges in both design and fabrication, but frequently these are also the most rewarding. Since the partial hand prosthesis is always in the basic form of a natural hand, good restoration of lifelike appearance is the second benefit that can be achieved.

When digits of good sensibility and useful motion have survived, they generally are brought through the prosthetic glove to be unrestricted in use. If a single digit remains but is so damaged as to be better covered

with the glove, it often is placed in the position of another finger of larger natural size (Fig. 94–18). For example, the surviving ring finger may be put into the middle finger of the prosthetic glove. This preserves the useful motion of the digit, but avoids having to make the prosthetic hand glove larger than the normal hand, as would be necessary to cover the finger if it were placed in its usual position. If the index finger has been amputated at the metacarpophalangeal joint level, resection of the second metacarpal facilitates such a shift and is helpful even if no digital shift is planned. However, if any of the proximal phalanx of the index finger exists, great judgment must be exercised for each patient in deciding whether to retain or delete the second metacarpal.

It is especially important for any surgeon treating severely mutilated hands to keep in mind the potentials of prosthetic fitting, as the optimal plan often is a combination of well-planned reconstructions and prosthetic fittings (see Fig. 94–6).

TOTAL PASSIVE HAND PROSTHESES

With complete hand loss, the passive prosthesis best meets the needs of many unilateral amputees, especially since it can be con-

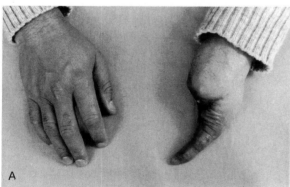

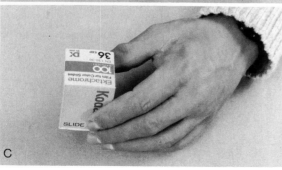

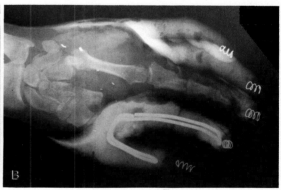

Figure 94–18. *A*, Only the small finger has survived a severe blast injury. *B*, Radiograph illustrates centralization of the small finger for better prehension and to permit use of a prosthetic glove equal in size to the normal hand. If the small finger were put into the corresponding position in the prosthesis, the prosthetic glove would have to be conspicuously larger than normal in order to fit over the finger. *C*, Useful prehension from the single finger in the partial hand prosthesis is illustrated. The prosthetic thumb can be passively positioned according to the size of the object to be held. (Courtesy of American Hand Prosthetics, Inc., New York, NY.)

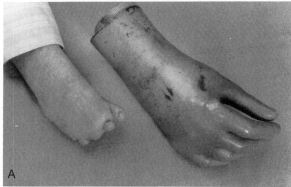

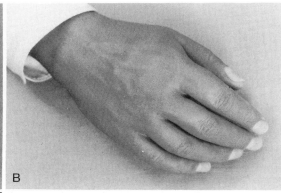

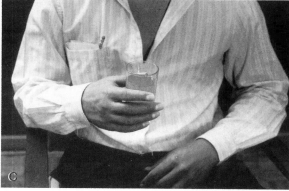

Figure 94–19. *A,* Congenital deformities of the right hand are shown along with a PVC prosthesis of unacceptable quality. It is esthetically more disturbing than the traditional black glove. *B,* A fine custom total hand prosthesis fitted with passively adjustable armatures to provide weak but useful holding capability. *C,* The resulting normal presentation avoids the hand being distracting during business and social life, the first priority of this patient. (Courtesy of American Hand Prosthetics, Inc., New York, NY.)

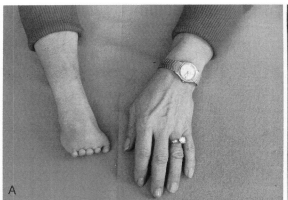

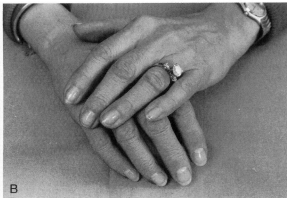

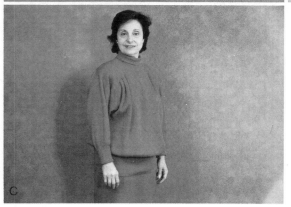

Figure 94–20. *A,* Agenesis at the carpal level. *B,* The wrist is advanced into the midpalm of the prosthesis for a more satisfactory fit and also for better physical assistance. *C,* The shortening of the arm caused by the advancement passes unnoticed and social presentation is essentially normal. (Courtesy of American Hand Prosthetics, Inc., New York, NY.)

structed to have a lifelike appearance. For holding light objects, armatures whose positions can be adjusted with the normal hand can be built into the prosthesis (Fig. 94–19). The holding power is small compared with active units, but it is useful. The armatures increase the weight of the prosthesis, but not excessively. An adult silicone total hand prosthesis weighs about 175 gm, and about 225 gm with armatures. Recognizing that a normal adult human hand weighs about 450 gm, this is not much, and most patients have no complaint about this small increase in weight.

The literature is replete with warnings against wrist disarticulations, stating that prosthetic fitting requires a split socket that can expand to pass over the condyle of the radius. The concept of elective sites of amputation, of which the old teaching was a part, has given way in general to preserving all length consistent with good soft tissue wound closure. This change is possible because of the development of soft and expandable silicone sockets and hand prostheses. With these, the condyle is even desirable as it contributes to good fixation with minimal coverage of the forearm. An exception to preserving maximal length is the case in which a myoelectric active prosthesis is to be fitted. For this, the forearm must be short enough to permit the prosthetic socket to contain a battery pack without the arm being too long. In cases of transcarpal amputation, the end may be advanced to fit in the prosthetic palm where it will contribute more to physical abilities (Fig. 94–20). A few centimeters of difference in arm length is not noticed and well justified by the advantage gained. When amputation is no more than about 5 cm proximal to the wrist, it often is best to fit the prosthesis on this, accepting the shortening as a trade-off against having to resort to a full forearm socket for fixation. When a forearm socket is used to attach the total hand, a passively adjustable rotation unit is used at the wrist level so that the direction the prosthesis faces can be changed according to whether the patient is sitting or walking.

PROSTHESES FOR MAJOR UPPER ARM AMPUTATIONS

When unilateral amputation is proximal to the elbow, few amputees gain enough from active prostheses to justify their disadvan-tages, as has been discussed. Most of these patients prefer to have passive, lightweight units primarily to restore good appearance (Fig. 94–21).

The new semiflexible silicone sockets can give secure suspension from the arm without straps if as little as 10 cm of arm distal to the axillary fold exist. In cases of shorter length, a shoulder cap must be used for suspension, but this too can be constructed of soft, flexible, nylon reinforced silicone. Unlike traditional fiberglass caps, it is light and comfortable and has a pleasant, tissue-like feeling to the touch. The latter is especially appreciated for social contacts such as dancing (Fig. 94–22).

SUMMARY

The success of treatment cannot be measured in terms of prehensile capability. It must be measured in terms of how well a patient achieves socioeconomic integration to be an independent, emotionally adjusted, and productive citizen.

The hand surgeon of today must be thoroughly knowledgeable about prosthetics, since optimal care requires their consideration in early comprehensive planning for many patients. Prostheses should be classified simply as active or passive. All are functional, but different ones meet different needs. Traditional teaching has contended that only active prostheses are important and of benefit to many patients. Today the absolute reverse of this is true. If we consider the frequency of partial hand and digital amputations as compared with total hand amputations and the rapid shifting of the work force from labor to service industries, it becomes evident that passive prostheses best meet the needs of the greater number of amputees today.

Prosthetic fitting will be a failure for the patient who is unrealistically expecting a true replacement of the lost parts. They are gone and gone forever.

The key to successful treatment lies in recognition that a prosthesis, and in fact major reconstructions, can meet only limited and specific objectives. There is no such thing as an artificial hand. The goal of active prostheses and many reconstructions is to restore a pinch mechanism with little regard for the esthetic result. Passive total hand prostheses cannot provide strong holding

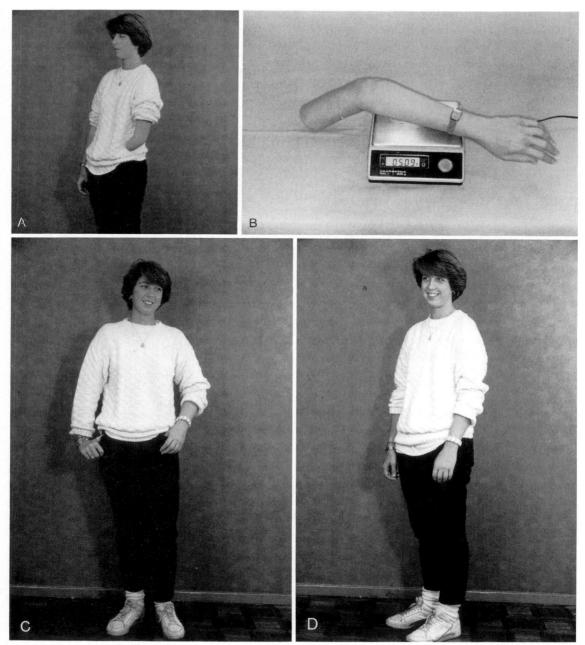

Figure 94–21. *A,* This adolescent had become extremely concerned about her disfigurement. Typically among patients with unilateral agenesis, she felt no physical impairment. *B,* New semiflexible silicone-nylon forearm socket is light in weight, tissue-like soft on contract, and absolutely secure without straps. The socket and the total hand prosthesis weighed only 509 gm (17 oz). *C, D,* Comfortable presentation with the lifelike passive prosthesis. (Courtesy of American Hand Prosthetics, Inc., New York, NY.)

power, but the trade-off is that they can be constructed to restore essentially lifelike appearance; in the case of partial hand and digital amputations they not only accomplish this but also often give dramatic improvement in physical capability.

The physician, often in conjunction with the hand therapist, must determine accurately the needs of each patient in order of priority. For the vast majority of upper limb amputees today, mechanically simple assisting devices of socially acceptable appearance

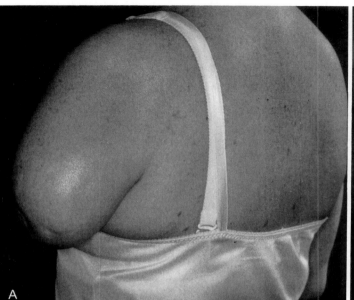

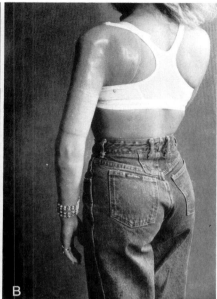

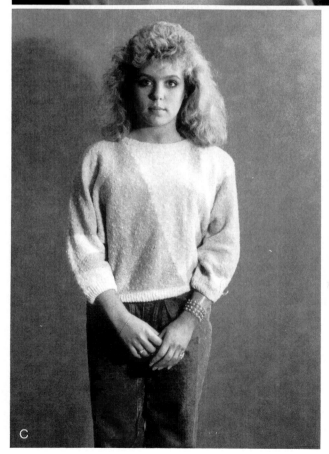

Figure 94–22. *A,* Arm amputations less than 10 cm distal to the axillary fold cannot be fitted with a socket, and a shoulder cap is required for secure suspension of the prosthesis. If the length is more than 10 cm beyond the fold, a socket without any straps is usually satisfactory. *B,* Rather than the traditional hard fiberglass shoulder cap with its heavy strap attachments, this patient wears a soft, pliable silicone-nylon cap that is secure with only a button to her bra. This arrangement is a great improvement for social contacts such as dancing and for comfort. *C,* The fine, passive hand prosthesis with a flexible hinge at the elbow level best meets the primary needs of this unilaterally amputated young woman. Unilateral, above elbow amputees almost never find lasting satisfaction from the active prostheses currently available. (Courtesy of American Hand Prosthetics, Inc., New York, NY.)

best meet their greatest needs. The lifelike appearance of passive prostheses prevents losses being distracting in business and casual social encounters. In a sense these prostheses are for the other people . . . not the patient.

To be satisfactory, prostheses must be thoughtfully prescribed to meet specific objectives, fabricated to the highest standards, and backed by prompt and efficient maintenance services. As with any mechanical device, the need for repairs from time to time is inevitable.

Acknowledgement: The author would like to acknowledge the valued assistance of Genevieve M. de Bese in the composition of this chapter.

REFERENCES

Aitken, G. T.: The child amputee, an overview. Orthop. Clin. North Am., 3:449, 1972.

Battye, C. K., Nightingale, A., and Whillis, J.: Use of myo-electric currents in the operation of prostheses. J. Bone Joint Surg., 37B:506, 1955.

Baumgartner, R.: Active and carrier-tool prostheses for upper limb amputations. Orthop. Clin. North Am., 12:955, 1981.

Beasley, R. W.: Reconstructive surgery in the management of congenital anomalies of the upper extremities. In Swingard, C. A. (Ed.): Limb Development and Deformity. Springfield, IL, Charles C Thomas, 1969, p. 476.

Beasley, R. W.: Hand Injuries. Philadelphia, W. B. Saunders Company, 1981, p. 6.

Beasley, R. W.: Cosmetic considerations in surgery of the hand. In Tubiana, R. (Ed.): The Hand. Vol. 2. Philadelphia, W. B. Saunders Company, 1985, pp. 96–103.

Beasley, R. W., and de Bese, G. M.: Upper limb amputations and prostheses. Orthop. Clin. North Am., 17:395, 1986.

Brown, P. W.: The rational selection of treatment for upper extremity amputations. Orthop. Clin. North Am., 12:843, 1981.

Goffman, E.: Stigma. Englewood Cliffs, NJ, Prentice-Hall, 1963, p. 7.

Kobrinski, A. E., et al.: Problems of bio-electric control in automatic and remote control. Proceedings of First International Congress of the International Federation of Automatic Control, Moscow, 1960. Vol. 2. London, Butterworth, 1961, p. 619.

Law, H. T.: Engineering of upper limb prostheses. Orthop. Clin. North Am., 12:929, 1981.

Modlin, H.: The post-accident anxiety syndrome: psychosocial aspects. Am. J. Psychiatry, 123:1008, 1967.

Sauter, W. F.: Prostheses for the child amputee. Orthop. Clin. North Am., 3:483, 1972.

Simpson, D. C.: The choice of control systems for multimovement prostheses. Extended physiologic proprioception. Proceedings of the International Symposium on the Control of Upper Extremity Prostheses and Orthoses, Goteborg, Sweden, 1971.

Harry J. Buncke

Thumb and Finger Reconstruction by Microvascular Second Toe and Joint Autotransplantation

In the entire body the second toe is the most expendable source of microvascular digit tissue for hand reconstruction. The donor area can be closed without a functional or cosmetic defect (Figs. 95–1 to 95–5). The principal disadvantage of the second toe is that it is short and narrow and not a good transfer for total finger reconstruction. With or without its proximal structures the second toe can be used to reconstruct the thumb (Figs. 95–6 to 95–8), portions of a single digit (Figs. 95–9, 95–10), multiple digits (Figs. 95–2 to 95–4, 95–8, 95–11 to 95–13), sensory island flaps, interphalangeal joints (Fig. 95–

10), metacarpophalangeal joints (Fig. 95–5), and the temporomandibular joint. The second metatarsal and the phalanges can be fashioned into an articulated vascularized bone graft carrying the overlying dorsalis pedis flap and the superficial peroneal nerve for sensory restoration. The short extensors with their motor nerve from the anterior tibial nerve can be added to create a dynamic vascularized myo-osteocutaneous autotransplant.

HISTORY

The history of second toe autotransplant for thumb or finger reconstruction began in 1898 when Nicoladoni, an Italian surgeon, first successfully transferred in multiple stages the second toe to replace a portion of the thumb (May and associates, 1978). Davis (1964) from Brazil modified the operation by rerouting the dorsalis pedis artery to a subcutaneous position, using macrovascular techniques. Clarkson (1962) reported several cases in which Nicoladoni's original technique was used. Immediate toe autotransplantation by means of microvascular techniques was accomplished on an experimental basis in the rhesus monkey in 1965 (Buncke, Buncke, and Schulz, 1966). Cobbett (1969) reported the first successful human toe to hand autotransplant in the western world. Although it is difficult to document in the

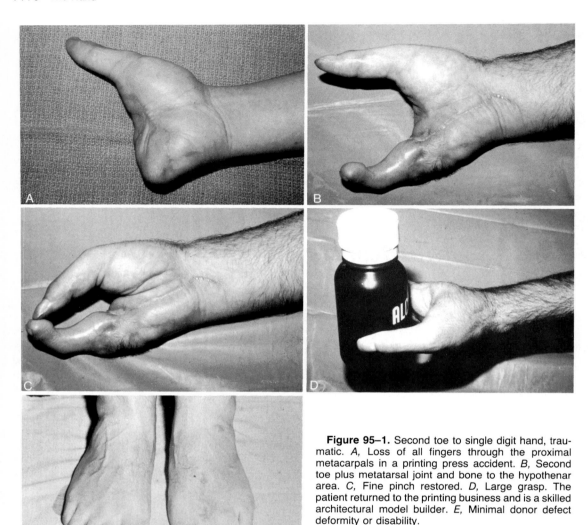

Figure 95–1. Second toe to single digit hand, traumatic. *A,* Loss of all fingers through the proximal metacarpals in a printing press accident. *B,* Second toe plus metatarsal joint and bone to the hypothenar area. *C,* Fine pinch restored. *D,* Large grasp. The patient returned to the printing business and is a skilled architectural model builder. *E,* Minimal donor defect deformity or disability.

world medical literature, surgeons at the First Medical College in Shanghai (First Teaching Hospital, 1973) successfully autotransplanted the second toe to reconstruct thumbs in five workers in 1966.

INDICATIONS FOR SECOND TOE AUTOTRANSPLANTATION

One to four digits on one or both hands can be restored utilizing the second toe from one or both feet (see Figs 95–2 to 95–4, 95–8, 95–9, 95–11 to 95–13), the second toe from one foot and two adjacent toes from the opposite foot (see Fig. 95–3), or two adjacent toes from

both (Holle and associates, 1982; Lichtman and associates, 1982; Wang, 1983; Gordon and associates, 1985). Loss of a single toe from one foot produces no functional defect; however, loss of two adjacent toes appreciably narrows the foot and compromises function (see Fig. 95–3). Single or multiple toe autotransplantation can be considered in congenital autoamputations of digits where all structures are present at the level of loss (Figs. 95–12, 95–14) (Gilbert, 1982). Toe autotransplantation is not indicated in congenital digital agenesis where proximal structures are not present. The second toe is particularly well suited to restoring the length of one or two digits amputated through

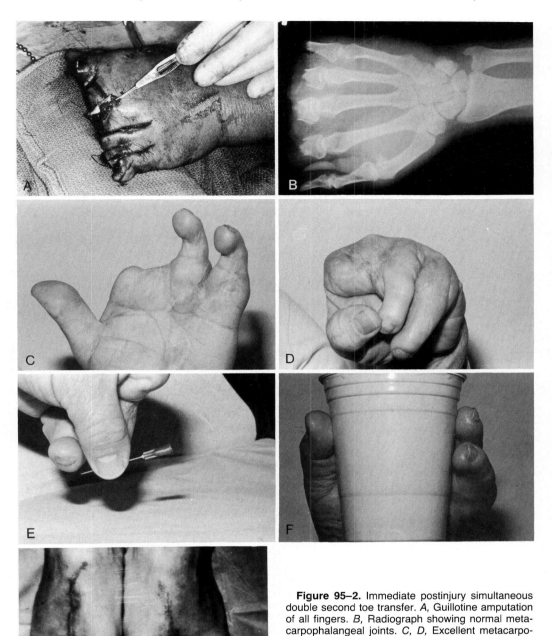

Figure 95–2. Immediate postinjury simultaneous double second toe transfer. *A,* Guillotine amputation of all fingers. *B,* Radiograph showing normal metacarpophalangeal joints. *C, D,* Excellent metacarpophalangeal function maintained by immediate reconstruction. *E,* Fine pulp to pulp pinch restored. *F,* Large grasp. The patient returned to work as a rigger in the oilfields. *G,* Donor defect at one month.

the middle phalanx (see Fig. 95–4). Unfortunately toes are considerably shorter than fingers and cannot therefore be used to rebuild full digital length, particularly when other normal fingers are present in the hand (Figs. 95–11, 95–15) (Rose and Buncke, 1980). Adequate tissue must be available in the recipient area if the entire toe is to be autotransplanted, since the proximal half of the proximal phalanx lies in the web space and is not covered by skin. This required cover can be provided in two operations with a

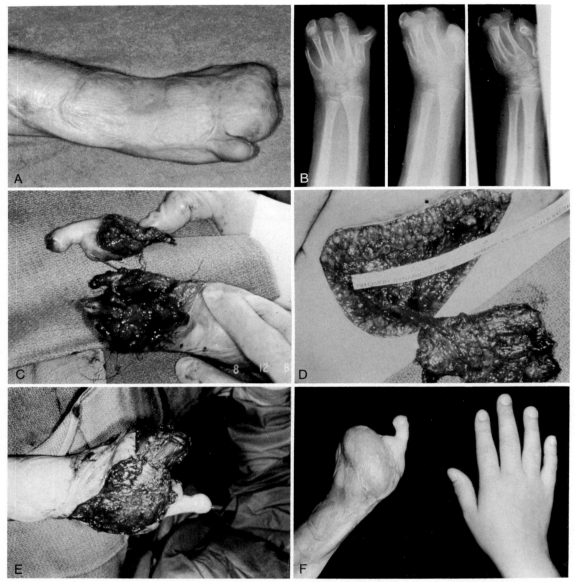

Figure 95–3. Triple toe and serratus muscle autotransplant to burned hand without digits. *A,* Preoperative condition. Nonfunctional mitten hand. *B,* Radiograph revealing the remnant of the proximal phalanx of the thumb. *C,* Scarred dorsal skin removed, the second toe next to the repositioned thumb proximal phalanx. *D,* Serratus muscle isolated. *E,* Serratus muscle wrapped around the base of the toe transfer and resurfacing the dorsum of the hand and metacarpal stumps. *F,* Early postoperative result of the first double auto-transplant—toe and muscle.

preliminary conventional groin flap, or in one operation as a double microvascular groin flap toe autotransplant (see Fig. 95–3) (Lister, Kalisman, and Tsao, 1983).

PREOPERATIVE EVALUATION

Single digit replacement is seldom a problem, but multiple digit replacement requires careful planning to restore maximal hand function. Three finger chuck pinch is the ultimate reconstructive goal on the radial side of the hand, while strong grip is the primary function of the digits on the ulnar side (see Figs. 95–1, 95–2, 95–11, 95–12). Preoperative arteriograms are needed when there has been extensive injury to the hand. The vascular anastomoses must be performed to normal vessels away from the zone of

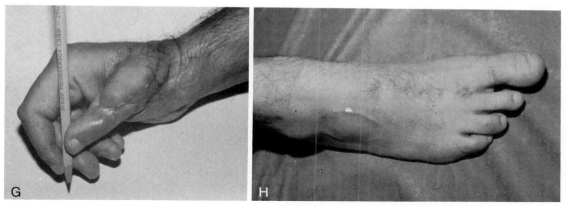

Figure 95–5 *Continued G,* Thumb stability and function restored. *H,* Minimal donor defect deformity or disability.

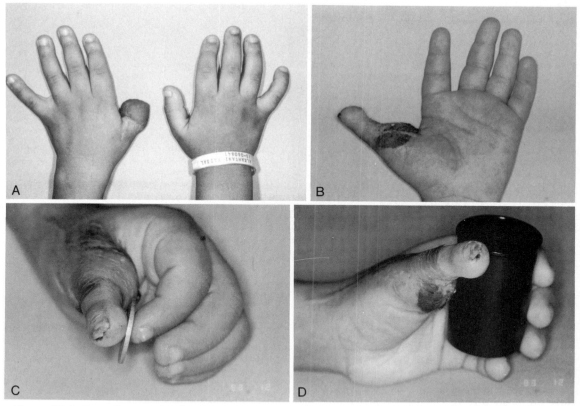

Figure 95–6. Second toe to thumb position—child, traumatic. *A,* Amputation of the thumb through the base of the proximal phalanx, partially salvaged with an abdominal tubed pedicle graft. *B,* Second toe in position. *C, D,* Pinch and grasp restored. Size discrepancy of the second toe is less apparent in children.

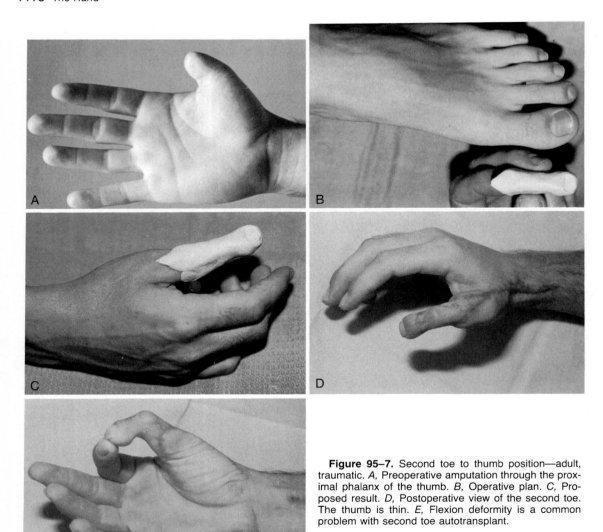

Figure 95–7. Second toe to thumb position—adult, traumatic. *A,* Preoperative amputation through the proximal phalanx of the thumb. *B,* Operative plan. *C,* Proposed result. *D,* Postoperative view of the second toe. The thumb is thin. *E,* Flexion deformity is a common problem with second toe autotransplant.

sal system, the penetrating or communicating branch at the base of the first metatarsal space should be mobilized for several centimeters to be used as a recipient vessel for the other toe autotransplant to its ulnar side (Sketch 95–2). In a similar fashion, a branch coming off the dorsal venous pedicle should be tied long so that it can be used as an internal shunt to drain the adjacent second toe.

The entire preoperative plan can be worked out on clay models of the digit or digits to be autotransplanted. One can visualize the syn-

ostoses, vascular pedicles, tendon, and nerve repairs, and flap orientation. The patient also has an opportunity to see the potential appearance and function of the autotransplanted digits (see Figs. 95–7, 95–12, 95–13).

OPERATIVE PLAN

Ideally, two operating teams work simultaneously, each with a full set of instruments. On occasion three teams are necessary for a double toe autotransplant, or for a toe auto-

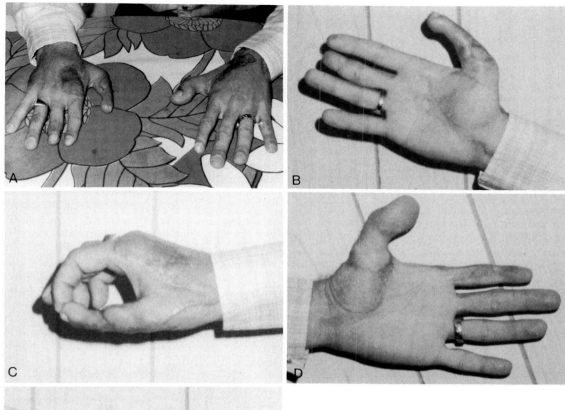

Figure 95–8. Double thumb reconstruction—two stage. *A*, Right thumb reconstruction with the second toe. Left thumb reconstruction with the large toe. *B, C,* The second toe is more slender than a normal thumb. *D, E,* The large toe, though somewhat large, is more "thumblike" in appearance.

Sketch 95–2. Internal vascular shunt for a double toe transfer to the ulnar side of the hand. *a,* The dorsal first metatarsal artery and dorsalis pedis arterial pedicle from the contralateral toe, now the ulnar digit is anastomosed to the proximal communicating branch of the ipsilateral toe, in the radial position. *b,* Dorsal first metatarsal artery of the ipsilateral toe. *c,* Dorsalis pedis artery of the ipsilateral toe anastomosed end to side. *d,* Dorsal radial artery in the anatomic snuffbox.

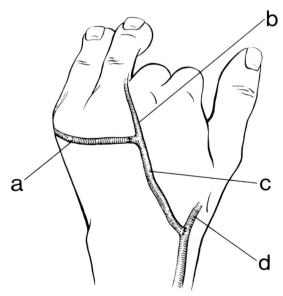

transplant combined with an additional microvascular flap or muscle to be used for proximal cover. Several extra hands are needed to prepare multiple operative and donor areas, and no member of the team should be above helping at this stage. Since the procedures are long, a heating pad helps to maintain patient body temperature. An eggcrate sponge rubber mattress helps to prevent pressure point problems during these long procedures. Pressure points should be checked repeatedly to prevent positional ischemia. All extremity dissections are performed under tourniquet control. Tourniquet time is monitored by the anesthesiologist, noted in the record, and reported to the operating team every 30 minutes. An indwelling urinary catheter is needed to prevent bladder distention and also to assist the anesthesiologist in evaluating fluid balance.

Hand Dissection

The preplanned flaps are marked and elevated in the hand, preserving the dorsal venous circulation. Branches from the dorsal radial sensory nerve are isolated to be later anastomosed to the branches of the deep and superficial peroneal systems in the foot. Each structure when isolated should be marked with a heavy silk tie. The dorsal radial artery with its venae comitantes is next isolated deep to the thumb long extensor, extensor brevis, and long abductor. The proximal bony juncture is then fashioned, preserving an articular surface if present, or tailoring the bone to receive a bone peg or side to side fixation. The digital nerves and their neuromas are then isolated on the palmar surface. They may have been avulsed in the primary injury back into the proximal palm, carpal canal, or distal wrist. When multiple digits are missing, the longest and most accessible digital nerves are used for the repair. In some instances, volar digital nerves cannot be found and sensation to the autotransplant must be provided through the dorsal radial system for the thumb and index, and the dorsal ulnar sensory nerve for ulnar digits. In high voltage electrical burns, long sural nerve grafts may be needed to reach healthy proximal recipient nerves in the forearm. The flexor tendons should be isolated so that repairs to the toe flexors can be performed in the palm or wrist away from the fibrocartilaginous tendon sheaths. It is preferable to repair only the long toe flexors, since post-

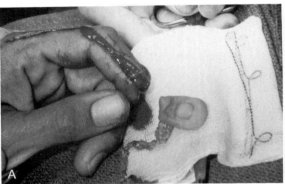
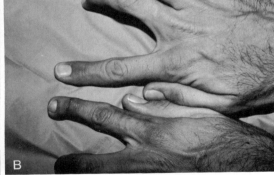
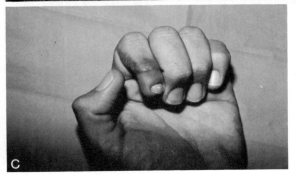

Figure 95–9. Second toe to index tip. *A,* Loss of the distal phalanx of the index. The distal phalanx of the second toe is ready to resurface the painful amputation stump. *B,* Digital length and functional pulp restored. The patient uses restored tip in his job as an accountant.

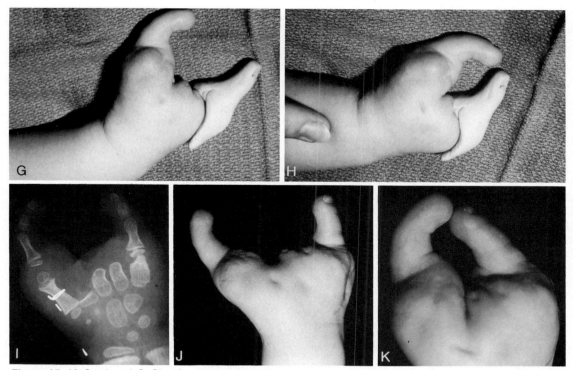

Figure 95–12 *Continued G,* Plan for second second toe transfer. *H,* Potential pinch between the first autotransplant and the second model. *I,* Postoperative radiograph of both autotransplants. *J,* Late follow-up. Wide grasp. *K,* Late follow-up. Pulp to pulp pinch.

fer, carefully preserving key structures that passed through it. Once the toe has been successfully perfused for 10 to 15 minutes, the vascular pedicles can be clamped and the digit transferred to the hand.

Toe Transfer

One member of the foot team should go with the toe to the hand to share knowledge of the toe structures with a remaining member of the hand team. The bony juncture is first wired, pinned, or screwed into position. The long flexor tendon is then sutured to a profundus tendon in the hand in an area least likely to develop restrictive adhesions. The arterial repair is performed next to keep ischemia time to a minimum. Interpositional grafts may be needed to permit tension-free repairs to undamaged proximal vessels. Vascular pedicles and grafts must be carefully stretched out to remove all twists. A twisted artery eventually spirals down to the distal anastomosis and becomes occluded; the same happens proximally with a twisted vein. Skin

closure may be difficult if several hours have passed and the flaps have become swollen and edematous. A small mesh graft placed over the vascular repairs is preferable to closure of the wound under tension. At the completion of the operation, both the hand and foot should be well elevated, loosely bandaged, and carefully splinted. Splints in the hand should be away from the vascular repairs and designed to immobilize the hand, wrist, and forearm comfortably.

POSTOPERATIVE MANAGEMENT

Dextran is started intraoperatively at the beginning of the microvascular repairs and continued at 500 units a day for five days. Aspirin, 150 mg a day, should be started five days before surgery and continued for two weeks postoperatively. Chlorpromazine is given postoperatively to relieve patients' apprehension and also for its antiserotonin effect; however, it is also a hypotensive agent (Buncke and Blackfield, 1963). The value of other vasodilating drugs is still not well documented. Respectable series of microvascular replants and autotransplants have been reported by groups who use no drug manipulation (Lister, Kalisman, and Tsao, 1983). Monitoring the circulation to the autotransplant is the single most important phase of postoperative management. This can be accomplished in a variety of ways, but nothing is more important than experienced nursing personnel and a dedicated house and attending staff. Capillary fill and perfusion are usually quite obvious in a robust autotransplant, but vascular spasm, hypotension, and slow perfusion can weaken this sign. A Doppler signal picked up over the artery distal to the anastomosis is a valuable sign. However, there may be a signal down to the level of a blocked anastomosis on the proximal side, or a misleading signal from an adjacent vessel

not entering the toe. Quantitative fluorescein studies performed every two hours provide a dependable, recordable, reproducible technique for monitoring capillary perfusion (Graham and associates, 1985). Except for technical difficulties with the machine, the author has found it to be the most sensitive and reliable index of vascular integrity.

The author prefers to follow all autotransplant patients on a one-to-one basis for 24 hours in a recovery room, intensive care, or coronary care unit. They are then returned to the microsurgical unit, where monitoring is continued on a four hourly basis for several days, depending on the clinical course. Most patients with an uncomplicated postoperative course can be sent home in seven to ten days. The donor foot is kept elevated for about two weeks, at which time sutures are removed and progressive ambulation is started in foot-

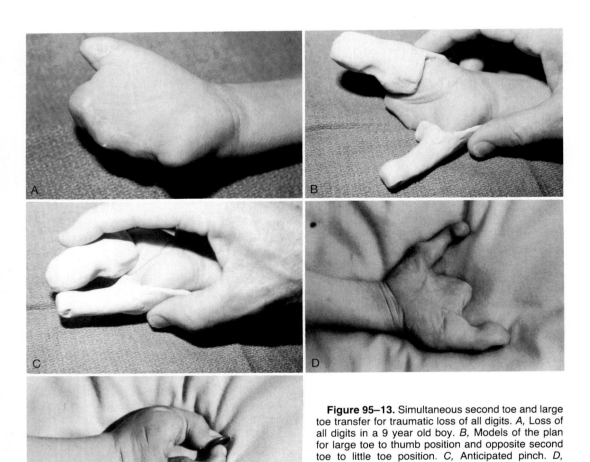

Figure 95–13. Simultaneous second toe and large toe transfer for traumatic loss of all digits. *A,* Loss of all digits in a 9 year old boy. *B,* Models of the plan for large toe to thumb position and opposite second toe to little toe position. *C,* Anticipated pinch. *D,* Postoperative span. *E,* Actual pulp to pulp pinch.

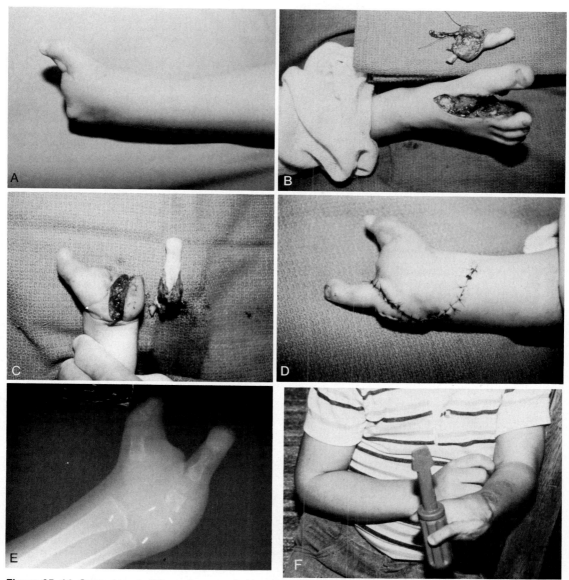

Figure 95–14. Second toe to fifth ray in congenital loss of all fingers. The thumb is hypoplastic. The patient is 3 years old. *A,* Preoperative condition. *B,* Second toe and metatarsal joint isolated. *C,* Toe transfer next to the fifth ray recipient wound. *D,* Second toe in place. *E,* Postoperative radiograph. *F,* Result two years after surgery.

wear. If the bony synostosis is solid, the transferred joints and tendons can be put through passive range of motion exercises by a skilled hand therapist several times a day, once the dextran has been stopped. Active motion of tendons is started at three weeks, protecting the bony juncture until it is solid clinically and radiographically. The most common problems with second toe autotransplants are flexion deformities at the interphalangeal joints, and lack of flexion at the

metatarsal or reconstructed metatarsal carpal joint (Fig. 97–7). Secondary tenolysis may be rewarding in some instances, but it produces minimal improvement in others. The more distal the digital reconstruction, the better is the result (see Fig. 95–9). A single digital autotransplant to a hand with only a thumb almost always produces a very useful pincher grasping unit as the thenar and hypothenar muscles hypertrophy (see Fig. 95–1). Double toe autotransplants to a similar

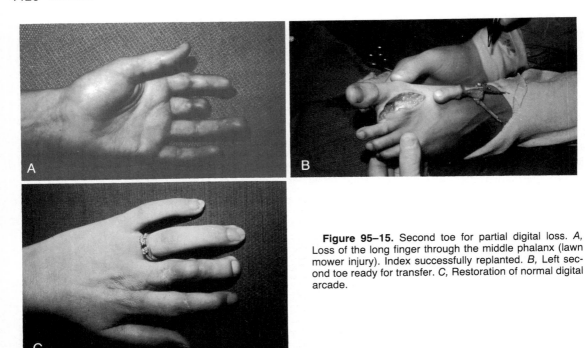

Figure 95–15. Second toe for partial digital loss. *A,* Loss of the long finger through the middle phalanx (lawn mower injury). Index successfully replanted. *B,* Left second toe ready for transfer. *C,* Restoration of normal digital arcade.

type of hand also quickly develop a chuck type of useful pinch and grasp (see Figs. 95–2 to 95–4, 95–8, 95–11 to 95–13). Single digit transfers to a hand containing normal fingers seldom perform as well as the adjacent normal digit. However, they restore the normal digital arcade and contribute to grasp and the overall function of the hand (see Fig. 95–

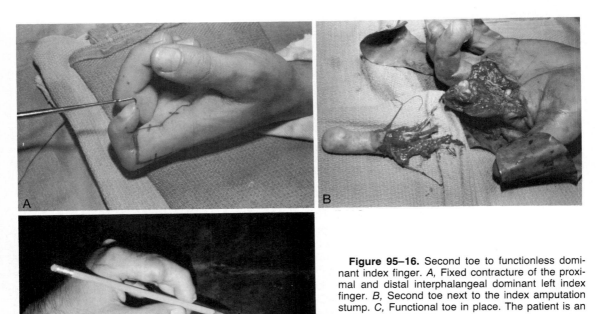

Figure 95–16. Second toe to functionless dominant index finger. *A,* Fixed contracture of the proximal and distal interphalangeal dominant left index finger. *B,* Second toe next to the index amputation stump. *C,* Functional toe in place. The patient is an architect and builder.

15). Single or multiple toe transfers to a severely injured hand often improve the function of the adjacent injured digits (see Figs. 95–4, 95–11) (Valauri and associates, 1986).

POSTOPERATIVE COMPLICATIONS

The most serious complication is thrombosis of the venous or arterial repairs, or both. With careful monitoring this can be picked up in minutes and the patient returned to the operating room for correction of the problem, usually by resection of the anastomosis, insertion of grafts, or direct repair of the vessels if adequate length is available. Prolonged ischemia leads to endothelial swelling and irreversible changes in a few hours (May and associates, 1978). Intra-arterial fibrinolysin (Thrombolysin) and streptokinase have been used in desperate situations, with occasional dramatic results. Hematoma is an early complication that responds dramatically to standard treatment. Vascular spasm may be precipitated by pain, cold, nicotine, or a variety of unknown causes, particularly in children. Local heat and regional bupivacaine blocks are tried before reexploration, but should be abandoned if response is not immediate. Many of these problems seem to develop in the hours between midnight and 6 AM, as a result of either hypotension, a decrease in body temperature, or other problems related to circulation monitoring at night time.

CONCLUSION

A second toe autotransplant, properly positioned and reinnervated on an injured hand, contributes to overall hand function in a dramatic fashion, without compromising foot function. In selected cases, second toe proximal interphalangeal or metacarpophalangeal joint transfer can significantly improve digital function.

REFERENCES

Buncke, H., and Blackfield, H.: The vasoplegic effect of chlorpromazine. Plast. Reconstr. Surg., *31*:353, 1963.

Buncke, H., Buncke, C., and Schulz, W.: Immediate Nicoladoni procedure in the rhesus monkey, or hallux-to-hand transplantation, utilizing microminiature vascular anastomoses. Br. J. Plast. Surg., *19*:332, 1966.

Buncke, G. M., Valauri, F. A., Buncke, H. J., Brooksher, R., Alpert, B. S., and Hing, D. N.: A review of 102 toe-to-hand transfers: correlation of preoperative angiograms and surgical anatomy. Presented to the American Society for Surgery of the Hand, New Orleans, February 16, 1986.

Clarkson, P.: On making thumbs. Plast. Reconstr. Surg., *29*:325, 1962.

Cobbett, J. R.: Free digital transfer. J. Bone Joint Surg., *51B*:677, 1969.

Davis, J. E.: Toe to hand transfer (pedochyrodactyloplasty). Plast. Reconstr. Surg., *331*:422, 1964.

First Teaching Hospital, Dept. of Surgery. Zhong-Shon Med. College: Some experiences on digital transfer. Nat. Med. J. China, *53*:335, 1973.

Gilbert, A.: Anatomy of the first intrametatarsal space. Symp. Microsurg., *14*:230, 1976.

Gilbert, A.: Toe transfer for congenital hand defects. J. Hand Surg., 7:118, 1982.

Gordon, L., Leitner, D., Buncke, H., and Alpert, B. S.: Hand reconstruction for multiple amputations by double microsurgical toe transplantation. J. Hand Surg., *10*:218, 1985.

Graham, B., Gordon, L., Alpert, B. S., Walton, R., Buncke, H., and Leitner, D.: Serial quantitative skin surface fluorescence: a new method for postoperative monitoring of vascular perfusion in revascularized digits. J. Hand Surg., *10A*:226, 1985.

Holle, J., Freilinger, G., Mandle, H., and Frey, M.: Grip reconstruction by double toe transplantation in case of a fingerless hand and handless arm. Plast. Reconstr. Surg., *69*:962, 1982.

Karkowski, J., and Buncke, H.: A simplified technique for free tissue transfer of groin flaps by use of a Doppler probe. Plast. Reconstr. Surg., *55*:6, 1975.

Leung, P. C.: Problems in toe-to-hand transfers. Ann. Acad. Med. Singapore, *12*:377, 1983.

Leung, P. C., Wong, W., and Kok, L.: Vessels of the first metatarsal web space. J. Bone Joint Surg., *65*:235, 1983.

Lichtman, D., Ahbel, D., Murphy, R., and Buncke, H.: Microvascular double toe transfer for opposite digits. J. Hand Surg., 7:279, 1982.

Lister, G., Kalisman, M., and Tsao, T.: Reconstruction of the hand with free microvascular toe-to-hand transfers, 54 toes. Plast. Reconstr. Surg., *71*:372, 1983.

May, J. Jr., Chait, L., Cohen, B., and O'Brien, B.: Free neurovascular flaps from the first web space of the foot in hand reconstruction. J. Hand Surg., 2:387, 1977.

May, J. Jr., Chait, L., O'Brien, B., and Hurley, J.: No reflow phenomenon in experimental free flaps. Plast. Reconstr. Surg., *61*:256, 1978.

Rose, E., and Buncke, H.: Simultaneous transfer of the right and left second toes for reconstruction of amputated index and middle fingers in the same hand. J. Hand Surg., 5:590, 1980.

Valauri, F. A., Buncke, G. M., Buncke, H. J., Brooksher, R., Alpert, B. S., and Hing, D. N.: Hand reconstruction with toe-to-hand transfers. A comprehensive review of 110 cases. Presented to the American Society for Reconstructive Microsurgery, New Orleans, February 14, 1986.

Wang, W.: Keys to successful second toe-to-hand transfer: a review of 30 cases. J. Hand Surg., 8:902, 1983.

Zhong-Wei, C., Meyer, V., and Beasley, R.: The versatile second toe microvascular transfer. Orthop. Clin. North Am., *12*:827, 1981.

Earl Z. Browne, Jr.

General Principles of Wound Management

Although the emphasis in this chapter is directed primarily toward soft tissue injuries, it is of utmost importance to keep in mind the concept of the hand as a functional organ when undertaking treatment of complex injuries. Unfortunately, patients are still frequently seen with stiff, poorly functioning hands after treatment by surgeons who have been too narrowly concerned with reconstruction of one specific area. Assessment of the injury must include evaluation not only of skin and soft tissue, but of the skeleton, joints, tendons, nerves, and vessels.

INITIAL WOUND CARE

The only absolute indication for immediate hand surgery is vascular insufficiency. Revascularization of ischemic parts must take priority over any other treatment, and is often carried out under less than ideal circumstances. If vascular integrity is satisfac-

tory, however, the primary goal of treatment should be to convert a contaminated wound into a tidy one. Much has been learned by hand surgeons in treating traumatic injuries during the various wars, especially during World War II, when regional hand centers were established under the direction of Dr. Sterling Bunnell (1955). It was estimated by him that, of the almost 600,000 Americans wounded during that war, approximately 15 per cent had hand injuries. The concept of initial evaluation, debridement, splinting, and dressing, followed by definitive treatment at a later stage, developed during this time. After initial treatment, the hand was elevated, antibiotics were administered, appropriate tetanus prophylaxis was employed, and the patient was transported to a secondary treatment facility where definitive hand care could be undertaken. It was recognized that it is possible to delay this definitive treatment for a few days to ensure that an ideal condition exists, free from devitalized tissue and bacterial colonization. When more rapid methods of evacuation to definitive centers became possible during the Korean and Vietnam wars, it was recognized that some patients with extensive injuries could be treated in the early phase if ideal conditions existed, but that the general principles of debridement and ensuring that bacterial colonization would not take place were essential. In general, wound closure can be successfully employed if a colonization of bacteria of less than 10^5 per gram of tissue is present (Krizek, Robson, and Kho, 1967).

Initial wound debridement should include generous irrigation and removal of all foreign material and definitely devitalized tissue. Skin debridement should be as minimal as possible, removing only tissue that is clearly nonviable. Small, completely free floating fragments of bone should be removed, but fragments that still have periosteal continuity should be maintained, and if possible some kind of skeletal stability should be achieved. In grossly contaminated wounds, this should be deferred for a few days until a second, more definitive, debridement is carried out and it can be determined that the wound is clean (Fig. 96–1). If possible, however, skeletal stability can be reestablished with K-wires that do not directly exit through the open wound. At this point it should be determined whether or not tendon and nerve repairs should be done. It is a cardinal principle that these structures should never be repaired unless complete closure with adequate skin and soft tissue can be established. Under extenuating circumstances some form of distant coverage, such as a skin flap, may be used for this purpose instead of primary closure. This is usually appropriate only when survival of deep structures is in jeopardy owing to lack of a suitable wound bed to nourish them (Fig. 96–2).

If it has been determined that skin closure can be safely accomplished, this should be followed by a dressing that is not occlusive, allowing for wound drainage to be absorbed. If the wound is not closed, care should be taken to make sure that the tissues do not dry out. Further necrosis can be expected, especially in partially devitalized tissue, if desiccation takes place. Although it is possible to prevent desiccation by placing occlusive dressings on the wound, it is preferable to

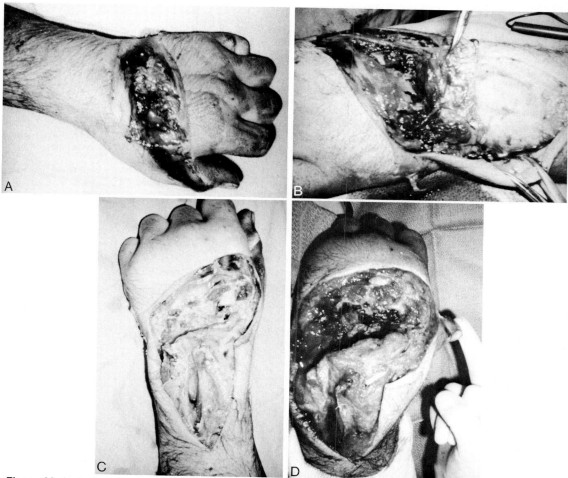

Figure 96–1. *A, B,* Filthy wound caused by a harvester in an agricultural injury. *C,* The wound appears clean after initial debridement. *D,* Three days later at subsequent debridement, infected tissue is found that would have certainly caused breakdown if the wound had been covered primarily.

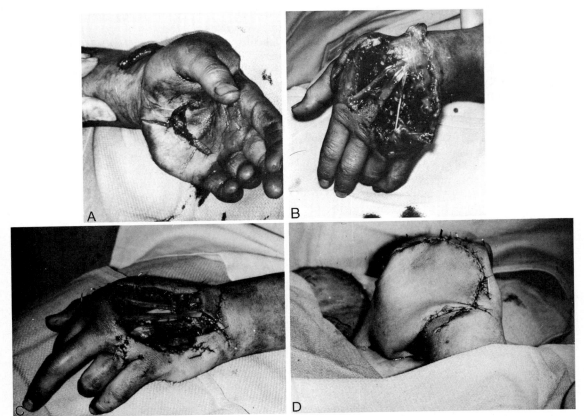

Figure 96–2. *A, B,* Severe injury caused by explosion of a home-made bomb. *C,* Multiple fractures and bone fragments pinned, and tendons repaired. *D,* Because no wound bed was present to nourish the stabilized structures, primary coverage was obtained with a nourishing flap.

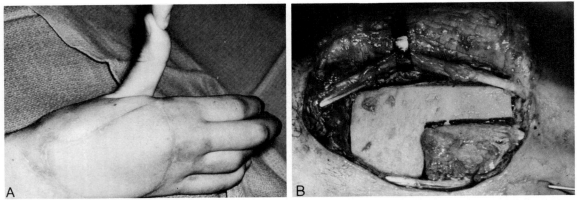

Figure 96–3. *A, B,* The patient whose hand was shown in Figure 96–2. The flap has resulted in good vascularity, so definitive reconstruction with a bone graft is performed several months after injury. Note that the extensor tendons have healed and survived.

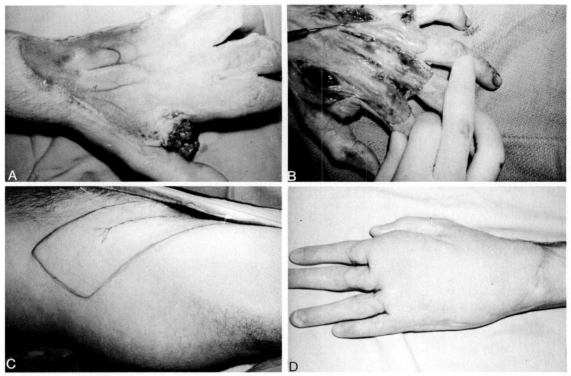

Figure 96–7. *A,* A mangle injury combining crush and burn. *B,* Debridement includes decompression of any muscle compartment compression. *C, D,* A primarily defatted groin flap results in thin pliable coverage that does not get in the way.

drainage an indwelling catheter for periodic or continuous installation of antibiotic solutions.

Graft Take

As previously noted, the most important aspect of success or failure of the graft is the bed upon which the graft is placed. When the skin graft is first applied to the wound, the graft survives by transudate from the wound, a process referred to as plasmatic circulation. For ultimate survival of the graft, there must be an ingrowth of blood vessels from the bed (inosculation), and anything that serves as a barrier, such as a hematoma, prevents this process and causes a slough. Therefore, there must be a well-vascularized bed present, no bleeding or exudation, and a lack of bacterial colonization (less than 10^5 organisms per gram of tissue). Bearing in mind the previous discussion on wound contraction, it is obvious that the sooner the graft can be applied to a vascularized wound, the better is the ultimate result. It is not necessary to have the beefy red granulation tissue present that is often thought to represent a healthy wound. In fact, a fine, lacy network of capillaries present in a thin wound is far superior (Fig. 96–8). Should excess granulation tissue develop in a wound, it is best to remove this tissue, since it can be the source of infection as well as continued contraction (Fig. 96–9).

Types of Grafts

In general, thinner grafts tend to take more readily than thick grafts. However, thin grafts do not slow down the continued wound contraction to so great an extent, do not afford as good quality of coverage, and contain fewer nerve endings that can subsequently be reinnervated by nerve ingrowth from the recipient area. In instances in which quality of coverage and need for return of reasonable sensibility are of consequence, a full-thick-

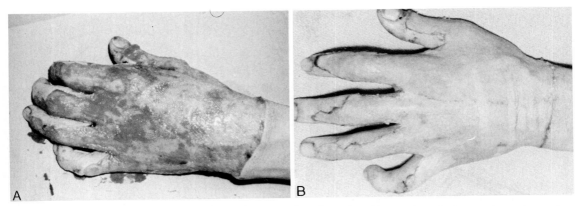

Figure 96–8. *A, B,* Thin, lacy network of vessels present in a three day old wound results in complete take at seven days, when early motion can be begun.

ness skin graft is the best choice. As a rule, volar grafts are most commonly full thickness, and dorsal grafts are split thickness.

Split-Thickness Grafts. Small pieces of skin may be taken to cover small avulsions, using a No. 10 knife blade or a Goulian knife. It is very convenient to remove these from the same arm that is being operated on, but it should be remembered that although the wound will epithelize, the loss of dermis is permanent. Sometimes the cosmetic effect of removing a piece of skin from the inner forearm is so bad that the patient complains more of the donor site than the recipient one (Fig. 96–10). An inconspicuous site such as the side of the hip or thigh is much better, since the quality of skin is no different and the donor area is thicker, thus healing better. Larger sheets of skin are more conveniently taken with a dermatome, such as the Padgett. Large sheets of skin, measuring approxi-

mately 0.010 to 0.020 inch in thickness, can be taken with this instrument. The technique of using these instruments is described in Chapters 99 and 129.

There will be times when the surgeon wishes to close the wound as soon as possible, but the bed is not judged to be optimum for successful graft take because of the risk of hematoma or infection. Under these circumstances, it may be convenient to convert the graft into a meshed one by passing it through a special mesh graft dermatome after harvesting. Various expansion ratios are possible with these instruments, but it is not appropriate to expand a graft very much for use on the hand. The principle in using this graft is to create a lot of interstices through which fluid exchange can occur, rather than to spread out the skin over a larger area. Although the open spaces do serve to allow fluid transudation, they are also spaces that are

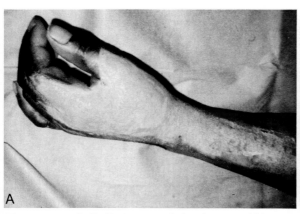
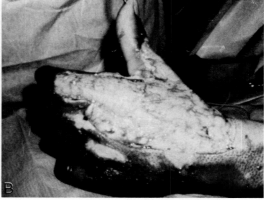

Figure 96–9. *A, B,* Excess granulation tissue could be completely excised so that a healthy bed could develop in a few days. Sharp excision is preferable to scraping.

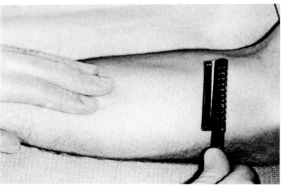

Figure 96–10. Although very convenient, the forearm is a poor place to use for a small graft, as shown about to be taken with a Goulian knife.

not being grafted. For these open areas to heal, there must be epithelization from the edges of the mesh. Therefore, all the tiny holes really are continuing contracting wounds. The quality of the graft ultimately is much better if the skin is simply meshed and placed on the wound with minimal, if any, expansion (Fig. 96–11). Transudation still takes place and the ultimate quality of the graft is much superior.

Full-Thickness Grafts. Full-thickness grafts may be taken from any convenient spot, but care should be exercised to prevent transfer of unwanted hair. This is especially true in the removal of inguinal grafts, particularly in children, who have not developed hair growth. Full-thickness grafts are measured to fit the defect, and are removed as ellipses, thus closing the donor site primarily. This has the advantage of producing a superior quality skin graft and also a donor site with very minimal morbidity (Fig. 96–12).

The best feature of a full-thickness graft is the transfer of sensory end organelles, which may be reinnervated in the recipient site. Clearly, the greater the density of appropriate end organelles, the better the type of sensibility that will be present. In critical areas, such as the fingertip, it is probably best to use glabrous skin. This can be conveniently taken from the hypothenar area of the hand. After removal of the graft, all extra subcutaneous tissue is removed with a scissors and the graft is sutured into place. Any skin graft should be immobilized carefully until vascularization takes place, but this is critical for full-thickness grafts. The most convenient method of anchoring these grafts is by use of a tie-over dressing that compresses the graft by means of a bolster. The bolster has the added advantage of causing some compression in the postoperative period, which minimizes the chance of seroma or hematoma formation. It also appears that by causing some pressure for a week or so after skin grafting, it is possible to minimize the extent of wound contraction that takes place under the graft, provided the quality of the bed is optimal. The hand should be splinted in a functional position until graft vascularization appears to be proceeding satisfactorily, and then gentle motion can be undertaken. Since the rate of vascularization that occurs is proportional to the thickness of the graft, this is usually done seven to ten days after placing the graft. It should be kept in mind that a skin graft is just like any other wound, and that there is very little tensile strength present until sufficient collagen deposition has occurred between the graft and the wound. Therefore, motion should be undertaken carefully, in order to prevent shear-

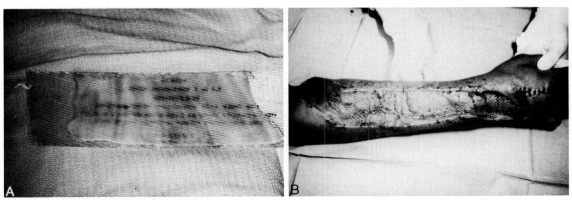

Figure 96–11. A, B, Split-thickness skin is meshed and used to cover a marginal wound. Minimal, if any, expansion is used and the holes still provide drainage.

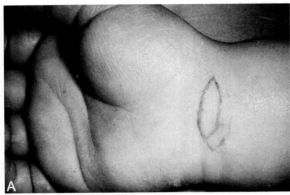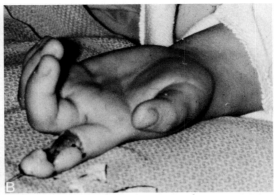

Figure 96–12. *A, B,* Full-thickness grafts provide superior coverage of volar wounds, and donor sites can be closed primarily; both are advantages in children.

ing forces that could separate the graft from the recipient bed.

REFERENCES

Browne, E. Z., Jr.: Skin grafts. *In* Green, D. P. (Ed.): Operative Hand Surgery. Vol. 2. New York, Churchill Livingstone, 1982, p. 1283.

Bunnell, S. (Ed.): Hand Surgery in World War II. Washington, DC, Office of Surgeon General, Department of Army, 1955.

Burkhalter, W. E.: Care of war injuries of the hand and upper extremity. Report of the War Injury Committee. J. Hand Surg., 8:810, 1983.

Converse, J. M., McCarthy, J. G., Brauer, R. O., and Ballantyne, D. L.: Transplantation of skin: grafts and flaps. *In* Converse, J. M. (Ed.): Reconstructive Plastic Surgery. 2nd Ed. Philadelphia, W. B. Saunders Company, 1977, pp. 152–239.

Corps, V. W. M.: The effect of graft thickness, donor site and graft bed on graft shrinkage in the hooded rat. Br. J. Plast. Surg., 22:135, 1969.

Fitzgerald, R. H., Cooney, W. P., Washington, J. A., Van Scoy, R. E., Linscheid, R. L., and Dobyns, J. H.: Bacterial colonization of mutilating hand injuries and its treatment. J. Hand Surg., 2:85, 1977.

Gabbiani, G., Hirschel, B. J., Ryan, G. B., Statkov, P. R., and Majino, G.: Granulation tissue as a contractile organ. A study of structure and function. J. Exp. Med., 135:719, 1972.

Goulian, D.: A new economical dermatome. Plast. Reconstr. Surg., 42:85, 1968.

Grinnell, F., Billingham, R. E., and Burgess, L.: Distribution of fibronectin during wound healing in vivo. J. Invest. Dermatol., 76:181, 1981.

Heggers, J. P., Robson, M. C., and Ristroph, J. D.: A rapid method of performing quantitative wound cultures. Milit. Med., 134:666, 1969.

Hunt, T. K.: Wound healing. *In* Dunphy, J. E., and Way, L. W. (Eds.): Current Surgical Diagnosis and Treatment. 5th Ed. Los Altos, Lange, 1981, p. 93.

Krizek, T. J., Robson, M. C., and Kho, E.: Bacterial growth and skin graft survival. Surg. Forum, 18:518, 1967.

Levine, N. S., Lindberg, R. B., Mason, A. D., and Pruitt, B. A.: The quantitative swab culture and smear: a quick, simple method for determining the number of viable aerobic bacteria on open wounds. J. Trauma, 16:89, 1976.

Peacock, E. E.: Wound Repair. 3rd Ed. Philadelphia, W. B. Saunders Company, 1984.

Rudolph, R.: Inhibition of myofibroblasts by skin grafts. Plast. Reconstr. Surg., 63:473, 1979.

Rudolph, R., Fisher, J. C., and Ninneman, J.: Skin Grafting. Boston, Little, Brown & Company, 1979.

Stone, P. A., and Madden, J. W.: Effect of primary and delayed skin grafting on wound contraction. Surg. Forum, 25:4, 1974.

are few because of the limited nature of the donor areas available. One must also keep in mind the specialized types of skin as they are contrasted in their elastic properties and function; e.g., the elastic and freely movable skin of the dorsum of the hand as opposed to the thick, poorly moving, and relatively immobile volar skin of the hand. Each serves specific functions and needs, and should be maintained for ideal reconstruction.

There are three basic types of local flaps: advancement, rotation, and transposition flaps. They all have in common a limited arc of motion because they are tethered by their bases, which contain their blood supply. Also, these local flaps are usually random in nature and do not have a specific arterial or axial blood supply. For this reason, these flaps are usually no longer than they are wide (i.e. length to width ratio of 1:1).

Z-Plasties

A specialized type of transposition flap is that of the Z-plasty, so named because two triangular flaps are transposed by way of a "Z"-shaped incision. The three limbs of the "Z" must be of equal length, and the net results of a Z-plasty are twofold: scar lengthening and positional or directional change of the scar. This entire concept of interposed triangular flaps was first mentioned by Horner in 1837. Subsequently, Berger (1904) used these types of flaps to relieve axillary contracture, and Morestin (1914) used sequential Z-plasties to lengthen a contracted scar in the hand. However, Limberg (1928) really placed Z-plasty in a geometric prospective and actually used this term. More recently, Furnas and Fischer (1971) worked out the biomechanical considerations in the laboratory on canine skin, and Roggendorf (1983) used pig skin in a stereometric-planimetric model.

A number of factors are involved in the design of Z-plasties. The basic design possibilities are: the length of the three "Z" limbs, the angles of the advancing flaps, and the decision whether to use one large Z-plasty or a series of smaller, multiple, connected Z-plasties.

As with any flap transposition, we are robbing Peter to pay Paul: nothing is free, and therefore there is a price to pay. Length is gained at the expense of width. Therefore, the longer the three limbs of the Z-plasty, the greater the scar can be lengthened; however, the cost of this increased length is a narrower width for more tension on horizontal closure.

Similarly, the acuteness of the advancing triangular transposition flaps determines the amount of increase in net length. The closer to 90 degrees these angles are designed, the greater length will result. However, 90-degree advancing tip angles frequently result in dog-ears at their bases. Narrow and acute angles at the advancing triangular Z-plasty tips may compromise blood supply in this area. The usual middle ground is that of an angle between 45 and 60 degrees, which works best in the clinical situation.

It is generally best to use one large Z-plasty instead of multiple, small, interconnected ones. The advantage is that there is a more robust blood supply to larger flaps because their bases are wider, the advancing angles of the tips of the flaps can be more obtuse, and larger esthetic and functional units are moved into better functioning positions. However, large flaps sometimes are not possible because of the anatomic constraints, and in these situations multiple, connected, sequential Z-plasties can be very helpful. The latter are frequently seen in the digits, and great care must be taken in digit Z-plasties because, if one large "Z" is used, it is possible to compromise the digit with constriction of horizontal width. In these cases, it is better to design several Z-plasties of small proportions, and their additive effect can result in a similar increase in length without a severe compromise of width.

The design of Z-plasties must be carefully planned envisioning a three-dimensional triangular flap, and the surgeon should feel comfortable that there are few compromises to the blood supply entering the base of this flap. Most cases requiring Z-plasties involve burned hands and fingers or traumatic and scarred contractures (Figs. 97–4, 97–5). In these situations, the surgeon must be completely cognizant of surrounding soft tissue and never base a Z-plasty triangular flap on scar. The transposition of this type of flap would obviously result in vascularly insufficient soft tissue and a poor result. Especially in the case of burned hand reconstructions, Z-plasty should be employed only if there is tissue laxity in the direction opposite the direction of skin to be lengthened (see Chap. 132).

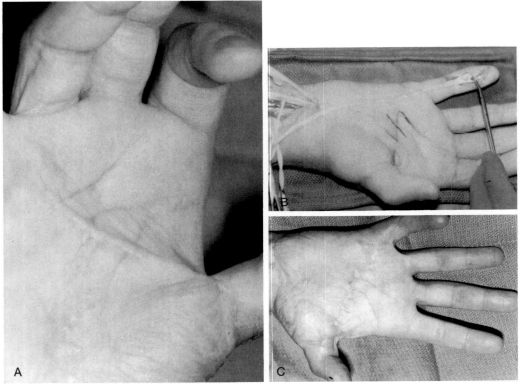

Figure 97–4. *A,* Horizontal scar contracture across the distal and middle palm. *B,* Sequential Z-plasties planned. *C,* The lengthened and healed result.

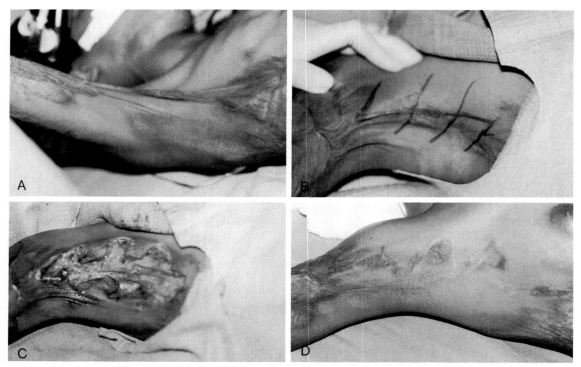

Figure 97–5. *A,* Burn scar contracture of the right axilla. *B,* Sequential Z-plasties planned. *C,* Incisions and interdigitations of flaps. *D,* Healed, lengthened, and transposed sequential Z-plasty flaps.

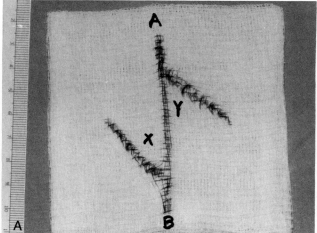

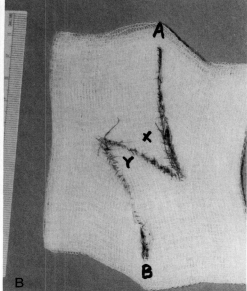

Figure 97–6. *A,* The scar line A–B is incised and will be lengthened Z-plasty transposition flaps X and Y are planned. This is best demonstrated on a gauze sponge that represents soft tissue. *B,* As flaps X and Y are transposed adjacent to one another, scar line A–B is lengthened. *C,* With the gauze sponge illustration, one can appreciate the lengthening of scar line A–B at the expense of width.

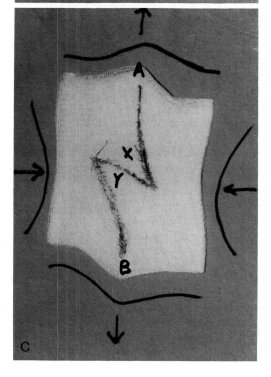

In preparing for the Z-plasty, the incision is made longitudinally along the axis of the actual contracture (Fig. 97–6*A*). The Z-plasty limbs should then come off this central line, usually in equilateral triangular segments (Fig. 97–6*B*). The design of the flap must take into account the fact that the base of each of these triangles must harbor healthy tissue so that vascular compromise is held to a minimum. The surgeon can also plan the resultant horizontal scar and the change of direction of the Z-plasty. The scar will be perpendicular to the central axis of contracture and will be in a horizontal position (Fig. 97–6*C*). This line can be predicted by connecting the lateralmost ends of the "Z" limbs with an im-

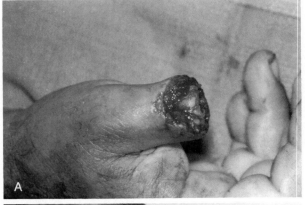
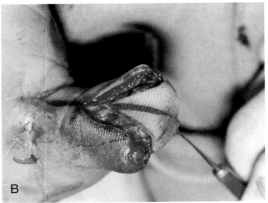
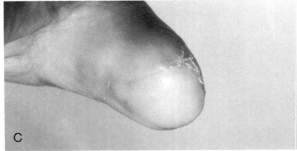

Figure 97–7. *A,* Amputation of the distal digit. *B,* Preservation of length with a V-Y advancement. *C,* The healed wound.

aginary line. This can be very helpful in planning Z-plasties so that on the volar aspect of digits one can produce the horizontal scar to lie in the flexion crease.

The Z-plasty can be very useful in preventing scar contraction if a laceration or elective incision (e.g., Dupuytren's) crosses a flexion crease.

Finally, Z-plasties can be used to deepen various web spaces or release contractures between the thumb and index finger. Two- or four-flap Z-plasties of the thumb web can enable the thumb to be abducted and opposed in a more functional fashion (Broadbent and Woolf, 1960).

Advancement Flaps

Advancement flaps take advantage of the elasticity of the skin. They are raised by undermining below the subdermal plexus of vessels in the subcutaneous plain. This releases the tethering effect of this tissue and allows for closure of defects that require minimal preparation. Rotation flaps, on the other hand, take into account a geometric design that requires a "cutback" at 90 degrees to the axis of rotation. This allows soft tissue to be "rotated" around a pivot point and usually allows for the entire wound to be closed primarily with some "fudging" in the suture line. Occasionally, skin grafts are needed to cover part of the donor site. Transposition flaps, on the other hand, are usually rectangular in nature and frequently interpose normal tissue between its donor and recipient sites. Transposition flaps are most often used in hand surgery; advancement and rotation flaps have less value because of their anatomic constraints.

The advancement flap is the most simple and most commonly used type of closure after a lenticular excision of a wound where skin is mobile and easily undermined. Any adjacent tissue undermining that takes advantage of the elastic stretching properties of the skin can, and properly should, be called an advancement flap. This most frequently is used on the dorsum of the hand where the skin is more elastic than the nongiving, relatively "fixed" tissue of the volar hand surface. Examples of specialized types of advancement flaps are a V-Y advancement from the volar aspect of the finger, as described by Atasoy and associates (1970) (Fig. 97–7) and the lateral bilateral V-Y advancement flaps, as described by Kutler (1947) for fingertip

elbow and soft tissue are missing, this distant flap can be used in a one-stage operation to provide soft tissue coverage and simultaneous elbow flexion with minimal donor morbidity. The latissimus dorsi muscle is dissected from its origin and insertion, along with a previously measured skin island, so that it is attached to the body only by its neurovascular bundle (the thoracodorsal artery, vein, and nerve). This flap is then transposed via the axilla to the flexor surface of the upper arm, and the donor site is closed primarily. A functional result is expected when the origin of the latissimus is attached to the proximal forearm or biceps tendon, and the insertion of the latissimus is sutured to the acromion or proximal biceps muscle. The patient can then be reeducated to obtain flexion of the elbow by conscious upper arm adduction.

A similar use of this myocutaneous flap is for soft tissue coverage of the posterior aspect of the arm superficial to or replacing the triceps muscle. Although this provides excellent soft tissue coverage, the functional aspects of the latissimus dorsi procedure to restore elbow extension are not absolutely necessary because this can be obtained by gravity.

The pectoralis major muscle can similarly be used either as a myocutaneous flap or as a muscle flap with covering skin graft to provide soft tissue coverage of the shoulder and upper humerus area. The dissection is straightforward, and the origins of the pectoralis major muscle from the sternum and

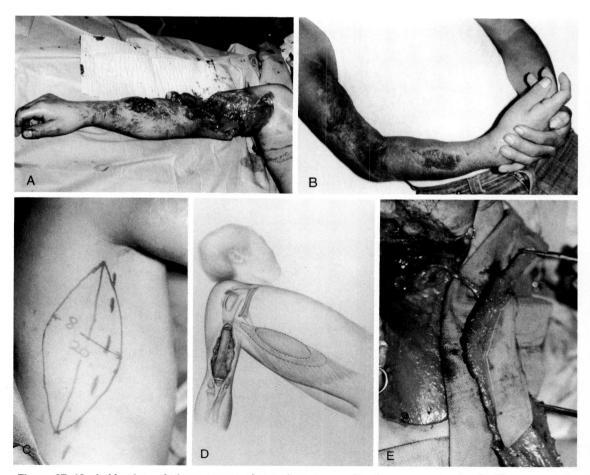

Figure 97–12. *A,* Massive soft tissue trauma after a shotgun wound to the upper extremity. *B,* After conservative wound closure and grafting, there is absent elbow flexion and poor soft tissue coverage. *C,* A latissimus dorsi myocutaneous flap is planned. *D,* The latissimus dorsi myocutaneous flap. *E,* Elevation of the flap with its neurovascular pedicle.

Illustration continued on following page

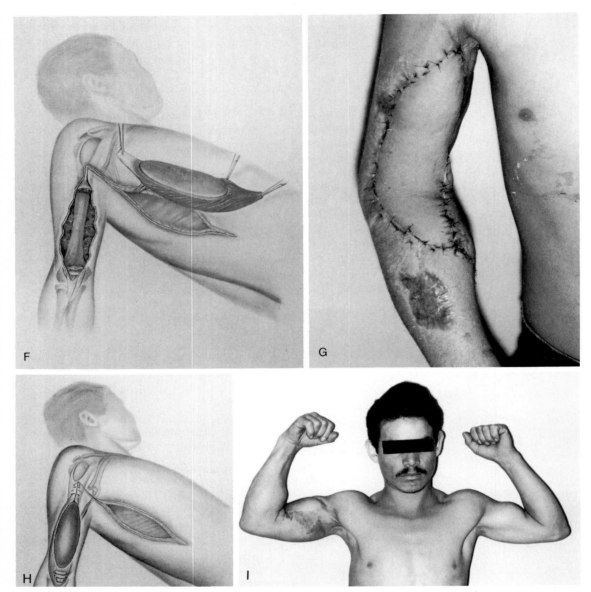

Figure 97–12 *Continued F,* Diagrammatic representation of the elevation of the flap and its pedicle, and division of its origin and insertion. *G,* Inset of the flap for improvement of soft tissue coverage and elbow flexion. *H,* Latissimus dorsi muscle transfer replaces the biceps and brachialis muscles. *I,* Excellent contour and approximately 10 lb of elbow flexion.

ribs must be divided so that lateral transposition can be effected. In this way the muscle is based on its major blood supply, the thoracoacromial artery and vein. Similarly, the pectoralis major muscle can be used for coverage of the axilla if so desired, but this use is obviously limited by the mobilization of the thoracoacromial vessels. Depending on functional needs and donor site morbidity, the latissimus dorsi muscle or the pectoralis major muscle offers the reconstructive surgeon two excellent choices for either of the above defects.

FASCIOCUTANEOUS FLAPS

Somewhat more obscure and infrequently used because of the relative unpredictability of the blood supply are the medial fasciocutaneous flap of the upper arm with its axial blood supply from the superior ulnar collateral artery, and the lateral fasciocutaneous flap based on the posterior radial collateral artery, which has cutaneous perforators at the level of the intermuscular septum. These can be designed as rectangular flaps for transpositional coverage. However, these two flaps leave large donor defects, involve tedious and challenging surgical dissections, and should be used only if other more accessible flaps have been ruled out.

RADIAL FOREARM FLAPS

A more popular axial cutaneous flap is that of the radial "Chinese" forearm flap, which is based on the radial artery and its venae comitantes. This flap was popularized in the Western world in the early 1980's (Song and associates, 1982) and has been used increasingly in recent years. It is an excellent free flap for transfer to other areas, but it carries the main disadvantage of leaving a large donor site scar. However, with tissue expansion, it is possible to minimize this handicap.

MUSCLE FLAPS

Although infrequently used, some forearm muscle flaps are transposed either as muscle flaps alone or as myocutaneous flaps. The flexor carpi ulnaris and brachioradialis can be used as muscle flap transfers for soft tissue coverage above and about the elbow. These muscles are supplied by branches of the ulnar and radial arteries, respectively, and cover relatively narrow defects, but can be useful to cover open elbow joint injuries. Once the muscle is in place, it can be skin grafted for coverage.

Chase (1984) described the abductor digiti minimi myocutaneous flap for functional and soft tissue coverage in the area of the thenar eminence. Because this muscle is useful in an opponensplasty, the overlying skin can provide excellent soft tissue coverage, while the donor site is skin grafted. This gives excellent esthetic contour to the thenar mass, albeit at the expense of a flattened hypothenar area.

Ideal coverage for soft tissue defects of the hand and upper extremity should be replaced with "like tissue." Local or distant flaps are excellent substitutions, but must (1) provide enough subcutaneous tissue for deep gliding structures; (2) supply subcutaneous tissue in bulk for coverage of vital neural, vascular, bone, and joint structures; and (3) be esthetically pleasing. With forethought, planning, and the use of plastic surgical principles, it is often possible to rob Peter to pay Paul by the use of distant or local flaps, and provide

for successful function and form in the upper extremity.

REFERENCES

Albee, F. H.: Synthetic transplantation of tissues to form new finger. Ann. Surg., 69:379, 1919.

Atasoy, E., Ioakimidis, E., Kasdan, M. L., et al.: Reconstruction of the amputated finger tip with a triangular volar flap. A new surgical procedure. J. Bone Joint Surg., 52A:921, 1970.

Bakamjian, V. Y.: A two stage method for pharyngoesophageal reconstruction with a primary pectoral skin flap. Plast. Reconstr. Surg., 36:173, 1965.

Berger, P.: Autoplastie par deboublement de la palmure et echange de lambeaux. In Berger, P., and Banzet, S. (Eds.): Chirurgie Orthopedique. Paris, Steinfeil, 1904.

Blair, V. P.: Surgery and Diseases of the Mouth and Jaws. St. Louis, C. V. Mosby Company, 1912.

Boyes, J. H.: Incisions in the hand. Am. J. Orthop., 4:308, 1962.

Broadbent, T. R., and Woolf, R. M.: Thumb reconstruction with contiguous skin-bone pedicle graft. Plast. Reconstr. Surg., 26:494, 1960.

Brones, M. F., Wheeler, E. S., and Lesavoy, M. A.: Restoration of elbow flexion and arm contour with the latissimus dorsi myocutaneous flap. Plast. Reconstr. Surg., 69:329, 1982.

Bruner, J. M.: Incisions for plastic and reconstructive (nonseptic) surgery of the hand. Br. J. Plast. Surg., 4:48, 1951.

Bruner, J. M.: The zig-zag volar-digital incision for flexor-tendon surgery. Plast. Reconstr. Surg., 40:571, 1967.

Bunnell, S.: Surgery of the Hand. 2nd Ed. Philadelphia, J. B. Lippincott Company, 1948.

Chase, R. A.: Atlas of Hand Surgery. Vol. II. Philadelphia, W. B. Saunders Company, 1984.

Chase, R. A.: Historical review of skin and soft tissue coverage of the upper extremity. Hand Clin., 1:599, 1985.

Cutler, C. W.: The Hand. Its Disabilities and Diseases. Philadelphia, W. B. Saunders Company, 1942.

d'Este, S.: La technique de l'amputation de la mamelle pour carcinome mammaire. Rev. Chir., 45:164, 1912.

Furnas, D. W., and Fischer, G. W.: The Z-plasty: biomechanics and mathematics. Br. J. Plast. Surg., 24:144, 1971.

Gillies, H. D., and Millard, D. R., Jr.: The Principles and Art of Plastic Surgery. Boston, Little, Brown & Company, 1957.

Hallock, G. G.: Island forearm flap for coverage of the anticubital fossa. Br. J. Plast. Surg., 39:533, 1986.

Horner, W. E.: Clinical report on the surgical department of Philadelphia Hospital, Blockley for the months of May, June, and July, 1837. Am. J. Med. Sci., 21:105, 1837.

Jin, Y., Guan, W., Shi, T., Quian, Y., Xu, L., and Chang, T.: Reversed island forearm fascial flap in hand surgery. Ann. Plast. Surg., 15:340, 1985.

Johnson, R. K., and Shrewsbury, M. M.: Anatomic course of the thenar branch of the median nerve. Usually in a separate tunnel through the transverse carpal ligament. J. Bone Joint Surg., 52A:269, 1970.

Kutler, W. A.: A new method of repair for finger tip amputation. J.A.M.A., 133:29, 1947.

Lesavoy, M. A.: The dorsal index finger neurovascular island flap. Orthop. Rev., *9:*91, 1980.

Lesavoy, M. A.: Reconstruction of the Head and Neck. Baltimore, Williams & Wilkins Company, 1981, p. 2.

Limberg, A. A.: Plastic interchange of triangular flaps. Odont. Stomat., *2:*74, 1928.

Lister, G. D.: The theory of the transposition flap and its practical application in the hand. Clin. Plast. Surg., *8:*115, 1981.

McFarlane, R. N., Heagy, F. C., Rodin, S., Aust, J. C., and Wermuth, R. G.: A study of the delay phenomenon in experimental pedicle flaps. Plast. Reconstr. Surg., *35:*245, 1965.

McGrath, M. H., Adelberg, D., and Finseth, F.: The intravenous fluorescein test: use in timing of groin flap division. J. Hand Surg., *4:*19, 1979.

McGregor, I. A., and Jackson, I. T.: The groin flap. Br. J. Plast. Surg., *25:*3, 1972.

Meals, R. A., and Lesavoy, M. A.: Hand Surgery Review. 2nd Ed. Massachusetts, PSG Publishing Company, 1985.

Millard, D. R.: Principlization of Plastic Surgery. Boston, Little, Brown & Company, 1986.

Morestin, M. H.: De la correction des flexions permanentes des doigts consecutives aux panaris et aux phlegmons de la paume de la main. Rev. Chir., *50:*1, 1914.

Myers, M. B.: Prediction of skin sloughs at the time of operation with the use of fluorescein dye. Surgery, *51:*158, 1962.

Myers, M. B., Cherry, G., and Milton, S.: Tissue gas levels as an index of the adequacy of circulation: the relation between ischemia and the development of collateral circulation (delay phenomenon). Surgery, *71:*15, 1972.

Reyes, F. A., and Burkhalter, W. E.: The fascial radial flap. J. Hand Surg., *13:*432, 1988.

Roggendorf, E.: The planimetric Z-plasty. Plast. Reconstr. Surg., *71:*834, 1983.

Shaw, D. T., and Payne, R. L.: One stage tubed abdominal flaps. Single pedicle tubes. Surg. Gynecol. Obstet., *83:*205, 1946.

Smith, R. C., and Furnas, D. W.: The hand sandwich. Plast. Reconstr. Surg., *57:*351, 1976.

Song, R., Gao, Y., Song, Y., Yu, Y., and Song, Y.: The forearm flap. Clin. Plast. Surg., *9:*21, 1982.

Tanzini: Spora il nito nuova processo di aupertozione della menuelle. Riforma Med., *22:*757, 1906.

Zeis, E.: The Zeis index and history of plastic surgery: 900 B.C.–1863 A.D. Vol. 1. Baltimore, Williams & Wilkins Company, 1977.

98

Leonard A. Sharzer

Free Flap Transfer in the Upper Extremity

Since the first successful free flap transfer was described by Daniel and Taylor (1973), this mode of soft tissue coverage has progressed from being an operation of last resort—one that was tried when all else had failed—to become, in many instances, the procedure of choice. It is undoubtedly a well-accepted component of the plastic surgeon's armamentarium.

It is not surprising that the first free flap described was used to cover a defect in the lower third of the lower extremity, nor is it surprising that most papers on the subject since then have related to its use in lower extremity reconstruction. In the lower extremity, particularly the distal one-third, there are few alternatives that provide satisfactory coverage.

In the upper extremity, however, the situation is somewhat different. Harii, Ohmori, and Ohmori (1974) reported the first successful free flap transfer to the upper extremity. Since then, there have been several articles relating specifically to the use of free tissue transfer in the upper extremity (Sharzer and associates, 1978; Daniel and Faibisoff, 1979; Shah, Garrett, and Buncke, 1979; Buncke and associates, 1981; Gilbert, 1981; Daniel and Weiland, 1982; Olson, Wood, and Irons, 1982; Wood, Cooney, and Irons, 1983; Wood and Irons, 1983; Stevenson and associates, 1984; Chase, 1984; Hing and associates, 1985) and numerous articles reporting series that include upper extremity patients (Harii, Ohmori, and Ohmori, 1974; Sharzer and associates, 1975; Ohmori and Harii, 1975; Morrison, O'Brien, and MacLeod, 1978; Harii, Yamada, and Torii, 1980; Dessapt and associates, 1981; Shaw, 1983). Nevertheless, the use of free flap transfers to obtain skin coverage in the upper extremity has failed to become standard, and remained controversial.

Free tissue transfers to the upper extremity have been of two types: (1) those to obtain soft tissue coverage and (2) those to restore functional deficits. The latter category includes such procedures as free muscle transfer; free transfer of vascularized tendon, nerve, or bone; and neurovascular transfer of sensate skin islands. These procedures have enabled the surgeon to restore function so satisfactorily that there is very little disagreement about their value (see Chaps. 95, 112, 115, and 125). Rather, it is in the former category, the provision of soft tissue coverage, that the use of free flap transfer remains controversial. It is to that group that this chapter is addressed.

GENERAL CONSIDERATIONS

Indications for Flap Coverage

General indications for flap coverage in the upper extremity are covered in detail elsewhere in the text and are reviewed only briefly here. Flap coverage is required when vital structures such as vessels, nerves, tendons, or bone are exposed. Often, flaps are necessary if secondary surgery (e.g., bone grafts, nerve grafts, tendon transfers) is to be performed. Finally, in chronic situations in which scarred or damaged skin prevents a satisfactory functional recovery, the injured area may need to be replaced with healthy, supple flap skin.

Advantages and Disadvantages of Free Flap Transfer

In the early years following the first successful free flap transfers, the graft survival rate in large, published series was approximately 80 per cent. At that time this rate was considerably less than that obtained using standard techniques of pedicle flap transfer. Furthermore, the procedures were very time-consuming, and although the second and third stages of the operation were often eliminated, the lengthy operative time was a problem. As experience has been gained with the technique, the success rate has risen considerably; it is now in the range of 90 per cent, and in experienced hands approaches the success rate of pedicle techniques (Serafin, Georgiade, and Smith, 1977; Daniel and May, 1978).

There are several specific advantages to the technique of free flap transfer. Coverage is complete in a single operation, avoiding the prolonged associated morbidity while the extremity is attached to an abdominal or groin flap. Furthermore, since attachment to a distant site is not necessary, the extremity may be elevated, edema reduced, and early motion begun. In the pedicle technique, the extremity is frequently dependent, and range of motion therapy can be applied only in limited fashion, if at all.

The free flap brings its own blood supply to the damaged area rather than acting as a parasite of the local tissue, as is the case with a pedicle flap. This property is particularly useful in a situation in which one of the main vessels in the extremity may have been destroyed distally, but may be used proximally as the recipient vessel for a free flap.

Many of the early free flaps were quite bulky and esthetically unsatisfactory compared with pedicle flaps, in which it was possible to obtain thin skin coverage from the outset. This situation has changed with the use of new flap donor sites, described later in this chapter.

Arteriography

Arteriography is rarely, if ever, necessary to evaluate the donor site. At the recipient site, however, its use is almost routine. Because of the variations in the vasculature of the upper extremity, it is important to know precisely which vessels are present and what they supply before proceeding with the free flap: e.g., the configuration of the palmar arch, and whether there are any connections between the radial and ulnar circulation, may determine which vessel is chosen, whether end to end or end to side arterial anastomosis is used, and which vessels may and may not be sacrificed. It has been the author's experience that the quality of the vessels cannot be determined by arteriography. The technique merely determines their presence, patency, and anatomic configuration.

The timing of arteriography in relation to flap transfer is of no consequence. In the acute situation the author has performed arteriography immediately before the transfer without adverse effect; in chronic situations arteriography has been performed at any time from the day before surgery to several months before operation without any problems related to the arteriogram.

Primary versus Delayed Coverage of Acute Wounds

The issue of primary versus delayed coverage of contaminated, traumatic wounds is controversial, and although there is a more complete discussion of the subject elsewhere in the text (see Chap. 90), several points

tages: a good color match to the skin of the hand, its thinness, and the potential for use as a composite flap with nerve, bone, or tendon. However, the procedure leaves a visible scar because the donor site usually needs to be grafted. This grafted area may later be converted to a linear scar through the use of soft tissue expansion.

This flap, if used as a local flap, may result in a steal syndrome, since it requires sacrifice of a major artery of the hand and possibly the need to reconstitute the circulation with a vein graft. For the vast majority of reconstructive needs in the hand, it is not the technique of choice.

Anatomy

The radial forearm flap (Fig. 98–10) is supplied by the radial artery, which, in the lower forearm, is located between the tendons

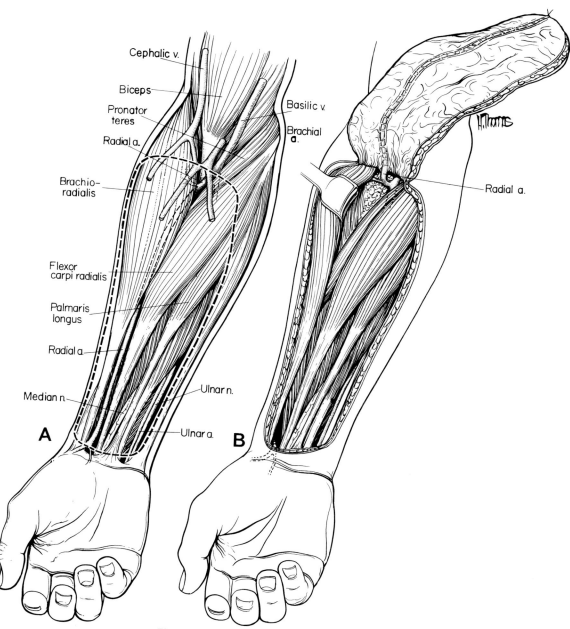

Figure 98–10. Radial artery forearm flap anatomy.

of the flexor carpi radialis and the brachio-radialis. Many cutaneous branches arise from the radial artery, supplying the skin of the lower forearm and anastomosing with the cutaneous branches of the ulnar and inter-osseous arteries. It is thought by some authors that lengths of the radial artery may be removed without affecting circulation to the hand as long as the ulnar artery is intact. The venous drainage of the flap is through the cephalic and radial veins.

Operative Technique

An Allen test or Doppler probe is used to assess the radial and ulnar circulation to the hand before embarking on this procedure. The course of the radial artery is marked on the forearm, and the flap is designed to over-lie it. Under tourniquet control the skin is incised down to the level of the fascia, and the cephalic vein and radial artery are divided at the distal end of the flap. Care is taken to preserve the superficial branch of the radial nerve. Dissecting in the plane between the deep fascia and muscle fascia, the flap is elevated, leaving behind the peri-tendinous tissue. After continuing to the flexor carpi radialis and brachioradialis tendons, the pedicle is dissected as far proximally as necessary. The tourniquet is released, and the flap and its pedicle are assessed for circulation. A split-thickness skin graft is used to close the donor site.

LATISSIMUS DORSI FLAP

Musculocutaneous flaps such as the latis-simus dorsi provide good skin coverage. These flaps, however, are quite thick, and even though the muscular component atrophies with time it is recommended for coverage of the forearm only. The flap is based on the thoracodorsal artery, which supplies a large cutaneous territory via the musculocutaneous perforators. If the latissimus flap is used as a muscle flap with skin graft, it may be har-vested through a small incision in the axilla, leaving a relatively hidden scar. The latissi-mus dorsi flap has been described by Mathes and Vasconez (1982), Bailey and Godfrey (1982), and Maxwell and associates (1978, 1979). A serratus anterior flap, composed of neighboring muscle, has also been described (Takayanagi and Tsukie, 1981).

Anatomy

The thoracodorsal artery, which provides the blood supply to the latissimus dorsi flap, is derived from the subscapular artery, the largest branch of the axillary artery. Running along the posterior axilla for 8 to 14 cm before entering the latissimus dorsi, the thoracodor-sal artery gives off one or two branches to the serratus anterior muscle and sometimes a cutaneous branch. A thoracodorsal nerve and a thoracodorsal vein (or, more rarely, veins) accompany the artery.

Operative Technique

Muscle location is defined preoperatively by having the patient place a hand on the hip and exerting pressure, outlining the an-terior border of the muscle. Skin paddles can be designed over the entire latissimus dorsi muscle or any part of it.

An incision is made from the axilla distally, cutting around the proposed skin island, if one is to be used. The skin is then elevated off the latissimus dorsi muscle medially and laterally. Sutures to anchor the skin paddle to the muscle fascia are helpful. The latissi-mus dorsi is then separated anteriorly from the serratus anterior, and the plane deep to the muscle dissected bluntly. The iliac origin of the latissimus dorsi is divided distally to the skin island, and the vertebral origin di-vided medially. The muscle is elevated off the chest wall and retracted cephalad, and the thoracodorsal artery is identified. The vas-cular pedicle is dissected into the axilla, di-viding small arterial and venous branches along the way. A pedicle length of up to 8 to 12 cm may be isolated, and the caliber of the artery may range from 1.5 to 2.5 mm. After complete mobilization of the pedicle, the in-sertion is divided. Division of the thoracodor-sal artery and vein completes the elevation of the flap.

Primary closure of the donor site is usually possible and suction drainage is mandatory.

GRACILIS FLAP

The gracilis flap is a musculocutaneous flap based on the profunda femoris artery. It is somewhat thick, making it undesirable for coverage in the hand but acceptable for cov-erage of large defects in the forearm. Its most important application in the upper extremity is its transfer as a functioning muscle-tendon unit. Its use in this manner is discussed in Chapter 115.

POSTERIOR CALF FASCIOCUTANEOUS FLAP

Described by Walton and Bunkis (1984), the posterior calf fasciocutaneous flap was developed as an alternative choice to the more commonly used groin and dorsalis pedis flaps. Although successfully accomplishing recipient site repair, this flap produces a visible donor site scar. The anatomy is variable and the donor arteries are of small caliber.

CONCLUSION

Use of free flaps for coverage problems in the upper extremity has limited application. The advantages include the single operation to obtain wound closure, the possibility of extremity elevation during recovery, and earlier rehabilitative therapy. The disadvantages are the added risk of flap loss and the technical difficulty of the procedure. Many possible donor sites for free flaps have been discussed. For defects in the hand, temporoparietal fascia with a skin graft or dorsalis pedis flap are the two procedures of choice. For forearm defects many good flaps are available including the groin flap, the scapular and parascapular flaps, and the latissimus dorsi flap. Several flaps from the upper extremity (including the medial and lateral arm and forearm) and lower extremity (calf) may be taken as fascia only and skin grafted. More experience is necessary with this technique to evaluate its proper role.

REFERENCES

Bailey, B. N., and Godfrey, A. M.: Latissimus dorsi muscle flaps. Br. J. Plast. Surg., *37*:47, 1982.

Budo, J., Finucan, T., and Clarke, J.: The inner arm fasciocutaneous flap. Plast. Reconstr. Surg., *73*:629, 1984.

Buncke, H. J.: Aesthetic aspects of hand surgery. Clin. Plast. Surg., *8*:349, 1985.

Chang, T. S., Wang, W., and Hsu, C. Y.: The free forearm flap—a report of 25 cases. Ann. Acad. Med. Singapore, *11*:236, 1982.

Chase, R. A.: Presidential address: The development of tissue transfer in hand surgery. J. Hand Surg., *9*:463, 1984.

Cormack, G. C., and Lamberty, B. G.: Fasciocutaneous vessels in the upper arm: application to the design of new fasciocutaneous flaps. Plast. Reconstr. Surg., *74*:244, 1984.

Daniel, R. K., and Faibisoff, B.: Free flap transfers for upper extremity reconstruction. Ann. Acad. Med., *8*:440, 1979.

Daniel, R. K., and May, J. W., Jr.: Free flaps: An overview. Clin. Orthop., *133*:122, 1978.

Daniel, R. K., and Taylor, I. G.: Distant transfer of an island flap by microvascular anastomoses. Plast. Reconstr. Surg., *52*:111, 1973.

Daniel, R. K., Terzis, J., and Midgley, R. D.: Restoration of sensation to an anesthetic hand by a free neurovascular flap from the foot. Plast. Reconstr. Surg., *57*:275, 1976.

Daniel, R. K., and Weiland, A. J.: Free tissue transfers from upper arm reconstruction. J. Hand Surg., *7*:66, 1982.

Dessapt, B., Saucier, T., Botta, Y., and Masson, C. L.: Microneurovascular free flaps. Int. Surg., *66*:23, 1981.

Dolmans, S., Guimerteau, J. C., et al.: The upper arm flap. J. Microsurg., *1*:162, 1979.

dos Santos, L. F.: The vascular anatomy and dissection of the free scapular flap. Plast. Reconstr. Surg., *73*:599, 1984.

Emerson, D. J., Sprigg, A., and Page, R. E.: Some observations on the radial artery island flap. Br. J. Plast. Surg., *38*:107, 1985.

Foucher, G., van Genechten, F., Merle, N., and Michon, J.: A compound radial artery forearm flap in hand surgery: an original modification of the Chinese forearm flap. Br. J. Plast. Surg., *37*:139, 1984.

Gilbert, A., and Teot, L.: The free scapular flap. Plast. Reconstr. Surg., *69*:601, 1982.

Gilbert, D. A.: An overview of flaps for hand and forearm reconstruction. Clin. Plast. Surg., *8*:129, 1981.

Godina, M.: Preferential use of end-to-side anastomoses in free flap transfers. Plast. Reconstr. Surg., *64*:673, 1979.

Harii, K., Ohmori, K., and Ohmori, S.: Successful clinical transfer of ten free flaps by microvascular anastomoses. Plast. Reconstr. Surg., *53*:259, 1974.

Harii, K., Yamada, A., and Torii, S.: Recent advances in flap coverage. Clin. Plast. Surg., *7*:495, 1980.

Hentz, V. R., Pearl, R. M., and Kaplan, E. N.: Use of the medial upper arm skin as an arterialised flap. Hand, *12*:241, 1980.

Hing, D. N., Buncke, H. J., Alpert, B. S., and Gordon, L.: Free flap coverage of the hand. Hand Clin., *1*:741, 1985.

Ikuta, Y., Watari, S., Kawamura, K., et al.: Free flap transfers by end-to-side arterial anastomosis. Br. J. Plast. Surg., *28*:1, 1975.

Kaplan, E. N., and Pearl, R. M.: An arterial medial arm flap—vascular anatomy and clinical applications. Ann. Plast. Surg., *4*:205, 1980.

Katsaros, J., Schusterman, M., Beppu, M., Banis, J. C., Jr., and Acland, R. D.: The lateral upper arm flap: anatomy and clinical applications. Ann. Plast. Surg., *12*:489, 1984.

MacGregor, I. A., and Jackson, I. T.: The groin flap. Br. J. Plast. Surg., *25*:3, 1972.

Man, D., and Acland, R. D.: The microarterial anatomy of the dorsalis pedis flap and its clinical applications. Plast. Reconstr. Surg., *65*:409, 1980.

Mathes, S. J., and Vasconez, L. O.: Free flaps (including toe transplantation). *In* Green, D. P. (Ed.): Operative Hand Surgery. Edinburgh, Churchill Livingstone, 1982.

Maxwell, G. P., Manson, P. N., and Hoopes, J. E.: Experience with thirteen latissimus dorsi myocutaneous free flaps. Plast. Reconstr. Surg., 64:1, 1979.

Maxwell, G. P., Stueber, K., and Hoopes, J. E.: A free latissimus dorsi myocutaneous flap: case report. Plast. Reconstr. Surg., 62:462, 1978.

May, J. W., Jr., Chait, L. A., Cohen, B. E., and O'Brien, B. M.: Free neurovascular flap from the first web of the foot in hand reconstruction. J. Hand Surg., 2:387, 1977.

May, J. W., Jr., Lukash, F. N., Gallico, G. G., III: Latissimus dorsi free muscle flap in lower extremity reconstruction. Case report. Plast. Reconstr. Surg., 68:603, 1981.

McCraw, J. B., and Furlow, L. T., Jr.: The dorsalis pedis arterialized flap. A clinical study. Plast. Reconstr. Surg., 55:177, 1975.

Morrison, W. A., O'Brien, B. M., and MacLeod, A.: Clinical experiences in free flap transfer. Clin. Orthop., 133:139, 1978.

Morrison, W. A., O'Brien, B. M., MacLeod, A., and Gilbert, A.: Neurovascular free flaps from the foot for innervation of the hand. J. Hand Surg., 3:235, 1978.

Nassif, T. M., Vidal, L., Bovet, J. L., and Baudet, J.: The parascapular flap: a new cutaneous microsurgical free flap. Plast. Reconstr. Surg., 69:591, 1982.

O'Brien, B. McC.: Microvascular Reconstructive Surgery. Edinburgh, Churchill Livingstone, 1977.

O'Brien, B. McC., and Shanmugan, N.: Experimental transfer of composite free flaps with microvascular anastomosis. Aust. N.Z. J. Surg., 43:285, 1973.

Ohmori, K., and Harii, K.: Free groin flaps: their vascular basis. Br. J. Plast. Surg., 28:238, 1975.

Ohmori, K., and Harii, K.: Free dorsalis pedis sensory flap to the hand, with microneurovascular anastomoses. Plast. Reconstr. Surg., 58:546, 1976.

Olson, R. M., Wood, M. B., and Irons, G. B.: Microvascular free-flap coverage of mechanical injuries to the upper extremity. Am. J. Surg., 144:593, 1982.

Robinson, D. W.: Microsurgical transfer of the dorsalis pedis neurovascular island flap. Br. J. Plast. Surg., 29:209, 1976.

Serafin, D., Georgiade, N. G., and Smith, D. H.: Comparison of free flaps with pedicled flaps for coverage of defects of the leg or foot. Plast. Reconstr. Surg., 59:492, 1977.

Shah, K. G., Garrett, J. C., and Buncke, H. J.: Free groin flap transfer to the upper extremity. Hand, 11:315, 1979.

Sharzer, L. A., Barker, D. T., and Adamson, J. E.: Free composite tissue transfer in the upper extremity. In Serafin, D., and Buncke, H. J., Jr. (Eds.): Microsurgical Composite Tissue Transplantation. St. Louis, C. V. Mosby Company, 1978.

Sharzer, L. A., O'Brien, B. M., Horton, C. L., et al.: Clinical applications of free flap transfer in the burn patient. J. Trauma, 15:766, 1975.

Shaw, W. W.: Microvascular free flaps: the first decade. Clin. Plast. Surg., 10:3, 1983.

Smith, P. J., Foley, B., McGregor, I. A., et al.: The anatomical basis of the groin flap. Plast. Reconstr. Surg., 49:41, 1972.

Song, R., Song, Y., Yu, Y., and Song, Y.: The upper arm free flap. Clin. Plast. Surg., 9:27, 1982.

Soutar, D. S., and Tanner, N. S.: The radial artery forearm flap. Br. J. Plast. Surg., 37:18, 1984.

Stevenson, T. R., Hester, T. R., Duus, E. C., and Dingman, R. O.: The superficial inferior epigastric artery arm flap for coverage of hand and forearm defects. Ann. Plast. Surg., 12:333, 1984.

Takayanagi, S., and Tsukie, T.: Free serratus anterior muscle and myocutaneous flaps. Ann. Plast. Surg., 8:277, 1981.

Taylor, G. I., and Townsend, P.: Composite free flap and tendon transfer: an anatomic study and clinical technique. Br. J. Plast. Surg., 32:170, 1979.

Upton, J., Rogers, C., Durham-Smith, G., and Swartz, W. M.: Clinical applications of temporoparietal flaps in hand reconstruction. J. Hand Surg., 11A:475, 1986.

Vila-Rovira, R., Ferreira, B. J., and Guinot, A.: Transfer of vascularized extensor tendons from the foot to the hand with a dorsalis pedis flap. Plast. Reconstr. Surg., 76:421, 1985.

Walton, R. L., and Bunkis, J.: The posterior calf fasciocutaneous free flap. Plast. Reconstr. Surg., 74:76, July 1984.

Wood, M. B., Cooney, W. P., III, and Irons, G. B., Jr.: Upper extremity reconstruction by free tissue transfer. Minn. Med., 66:503, 1983.

Wood, M. B., and Irons, G. B.: Upper-extremity free skin flap transfer: results and utility as compared with distant pedicle skin flaps. Ann. Plast. Surg., 11:523, 1983.

Yang, G., Baoqui, C., and Yuzhi, G.: Free forearm skin transplantation. Natl. Med. J. China, 61:139, 1981.

99

Robert C. Russell

Fingertip Injuries

The hand, more than any other organ system, enables us to manipulate and control our environment. From the dawn of human existence, man's place on earth has been hand carved. Primitive man fashioned weapons and later tools by hand. Through the centuries art, literature, music, and science have been drawn, written, composed, and discovered by hand. Civilizations have been created, destroyed, and rebuilt by human hands. We are a product of our hand function, and when hand injuries occur, the quality of human life is altered.

Approximately one-third of all traumatic injuries in the United States involve the upper extremities (Kelsey and associates, 1980). The fingertips are the terminal extensions of the hand and are the part most frequently injured. Exact statistics on the number of fingertip injuries in the United States are not available. However, there are an estimated 6 million emergency room visits and another 12 million physicians' office visits for upper extremity injuries each year. Approximately 90 million days of restricted activity and 16 million days lost from work are due to hand injuries annually. The yearly cost to American society for all upper extremity problems, including time lost from work, is approximately 10 billion dollars.

Fingertip injuries occur in patients of all ages from infants in neonatal nurseries to nursing home residents. The choice of surgical treatment must be made after considering many factors. The patient's age, occupation, sex, and hand dominance, as well as the mechanism of injury, associated medical problems, and anticipated future hand use, must be considered in choosing any type of reconstruction. Successful repair of fingertip injuries requires a knowledge of anatomy and the techniques of reconstruction, and sound surgical judgment.

ANATOMY

The skin of the fingertip and palm is stabilized for pinch and grasp by a specialized layer of thick, cornified, stratified, squamous epithelium that becomes thicker with use (Barron, 1970). A series of ridges and grooves uniquely patterned to each individual are visible as fingerprints. They help to stabilize pinch and grasp, creating a textured, nonslip surface. Numerous fibrous septa, including Clelland's and Grayson's ligaments, connect the volar digital skin to the underlying bone and tendon sheath, further stabilizing pinch and grasp (Figs. 99–1, 99–2) (Jones, 1942; Johnson and Cohen, 1975). The subcutaneous tissue between fibrous septa transmits the

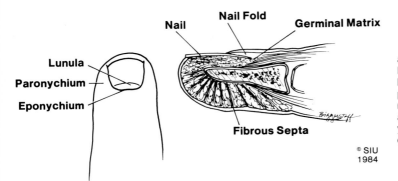

Figure 99–1. The nail bed is closely adherent to the underlying distal phalanx while numerous fibrous septa stabilize the volar fingertip skin during pinch. The nail originates from the germinal matrix in the base of the nail fold, and is bordered proximally by the eponychium and laterally by the paronychium.

digital arteries and nerves. Dorsal hand skin is thinner and loosely adherent, with little subcutaneous tissue, and is more easily avulsed or injured in severe hand trauma.

The fingernail is a specialized epidermal structure like hair, originating from the germinal matrix in the base of the nail fold (Zook and associates, 1980b) (Fig. 99–1). The nail grows out along the nail bed as a single unit with the bed and, at its interface, is thickened as the nail grows distally. The deep surface of the nail bed is closely adherent to the periosteum of the distal phalanx, with very little subcutaneous tissue. The lunula is the white semicircle at the base of the nail. The eponychium or cuticle is the epidermal shelf at the base of the nail; the paronychium is the skin surrounding the nail. The perionychium includes the entire complex of nail, nail bed (sterile and germinal matrix), and surrounding paronychium.

The fingertip is the end organ for touch

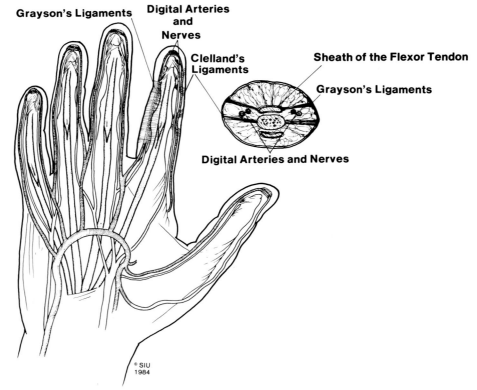

Figure 99–2. Bilateral digital arteries and nerves course between dorsal Clelland's and volar Grayson's ligaments. Digital nerves course volar to arteries in the digit, but reverse in the palm to lie dorsal to the common digital vessels.

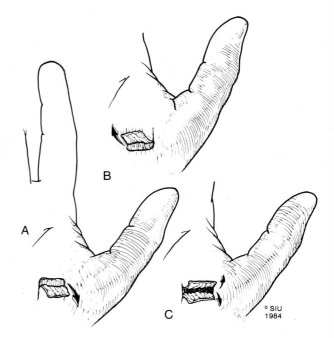

Figure 99–19. Thenar flaps including skin and subcutaneous tissue from over the thenar eminence can be based *(A)* proximally, *(B)* distally, or *(C)* both, depending on the orientation of the fingertip defect. The donor site is skin grafted or closed primarily.

(Fig. 99–20*B*). Less flexion of the injured digit is required than with a standard thenar flap (Fig. 99–20*C*).

Division and inset is accomplished after 14 to 21 days, and immediate active range of motion exercises of both the digit and the thumb are initiated. Stretching of the thumb skin occurs with use, and full extension is normally regained. Residual digital stiffness is a possible complication of all thenar flap techniques, which are best used in children or young adults with supple digits.

The 13 year old child pictured in Figure 99–21 sustained dorsally directed index and long fingertip amputations with exposed distal phalanges. The tip defects were closed with a thenar crease and a side finger flap, with the donor sites closed primarily (Fig. 99–21*B*). One year later the fingertips show good contour with no visible donor site deformity (Fig. 21*C,D*).

DORSAL DIGITAL INJURIES

Dorsal digital avulsion injuries involving multiple fingers with exposed tendon or bone stripped of perivascular connective tissue, or

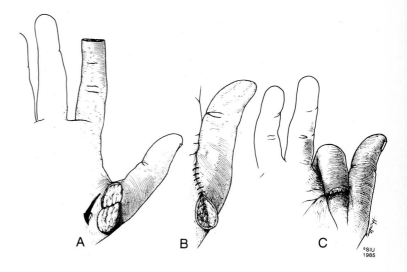

Figure 99–20. Thenar crease flap. *A,* A modified thenar flap is radially based and elevated from the metacarpophalangeal joint flexion crease of the thumb. *B,* The donor site is closed primarily by flexing the thumb. *C,* The fingertip is flexed into the flap.

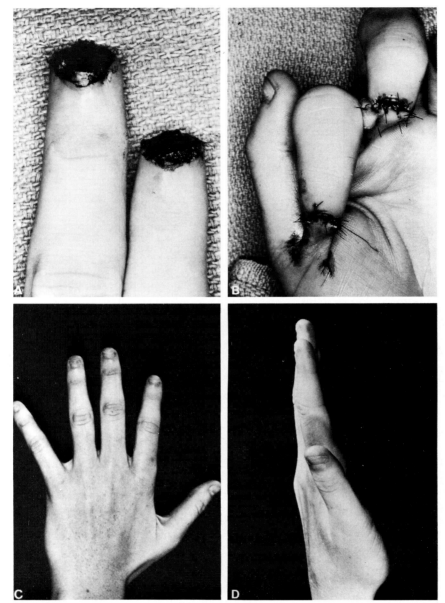

Figure 99–21. Thenar/side finger flaps. *A,* Dorsally directed index and long fingertip amputations in 13 year old girl. *B,* The tip defects covered with a thenar crease and a side finger flap. *C,* No donor site deformity is visible on the dorsum of the hand. *D,* Good fingertip contour has been sutured.

with open joint surfaces, cannot be covered by a skin graft. When large areas of dorsal loss have occurred, a distant pedicle flap from the chest (Chase, 1973), abdomen (Milford, 1971), groin (McGregor and Jackson, 1972), or opposite arm (Smith and Furnas, 1976; Dolich, Olshansky, and Barbar, 1978) can be used to cover the entire defect. The flap is elevated usually at the level of the deep muscle fascia and sutured to the cut skin edges of the digital defects. A temporary syndactyly is normally created between digits before flap coverage, to obtain a totally closed wound. The syndactyly is released after dividing and insetting the flap at a third operative procedure. The disadvantages of distant flap coverage include prolonged hand and extremity immobilization, bulkiness of the

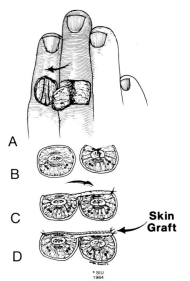

Figure 99–22. Upside-down cross finger flap. *A,* A dorsal digital defect with exposed tendon or joint surfaces. *B,* A standard cross finger flap is deeply deepithelized with a scalpel. *C,* The flap is elevated and turned 180 degrees upside down over the dorsal defect of the adjacent finger. *D,* The donor site and the undersurface of the flap are skin grafted.

and most expeditious method of wound coverage for large dorsal hand and/or multiple finger defects. Two types of alternative hand flaps can also be used to cover less extensive dorsal digital avulsion injuries, or in special circumstances when adjacent fingers are not available as donor sites.

Upside-Down Cross Finger Flap. A modification of the standard cross finger flap (Pakiam, 1978; Russell and associates, 1981) used to cover small dorsal digital avulsion injuries that cannot be grafted is the deepithelized upside-down cross finger flap (Fig. 99–22). A standard cross finger flap from the dorsum of the middle phalanx of an adjoining finger is outlined and deeply deepithelized with a scalpel. The flap is elevated in the standard fashion but turned over 180 degrees like a book page to cover the dorsal defect of the injured finger. The donor defect and the undersurface of the upside-down flap are covered with a thick split-thickness skin graft and stent dressing. The technique does not minimize donor site deformity but does provide skin and subcutaneous tissue cover for a single finger in a simple fashion, eliminating the whole extremity immobilization required for a distant flap. Deep dermal deepithelization must be carried out to prevent later epidermal inclusion cyst formation. The

flap, digital and/or extremity stiffness, multiple surgical procedures, and poor return of flap sensibility. Despite these limitations, distant pedicle flaps may still offer the safest

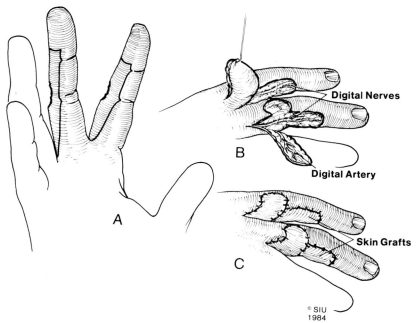

Figure 99–23. Arterialized side finger flap. *A,* Dorsal digital defects over the proximal interphalangeal joints of the long and index fingers. Arterialized side finger flaps are drawn to just past the distal interphalangeal joint flexion crease and darted to prevent a straight midline scar. *B,* The flaps elevated to include the digital artery but sparing the digital nerve. *C,* The flaps turned dorsally over the proximal interphalangeal joint, with the donor sites skin grafted.

complications described with this procedure include incomplete skin graft take, a noticeable donor site deformity, digital stiffness, and inclusion cyst formation. The technique is best utilized for small defects of a single digit requiring full-thickness cover that would otherwise necessitate a distant pedicle flap.

Arterialized Side Finger Flap. An alternative flap that can also be used to cover the dorsal proximal interphalangeal joint, when adjacent digits are not available as donor sites for cross finger flaps, is the arterialized side finger flap (Russell and associates, 1981) (Fig. 99–23). Localized trauma can cause disruption of soft tissue over the proximal interphalangeal joints of adjacent digits, or can result after breakdown of a previously placed dorsal skin graft in the healed burned hand. In such cases, adjacent fingers are not usually available as donor sites but flap coverage is still required. An arterialized side finger flap from the lateral volar surface of the injured digit can be used to avoid distant flap coverage.

The flap is outlined on the lateral volar nondominant side of the digit from just distal to the distal interphalangeal joint flexion crease to the web space proximally (Fig. 99–23A). The volar incision is darted at the interphalangeal joint flexion creases to prevent a midline volar scar. The flap is elevated to include a digital artery but spares the digital nerve, which is left intact (Fig. 99–23B). All superficial veins in the base of the flap are preserved. The flap is then rotated dorsally to cover the dorsal digital defect, and the donor site is covered with a full-thickness skin graft from the groin with a stent dressing (Fig. 99–23C). Tip sensibility is not disturbed by this technique and the skin graft becomes reinnervated. A digital Allen test or Doppler examination to determine the patency of both digital arteries is necessary before the transfer. The flap has excellent vascularity and can be reelevated at a later date for extensor tendon reconstruction. Rose (1983) successfully modified the technique by elevating digital soft tissue on a single digital artery and venae comitantes as an island flap for coverage of more proximal defects.

SUMMARY

Fingertip injuries are the most common type of upper extremity trauma. Injuries oc-

cur to patients of all ages but are most often seen in working men. All patients should be evaluated on an individual basis considering their overall physical condition, the medical history, the etiology and time of injury, and the anticipated future hand use. The type and timing of fingertip reconstruction must be planned accordingly. The ideal reconstruction should be stable during use, sensible but pain free to touch and pressure, and durable enough for strenuous hand activity. The patient's anticipated future functional use of the injured digit and the entire extremity is the guiding consideration in choosing any type of reconstruction.

For further information on innervated free flaps and soft tissue reconstruction of the thumb, see Chapters 112 and 122.

REFERENCES

Ashbell, T. S., Kleinert, H. E., Putcha, S. M., and Kutz, J. E.: The deformed fingernail, a frequent result of failure to repair nail bed injuries. J. Trauma, 7:177, 1967.

Atasoy, E., Ioakimidis, E., Kasdan, M. L., Kutz, J. E., and Kleinert, H. E.: Reconstruction of the amputated finger tip with a triangular volar flap—a new surgical procedure. J. Bone Joint Surg., 52A:921, 1970.

Barron, J. N.: The structure and function of the skin of the hand. Hand, 2:93, 1970.

Barton, N. J.: A modified thenar flap. Hand, 7:150, 1975.

Beasley, R. W.: Principles and techniques of resurfacing operations for hand surgery. Surg. Clin. North Am., 47:389, 1967.

Bennett, J. E.: Upper arm tourniquet tolerance in unanesthetized adults. Surg. Forum, 15:463, 1964.

Bennett, J. E., and Mohler, L.: Arm tourniquet tolerance in unanesthetized adults. Surg. Forum, 15:463, 1964.

Bojsen-Moller, J., Pers, M., and Schmidt, A.: Finger tip injuries: late results. Acta Chir. Scand., 122:177, 1961.

Bossley, C. J.: Conservative treatment of digit amputations. N.Z. Med. J., 82:379, 1975.

Chase, R. A.: Early salvage in acute hand injuries with a primary island flap. Plast. Reconstr. Surg., 48:521, 1971.

Chase, R. A.: Atlas of Hand Surgery. Vol. 1. Philadelphia, W. B. Saunders Company, 1973.

Cohen, B. E., and Cronin, E. D.: An innervated cross-finger flap for fingertip reconstruction. Plast. Reconstr. Surg., 72:688, 1983.

Cronin, T. D.: The cross-finger flap—a new method of repair. Am. Surg., 17:419, 1951.

Curtis, R. M.: Cross-finger pedicle flap in hand surgery. Ann. Surg., 145:650, 1957.

Das, S. K., and Brown, H. G.: Management of lost finger tips in children. Hand, 10:16, 1978.

Dellon, A. L.: Evaluation of Sensibility and Reduction of Sensation in the Hand. Baltimore, Williams & Wilkins Company, 1981.

Dolich, B. H., Olshansky, K. J., and Barbar, A. H.: Use of a cross-forearm neurocutaneous flap to provide sensation and coverage in hand reconstruction. Plast. Reconstr. Surg., 62:550, 1978.

Douglas, B. S.: Conservative management of guillotine amputation of the finger in children. Aust. Paediatr. J., 8:86, 1972.

Fisher, R. H.: The Kutler method of repair of fingertip amputations. J. Bone Joint Surg., 49A:317, 1967.

Flatt, A. E.: The thenar flap. J. Bone Joint Surg., 39B:80, 1957.

Flatt, A. E.: The Care of Minor Hand Injuries. 3rd Ed. St. Louis, MO, C. V. Mosby Company, 1972, p. 137.

Frandsen, P. A.: V-Y plasty as treatment of finger tip amputations. Acta Orthop. Scand., 49:255, 1978.

Freiberg, A., and Manktelow, R.: The Kutler repair of finger tip amputations. Plast. Reconstr. Surg., 50:371, 1972.

Frykman, G. K.: Iatrogenic digital nerve compression. American Society for Surgery of the Hand Correspondence Club Newsletter, Nov. 1, 1979.

Gatewood: A plastic repair of finger defects without hospitalization. J.A.M.A., 87:1479, 1926.

Graham, W. P.: Incisions, amputations and skin grafting in the hand. Orthop. Clin. North Am., 1:213, 1970.

Gurdin, M., and Pangman, W. J.: The repair of surface defects of fingers by transdigital flaps. Plast. Reconstr. Surg., 5:368, 1950.

Haddad, R. J.: The Kutler repair of finger tip amputation. South Med. J., 61:1264, 1968.

Holm, A., and Zachariae, L.: Finger tip lesions: an evaluation of conservative treatment versus free skin grafting. Acta Orthop. Scand., 45:382, 1974.

Hoskins, H. D.: The versatile cross-finger pedicle flap—a report of twenty-six cases. J. Bone Joint Surg., 42A:261, 1960.

Hutchinson, J., Tough, J. S., and Wyburn, G. M.: Regeneration of sensation in grafted skin. Br. J. Plast. Surg., 2:82, 1949.

Illingworth, C. M.: Trapped fingers and amputated finger tips in children. J. Pediatr. Surg., 9:853, 1974.

Johnson, M. K., and Cohen, M. J.: The fingers. In The Hand Atlas. Springfield, IL, Charles C Thomas, 1975.

Johnson, R. K., and Iverson, R. E.: Cross finger pedicle flaps in the hand. J. Bone Joint Surg., 53A:913, 1971.

Jones, F. W.: The Principles of Anatomy as Seen in the Hand. 2nd Ed. London, Bailliere Tindall Cox, 1942.

Keim, H. A., and Grantham, S. A.: Volar-flap advancement for thumb and fingertip injuries. Clin. Orthop., 66:109, 1969.

Kelsey, J. L., Pastides, H., Kreiger, N., Harris, C., and Chernow, R. A.: Upper extremity disorders: a survey of their frequency and cost in the United States. St. Louis, MO, C. V. Mosby Company, 1980.

Kleinert, H. E.: Finger tip injuries and their management. Am. Surg. 25:41, 1959.

Kleinert, H. E., McAlister, C. G., McDonald, C. J., and Kutz, J. E.: A critical evaluation of cross-finger flaps. J. Trauma, 14:756, 1974.

Kutler, W.: A new method for finger tip amputation. J.A.M.A., 133:29, 1947.

Lie, K. K., Magargle, R. K., and Posch, J. L.: Free full thickness skin grafts from the palm to cover defects of the fingers. J. Bone Joint Surg., 52A:559, 1970.

Littler, J. W.: Neurovascular pedicle transfer of tissue in reconstructive surgery of the hand. J. Bone Joint Surg., 38A:917, 1956.

Louis, D., Palmer, A., and Burney, R.: Open treatment of digital tip injuries. J.A.M.A., 244:7, 1980.

Macht, S. D., and Watson, K. H.: The Moberg volar advancement flap for digital reconstruction. J. Hand Surg., 5:372, 1980.

Mandal, A. C.: Thiersch grafts for lesions of the finger tip. Acta Chir. Scand., 129:325, 1965.

McCash, C. R.: Free nail grafting. Br. J. Plast. Surg., 8:19, 1955.

McGregor, I. A., and Jackson, I. T.: The groin flap. Br. J. Plast. Surg., 25:3, 1972.

Micks, J. E., and Wilson, J. N.: Full thickness sole-skin grafts for resurfacing the hand. J. Bone Joint Surg., 49A:1128, 1967.

Milford, L.: The hand. In Crenshaw, E. H. (Ed.): Campbell's Operative Orthopaedics. St. Louis, MO, C. V. Mosby Company, 1971.

Miller, A. J.: Single fingertip injuries treated by thenar flap. Hand, 6:311, 1974.

Moberg, E.: Aspects of sensation in reconstructive surgery of the upper extremity. J. Bone Joint Surg., 46A:817, 1964.

Moynihan, F. J.: Long-term results of split-skin grafting in finger-tip injuries. Br. Med. J., 5255:802, 1961.

Napier, J. R.: The return of pain sensibility in full thickness skin grafts. Brain, 75:147, 1952.

O'Brien, B.: Neurovascular island pedicle flaps for terminal amputations and digital scars. Br. J. Plast. Surg., 21:258, 1968.

O'Malley, T. S.: Full thickness skin grafts in finger amputation. Wis. Med. J., 33:337, 1934.

Pakiam, A. I.: The reversed dermis flap. Br. J. Plast. Surg., 31:131, 1978.

Patton, H. S.: Split skin graft from the hypothenar area for fingertip avulsions. Plast. Reconstr. Surg., 43:426, 1969.

Ponten, B.: Grafted skin, observations on innervation and other qualities. Acta Chir. Scand. Suppl., 257:1, 1960.

Porter, R. W.: Functional assessment of transplanted skin in volar defects of the digits. A comparison between free grafts and flaps. J. Bone Joint Surg., 50A:955, 1968.

Posner, M. A., and Smith, R. J.: The advancement pedicle flap for thumb injuries. J. Bone Joint Surg., 53A:1618, 1971.

Quilliam, T. A., and Ridley, A.: The receptor community in the finger tip. J. Physiol., 216:15P, 1971.

Reed, J. V., and Harcourt, A. K.: Immediate full thickness grafts to finger tips. Surg. Gynecol. Obstet., 68:925, 1939.

Ridley, A.: A biopsy study of the innervation of forearm skin grafted to the finger tip. Brain, 93:547, 1970.

Rose, E. H.: Local arterialized island flap coverage of difficult hand defects preserving donor digit sensibility. Plast. Reconstr. Surg., 72:848, 1983.

Russell, R. C., VanBeek, A. L., Wavak, P., and Zook, E. G.: Alternative hand flaps for amputations and digital defects. J. Hand Surg., 6:399, 1981.

Saito, H.: Free nailbed graft for treatment of nailbed injuries of the hand. J. Hand Surg., 8:171, 1983.

Salaman, J. R.: Partial thickness skin grafting of finger tip injuries. Lancet, 1:705, 1967.

Santoni-Rugiu, P.: An experimental study on the reinnervation of free skin grafts and pedicle flaps. Plast. Reconstr. Surg., 38:98, 1966.

Schenek, R. R., and Cheema, T. A.: Hypothenar skin grafts for fingertip reconstruction. J. Hand Surg., 9A:750, 1984.

Shaw, M. H.: Neurovascular island pedicled flaps for terminal digital scars—a hazard. Br. J. Plast. Surg., *24*:161, 1971.

Shepard, G. H.: Treatment of nail bed avulsions with split-thickness nail bed grafts. J. Hand Surg., *8*:49, 1983.

Showalter, J. T.: Results of replacement of finger tip tissue. Int. Surg., *50*:306, 1968.

Smith, R. C., and Furnas, D. W.: The hand sandwich. Plast. Reconstr. Surg., *57*:351, 1976.

Smith, R. J., and Albin, R.: Thenar "H-flap" for fingertip injuries. J Trauma, *16*:778, 1976.

Snow, J. W.: The use of a volar flap for repair of fingertip amputation: a preliminary report. Plast. Reconstr. Surg., *40*:163, 1967.

Sturman, M. J., and Duran, R. J.: The late results of finger tip injuries. J. Bone Joint Surg., *45A*:289, 1963.

Tempest, M. N.: Cross-finger flaps in the treatment of injuries to the finger tip. Plast. Reconstr. Surg., *9*:205, 1952.

Tranquilli-Leali, E.: Ricostruzione dell'apice delle falangi ungueali mediante autoplastica volare peduncolata per scorrimento. Infortun. Traum. Lav., *1*:186, 1935.

Wavak, P., and Zook, E. G.: A simple method of exsanguinating the finger prior to surgery. JACEP, 7:124, 1978.

Wilgis, E. F. S., and Maxwell, G. P.: Distal digital nerve grafts: clinical and anatomical studies. J. Hand Surg., *4*:439, 1979.

Wood, R. W.: Multiple cross finger flaps—"piggy back" techniques. Plast. Reconstr. Surg., *41*:54, 1968.

Woolf, R. M., and Broadbent, T. R.: Injuries to the fingertips: treatment with cross-finger flaps. Rocky Mt. Med. J., *64*:35, 1967.

Zadik, F. R.: Immediate skin grafting for traumatic amputation of finger tips. Lancet, *1*:335, 1943.

Zook, E. G., Guy, R. J., and Russell, R. C.: A study of nailbed injuries: causes, treatment, and prognosis. J. Hand Surg., *9*:247, 1984.

Zook, E. G., Miller, M., VanBeek, A. L., and Wavak, P.: Successful treatment protocol for canine fang injuries. J. Trauma, *20*:243, 1980a.

Zook, E. G., VanBeek, A. L., Russell, R. C., and Beatty, M. E.: Anatomy and physiology of the perionychium: a review of the literature and anatomic study. J. Hand Surg., *5*:528, 1980b.

Elvin G. Zook

Surgically Treatable Problems of the Perionychium

ANATOMY AND PHYSIOLOGY

Embryology

A mushroom-shaped plume of dorsal tissue develops on the dorsum of the finger at approximately 10 weeks of fetal life (Jones, 1941; Hanrahan, 1946; Lewis, 1954). It is made up of 10 to 12 layers of spindle-shaped, partially keratinized cells over an area of keratohyaline-like granule activity. At 12 weeks the nail fold develops by formation of a shallow depression in the skin on the dorsum of the finger. At 16 weeks the nail lays beneath a thin sheet of laminated keratin. By 20 weeks two identifiable layers of nail are present (Lewis, 1954). The overlying keratin sheath breaks down before normal ges-

tational birth and the nail is exposed to the environment.

Anatomy

A knowledge of the anatomy and physiology of the perionychium is an essential prerequisite for surgical care of this area. The literature includes a large array of varying terms for the same anatomic structures, which causes confusion in reporting and discussion (Hamrick, 1946; Hanrahan, 1946; McCash, 1955; Buncke and Gonzales, 1962; Horner and Cohen, 1966; Ashbell and associates, 1967; Tajima, 1974). A standard nomenclature is available and is used in this chapter (Zook and associates, 1980) (Fig. 100–1).

The perionychium consists of the nail, the nail bed (sterile and germinal matrix), and the surrounding paronychium. The proximal nail is enclosed in a pocket called the nail fold. The skin over the dorsal aspect of the nail fold is the nail wall, and the extension of the skin over the proximal nail is the eponychium. The nail root is a protrusion of cornified material between the eponychium and the nail, and is the portion pushed proximally with manicuring. The nail divides the nail fold into the dorsal roof and the ventral floor. The hyponychium is a mass of keratin between the ventral surface of the free edge of the nail and the epidermis of the tip. A large number of lymphocytes and other white cell components are present here and serve as a barrier against fungi and bacteria that would otherwise intrude beneath the nail.

The lunula is the white arc in the nail just distal to the eponychium. The white color is due to incompletely cornified nail cells and

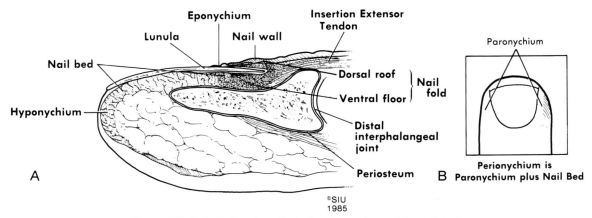

Figure 100–1. *A, B,* Drawings illustrating the anatomy of the nail bed.

retained keratohyaline granules in the nail cells, or variance of nail adherence and light reflection (Burrows, 1919; Jones, 1941; Pardo-Castello, 1960). The shape of the lunula varies from primate to primate, but as a rule has a shape similar to the distal border of the nail (Zias, 1980).

The proper volar digital artery crosses the distal interphalangeal joint in the midlateral line. It sends a branch dorsally to the nail fold, and after progressing a short distance sends a branch to the nail bed and one to the pad of the finger (Zook and associates, 1980). The branch to the side of the nail bed communicates with the branch to the nail fold in a network that supplies the paronychium. They join in primary arches parallel to the lunula and at the free edge of the nail (Samman, 1978). Blood sinuses are formed that are surrounded by muscle fibers and nonmedullated nerve fibers, forming a pulsatile glomus that plays a part in the regulation of blood pressure and flow to the extremity (Pardo-Castello, 1960).

The venous components of the nail bed coalesce proximal to the nail fold and remain very small distal to the distal interphalangeal joint level.

Near the free edge of the nail the lymphatics are more numerous than in any other dermal area of the body. This is the probable reason why, unless the hyponychium is softened by soaking or chemicals, subungual infections at the distal border of the nail are rare.

Dorsal branches of the paired proper digital nerves supply the nail bed and form a dense network of nerves around the vascular plexuses (Wilgis and Maxwell, 1979; Zook and associates, 1980).

Physiology

Three areas are involved in production of the nail (Lewis, 1954) (Fig. 100–2). The proximal half of the dorsal roof of the nail fold and the proximal portion of the fold produce

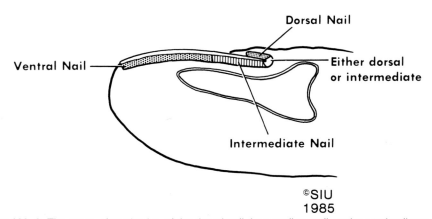

Figure 100–2. The areas of production of the dorsal nail, intermediate nail, and ventral nail are shown.

scribed by Barre and Masson in 1924. Proliferation of angiomatous tissue presses on the nerve plexuses, causing exquisite pain. The nail may also be tender to pressure and temperature changes. Examination of the nail may reveal a small bluish discoloration. The entire nail bed of the suspected finger must be examined carefully, because glomus tumors may be multiple.

Treatment consists of removal of the nail, identification of the glomus tumor or tumors, and tumor removal. If the glomus is in the sterile matrix and the defect cannot be closed primarily, a split-thickness nail bed graft from another portion of the involved fingernail or toenail bed can be used. A full-thickness sterile matrix graft from the toe may also be used, but this causes subsequent deformity of the toenail.

Cysts (see also Chap. 6). Inclusion cysts of the nail bed or distal phalanx, or enchondromas, cause progressive nail deformity and require radiography for diagnosis (Fig. 100–17A,B). Access to the cyst is usually best carried out through a "fishmouth" type of incision, elevating the nail bed from the underlying bone (Fig. 100–17C). Removal of the nail is necessary to allow the nail bed to assume a normal position after the cyst has been removed. The thin dorsal cortex is removed and the endochondroma or inclusion cyst curetted. The resultant cavity should be filled with medullary bone graft (Fig. 100–17D) to allow the replaced nail bed to lie flat and permit normal nail growth (Fig. 100–17E).

Nail cysts may occur after fingertip amputation when fragments of nail bed are trapped in the subcutaneous tissue, and may be painful or tender. Treatment consists of complete excision of the cyst and cyst wall.

Ganglions (see also Chap. 16). Cysts on the dorsum of the finger proximal to the nail have been called clear cysts, mucous cysts, and many other terms (Lewis, 1954; Pardo-Castello, 1960). Kleinert and associates (1972) reported a communication between the cysts and the DIP joint when microscopic dissection was used. They found the joint exit site of the ganglion in proximity to an osteoarthritic osteophyte.

When the cystic expansion of a ganglion is above the nail fold it causes elevation of the nail wall and pressure on the dorsum of the forming nail (Fig. 100–18). The nail may be grooved, thinned or roughened. When the expansion is between the floor of the nail fold and the periosteum, nail deformity is a localized upward ridge or curve, of the entire nail, or a ragged nail (Fig. 100–19).

Steroid injections have been recommended (Zias, 1980), but there is no reason why these should be more successful than they are with any ganglion. The author prefers a T-incision, with the body of the "T" in the transverse fold of the distal interphalangeal joint dorsally and the crossarm in the lateral line on the same side of the finger as the ganglion. If the ganglion is midline, the crossarm is placed on the base of the "T" on the opposite side, to create an "H." This allows excellent exposure of the entire joint. The cyst is dis-

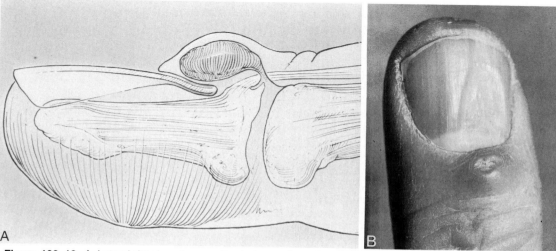

Figure 100–18. *A,* Lateral drawing of a ganglion between the nail wall and the dorsal roof of the nail fold. *B,* Clinical picture of the deformity frequently caused by this ganglion location.

Figure 100–19. *A,* Illustration of the ganglion dissecting beneath the germinal matrix and the periosteum of the bone. *B,* This deformity is usually the result of a ganglion in this location.

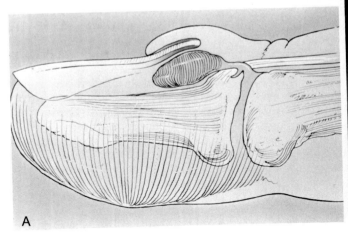

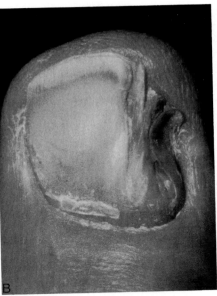

A

B

sected from the overlying skin, using magnification. This can almost always be accomplished without disrupting the cyst or perforating the thin skin over it. The author prefers this incision to one over the cyst (Angelides, 1982). The joint osteophytes are carefully removed with a fine rongeur. It is necessary to remove the nail from the nail bed after the cyst has been removed, to allow the nail bed to return to its normal position; otherwise, the empty area where the cyst was removed will fill with seroma or hematoma and a nail deformity will persist.

Ganglions occasionally rupture and drain through the nail fold or the overlying skin. If infection occurs, permanent nail deformity may result. A rupture should be treated with antibiotics until healed, and the surgeon should then resect before the rupture recurs. Removal of a draining ganglion may lead to an infection of the perionychium and joint, and subsequent deformity.

If the ganglion is beneath the nail bed and midline, the deformity can resemble a "pincher nail" (Fig. 100–20).

Giant Cell Tumor (Nodular Synovitis) (see also Chap. 16). Growth of the giant cell tumor may cause pressure on the nail-forming elements, with resultant nail deformity. Treatment consists of complete removal of the giant cell tumor and nail, to allow the nail bed to return to its original position.

Inflammatory Lesions. Some acute or chronic nail deformities defy preoperative di-

agnosis. It is necessary to remove the nail and explore the nail bed for diagnosis and treatment. Exposure of the nail fold is carried out by incisions 6 to 8 mm in length running perpendicular to the eponychial edge at both corners of the eponychium. The dorsal roof of the nail fold is turned proximally and the nail removed, to permit identification and treatment of the nail bed lesion. Treatment consists of biopsy and/or resection of the lesion. If the defect is small, it may be closed primarily, but if it is not possible to close it without tension, a split nail bed graft or local rotation flap (if in the sterile matrix) or full-thickness germinal matrix graft or flap (if in the germinal matrix) should be used. A piece of 0.020 silicone sheet is used to keep the nail fold open during healing.

Malignant Tumors

Basal Cell Carcinoma (see also Chap. 16). Basal cell carcinoma is rare on the hand and rarer still on the finger (Alport, Zak, and Werthamer, 1972; Hoffman, 1973). Complete resection is indicated, with frozen section examination of the margins to ensure complete removal. If there is bony involvement, amputation at the next joint must be considered.

Squamous Cell Carcinoma (see also Chap. 16). Although infrequent, squamous cell carcinoma is probably the most common

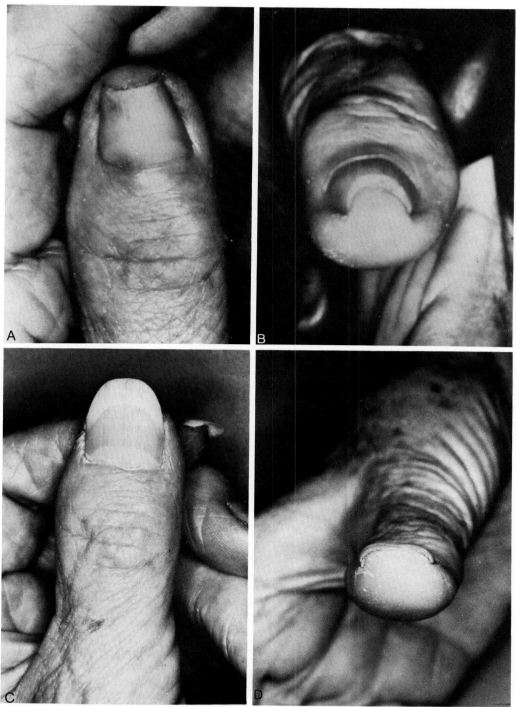

Figure 100–20. *A,* A 65 year old woman who has had progressive deformity of the thumbnail over a period of several months. *B,* The nail is curving much as it would in a "pincher nail." *C,* After removal of a midline ganglion between the ventral floor of the nail fold and the periosteum, the nail returned to normal. *D,* The nail has flattened after the operation. (Courtesy of David P. Green, M.D.)

malignancy of the perionychium. It may be primary or secondary to radiation exposure (Shapiro and Baraf, 1970; Alport, Zak, and Werthamer, 1972; Carroll, 1976).

Squamous cell carcinomas are frequently misdiagnosed as paronychia and have been inadequately treated (Fig. 100–21). The thumb is the most commonly involved digit and it occurs most often in males (Carroll, 1976). The average length of time between occurrence and treatment is four years. These carcinomas are most often found in the hands of dentists who have been exposed to chronic irradiation, and pain has always been present (Shapiro and Baraf, 1970).

A small paronychial squamous cell carcinoma with no bone involvement requires resection of the entire lesion, with adequate margins and skin graft. If the carcinoma is of long-term existence, and/or if large or bony changes are present, amputation of the distal or more proximal phalanx is indicated, as necessary. Node dissection is indicated only if nodes do not disappear after amputation, since most nodal enlargements appear to be inflammatory (Ellis, 1948; John, 1956; Shapiro and Baraf, 1970).

Melanoma (see also Chap. 16). Melanomas of the hands and feet, although uncommon, have a poorer prognosis than those anywhere else on the body (Day and associates, 1982). Many common paronychial conditions mimic melanoma in appearance and symptomatol-

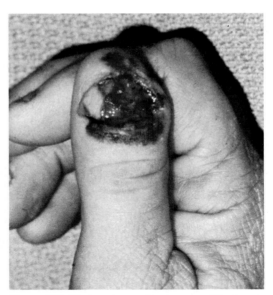

Figure 100–22. An advanced melanoma of the thumbnail of a 55 year old woman.

ogy, which delays diagnosis (Goldsmith, 1979). The classic appearance is of a pigmented area occurring in or beneath the nail that enlarges, darkens, or causes change in the nail (Fig. 100–22).

Seventy-two cases of subungual melanoma were reported by Pack and Oropeza (1967), 32 in the toes and 40 in the fingers; almost two-thirds were in the thumb or large toe. Almost all white patients had fair complexions, red or sandy hair, and blue or hazel eyes; 18.5 per cent of cases occurred in blacks. A pigmented area had been present for many years in 29 per cent of patients. There was nodal involvement on the first visit in 38.8 per cent of patients, and at resection there was no melanoma in only 2 per cent of those.

The recommended treatment for Stage I subungual melanoma is metacarpal or metatarsal amputation (Pack and Oropeza, 1967; Goldsmith, 1979). Authors vary on the advisability of nodal dissection and the timing of regional node dissection (Booher and Pack, 1957; Fortner, Booher, and Pack, 1964; Pack and Oropeza, 1967). Node dissection (Pack and Oropeza, 1967) carried out in patients with nonpalpable nodes but microscopic tumor produced a cure rate twice that in those in whom dissection was not performed. Pack and Oropeza also recommend amputation at one joint level above the lesion and node dissections when nodes are palpable.

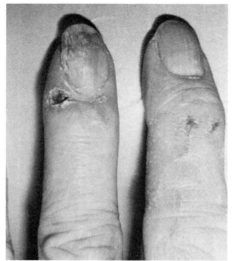

Figure 100–21. A squamous cell carcinoma of the perionychium of a veterinarian who had been exposed to irradiation.

REFERENCES

Alport, L. I., Zak, F. G., and Werthamer, S.: Subungual basal cell epithelioma. Arch Dermatol., *106*:599, 1972.

Angelides, A. C.: Ganglion of the hand and wrist. *In* Green, D. P. (Ed.): Operative Hand Surgery. Vol. II. New York, Churchill Livingstone, 1982, p. 1635.

Ashbell, T. S., Kleinert, H. E., Putcha, S. M., and Kutz, J. E.: The deformed fingernail, a frequent result of failure to repair nail bed injuries. J. Trauma, 7:177, 1967.

Baden, H. P.: Regeneration of the nail. Arch. Dermatol., *91*:619, 1965.

Barre, J. A. and Masson, P. V.: Anatomo-clinical study of certain painful subungual tumors (tumors of the neuro-myoarterial glomus of the extremities). Bull. Soc. Franc. Dermat. Symph., *31*:148, 1924.

Barron, J. N.: The structure and function of the skin of the hand. Hand, 2:93, 1970.

Booher, R. J., and Pack, G. T.: Malignant melanoma of the feet and hands. Surgery, *42*:1084, 1957.

Buncke, H. J., and Gonzales, R. I.: Fingernail reconstruction. Plast. Reconstr. Surg., *30*:452, 1962.

Burrows, M. T.: The significance of the lunula of the nail. Johns Hopkins Hosp. Rep., *18*:357, 1919.

Carroll, R. E.: Squamous cell carcinoma of the nailbed. J. Hand. Surg., *1*:92, 1976.

Clark, W. E., and Buxton, L. H. D.: Studies in nail growth. Br. J. Dermatol., *50*:221, 1938.

Day, C. L., Lew, R. A., Mihm, M. C., et al.: A multivariate analysis of prognostic factors for melanoma patients with lesions more than 3.65 mm in thickness. Ann. Surg., *195*:44, 1982.

Ellis, V. H.: Squamous cell carcinoma of the nail bed. J. Bone Joint Surg., *30B*:656, 1948.

Flatt, A. E.: Nailbed injuries. Br. J. Plast. Surg., *8*:34, 1955a.

Flatt, A. E.: Minor hand injuries. J. Bone Joint Surg., *37B*:117, 1955b.

Fleegler, E., and Clark, W.: Personal communication, 1984.

Fortner, J. G., Booher, R. J., and Pack, G. T.: Results of groin dissection for malignant melanoma in 220 patients. Surgery, *55*:485, 1964.

Goldsmith, H. S.: Melanoma: an overview. CA, *29*:194, 1979.

Halpern, L. K., and Lane, C. W.: Treatment of periungual warts. Mo. Med., *50*:765, 1953.

Hamrick, W. H.: Suture of the fingernail in crushing injuries. U.S. Naval Med. Bull., *46*:255, 1946.

Hanrahan, E. M.: The split thickness skin graft as a cover following removal of a fingernail. Surgery, *20*:398, 1946.

Hoffman, S.: Basal cell carcinoma of the nail bed. Arch. Dermatol., *108*:828, 1973.

Horner, R. L., and Cohen, B. I.: Injuries to the fingernail. Rocky Mt. Med. J. *63*:60, 1966.

John, H. T.: Primary skin cancer of the fingers simulating chronic infection. Lancet., *1*:662, 1956.

Jones, F. W.: The Principles of Anatomy as Seen in the Hand. 2nd Ed. London, Bailliere, Tindall & Cox, 1941.

Keyser, J. J., and Eaton, R. G.: Surgical cure of chronic paronychia by eponychial marsupialization. Plast. Reconstr. Surg., *58*:66, 1976.

Kleinert, H. E., Kutz, J. E., Fishman, J. H., and McGraw, L. H.: Etiology and treatment of the so called mucous cyst of the finger. J. Bone Joint Surg., *54A*:1455, 1972.

Kligman, A. M.: Why do nails grow out instead of up? Arch. Dermatol., *84*:313, 1961.

Lewis, B. L.: Microscopic studies of fetal and mature nail and surrounding soft tissue. A.M.A. Arch. Dermatol. Syphilol., *70*:732, 1954.

McCash, C. R.: Free nail grafting. Br. J. Plast. Surg., *8*:19, 1955.

Newmeyer, W. L., and Kilgore, E. S.: Common injuries of the fingernail and nail bed. Am. Fam. Phys., *16*:93, 1977.

Pack, G. T., and Oropeza, R.: Subungual melanoma. Surg. Gynecol. Obstet., *124*:571, 1967.

Pardo-Castello, V.: Diseases of the Nail. 3rd Ed. Springfield, IL, Charles C Thomas, 1960.

Saito, H., Suzuki, Y., Tujino, K., and Tajima, T.: Free nail bed graft for treatment of nail bed injuries of the hand. J. Hand Surg., *8*:171, 1983.

Samman, P. D.: The Nails in Disease. 3rd Ed. Chicago, Year Book Medical Publishers, 1978.

Schiller, C.: Nail replacement in fingertip injuries. Plast. Reconstr. Surg., *19*:521, 1957.

Shapiro, L., and Baraf, C. S.: Subungual epidermoid carcinoma and keratoacanthoma. Cancer, *25*:141, 1970.

Shepard, G. H.: Treatment of nail bed avulsions with split-thickness nail bed grafts. J. Hand Surg., *8*:49, 1983.

Shoemaker, J. V.: Some notes on the nails. J.A.M.A., *15*:427, 1890.

Swanker, W. A.: Reconstructive surgery of the injured nail. Am. J. Surg., *74*:341, 1947.

Tajima, T.: Treatment of open crushing type industrial injuries of the hand and forearm: degloving, open circumferential, heat press and nail bed injuries. J. Trauma, *14*:995, 1974.

Weckesser, E. C.: Treatment of Hand Injuries: Preservation and Restoration of Function. Chicago, Year Book Medical Publishers, 1974.

Wilgis, E. F. S., and Maxwell, G. P.: Distal digital nerve graft: clinical and anatomical studies. J. Hand Surg., *4*:439, 1979.

Zias, N.: The Nail in Health and Disease. New York, S. P. Medical & Scientific Books, 1980.

Zook, E. G.: The perionychium: anatomy, physiology and care of injuries. Clin. Plast. Surg., *8*:21, 1981.

Zook, E. G.: Fingernail injuries. *In* Strickland, J. W., and Steichen, J. B. (Ed.): Difficult Problems In Hand Surgery. St. Louis, MO, C. V. Mosby Company, 1982a, p. 22.

Zook, E. G.: Injuries of the fingernail. *In* Green, D. P. (Ed.): Operative Hand Surgery. Vol. I. New York, Churchill Livingstone, 1982b, p. 895.

Zook, E. G., Guy, R. J., and Russell, R. C.: A study of nailbed injuries: causes, treatment, and prognosis. J. Hand Surg., *9A*:247, 1984.

Zook, E. G., Van Beek, A. L., Russell, R. C., and Beatty, M. E.: Anatomy and physiology of the perionychium: a review of the literature and anatomic study. J. Hand Surg., *5*:528, 1980.

Flexor Tendon

The flexor tendon continues to fascinate. It does so for three reasons: it is essential for efficient manual handling, it is the source of continued scientific controversy, and its repair demands a level of surgical skill that even acknowledged craftsmen cannot always achieve. The first fact is self-evident, especially to anyone who has had the misfortune to have one finger immobilized for any length of time. The second has been the subject of many excellent publications (Strickland,

1985a to d), which have also reviewed the history of flexor tendon surgery and the disputes that have surrounded it, from the time of Galen up to the present day. For this reason, this chapter, while not ignoring the essential science of anatomy, nutrition, and healing, is concerned primarily with matters technical, taking the reader step by step through primary tendon repair and secondary reconstruction, the construction of the controlled mobilization splint, and the simple, though demanding and mandatory, therapy program.

NUTRITION

It is now recognized that the flexor tendon within the digital theca receives nutrition from two distinct sources, vascular and synovial (Manske and Lesker, 1985). The blood supply enters the tendon distally from the bony insertion, proximally from the palm and along its length via the vincula (Berkenbusch, 1887; Lundborg, Myrhage, and Rydevik, 1977). Four digital arches are created by the anastomoses of branches from the two proper digital arteries. These arches are located at the base and the neck of both the proximal and middle phalanges (Fig. 101–1). A vinculum arises from each of these arches, named V1 to V4 from proximal to distal (Armenta and Lehrman, 1980). V1 and V2 supply primarily the flexor digitorum superficialis (FDS), V3 and V4 the flexor digitorum profundus (FDP). The arches, which form V2 and V4 and are at the necks of the phalanges, lie between the check-rein ligaments and the bone. The vinculum arising from each of these arches emerges from the recess between the two check-rein ligaments to gain the dorsal,

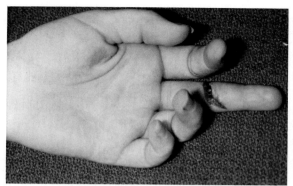

Figure 101–5. Flexor tendon laceration. The postural change that results from laceration of both tendons over the middle phalanx can be seen.

injury present late, on average over two months after the trauma (see p. 4536).

Division of the flexor pollicis longus results in full extension of the interphalangeal joint of the thumb, which may appear hyperextended.

It is important to appreciate that, despite all that has been said about reaching a diagnosis on the basis of posture, *division of superficialis tendons without injury to the profundus* results in *no* detectable change in posture. For this reason it is important always to test the tendons individually (Lister, 1984). If this is done against resistance, partial lacerations may be suggested by pain experienced by the patient. Exploration of the wound remains the final arbiter.

Technique

Suturing of freshly severed tendons will give a far better result than repairing such cases when old.

BUNNELL, *1918*

Once the sheath is exposed, the end of the tendon may be seen beneath the retinacular part as a junction between the white of tendon and the red of blood in the sheath. If it lies beneath the annular portion, manipulation of the distal joints into flexion should bring it into view. The retinacular portion through which the distal end is seen should now be opened by reflecting it as a flap, taking care to leave sufficient margin—approximately 2 mm—to permit later suturing (Lister, 1983). This can best be done with scissors, the blade within the sheath determining its lateral extent before the incision is made (Fig. 101–

6). Closure of the sheath is eased if only one transverse cut is made, creating an L-shaped flap. If such a design is possible in the primary window, the transverse cut is more often than not the original laceration. If an inviolate retinacular window is being opened, the transverse incision should be made adjacent to the edge of the annular pulley but separated from it by the same distance as was left as a lateral rim, i.e., approximately 2 mm. When it is apparent that a tendon end is going to be passed beneath a pulley *after* placement of one-half the core suture (see below), the transverse cut of the L should always be made on the aspect of the retinacular window *away* from that pulley, thereby creating a channel into which the cut end can be more easily funneled. The flimsy retinacular flap so created should be laid back. Care must be taken not to damage it during subsequent tendon repair.

The appropriate manipulation of tendons and placement of sutures is usually left until the proximal end has been retrieved.

Retrieval of a retracted proximal tendon end can be one of the more frustrating exercises in hand surgery. Special instruments have been devised, and suction has been recommended (Pennington, 1977), but there appears to be little substitute for an experienced touch, and by definition experience cannot be taught. A few tips can be passed on.

Before commencing location and retrieval of the proximal end, the surgeon should have

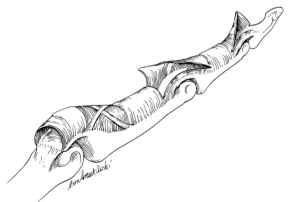

Figure 101–6. The retinacular windows commonly employed are demonstrated. It is seen that A$_2$ and A$_4$ are left untouched. Commonly the window over the proximal interphalangeal and distal interphalangeal joints is opened. Care is taken to preserve a margin of the window for later suture. The window is opened on only two sides in order to create an L-shaped "funnel" cut through which the flexor tendon can easily be passed.

a 23 gauge hypodermic needle available for transfixion. Failure to observe this step has let many tendons slip away, and results in unnecessary additional injury to the tendon end.

By seeing the relationship between the cut distal end and the laceration in the sheath, the surgeon can confirm what he previously deduced from the history of the position of the digit at the time of injury.

The first step in tendon retrieval is to fully flex the wrist. When the fist has been fully clenched at the time of injury, the tendon's end may appear in the wound with this simple maneuver. This permits ideal handling of the end (discussed later). If the tendon does not appear, the surgeon should look down the sheath, as the tendon may be sitting close to the laceration. When success has not attended either of these steps, the surgeon must use instruments. In doing so, he should remember: (1) the end is usually nearer than you think, (2) contact will be hard to appreciate, and (3) the instrument can pass the tendon or push it proximally.

Using a fine mosquito hemostat with the tips of the index finger and thumb in the rings of the instrument and the hinge supported by the distal phalanx of the middle finger, the surgeon should explore the sheath proximally (Fig. 101–7). The open jaws are advanced, closed, and withdrawn. Little or no longitudinal resistance will be encountered either on touching the tendon end or on successfully grasping it until it has been withdrawn almost to original length. Depend-ing on the amount of tendon grasped, some transverse resistance *may* be felt by the index finger and thumb on closure of the hemostat. Thus, contact with the tendon end can scarcely be detected by the gentle, trained hand and certainly not by any coarser movement. It follows that when the tendon end is caught, its appearance from the sheath in the instrument is often a surprise, so freely does it move. Further, if any resistance to longitudinal traction is met with, the instrument must be opened immediately, since it has hold of the sheath, and traction can inflict potentially serious injury.

If after three attempts (they should be counted) no tendon has been located, consideration should be given to the next step. Proximal to distal massage of the palm has been recommended by reputable authorities. The author has had infrequent success with this technique and suspects that pressure may as often drive the tendon proximally as distally. Finally, if all else fails, proximal incision and exploration is required (Fig. 101–8).

The proximal incision is best made formally at the distal palmar crease, bearing in mind the possibility of future tendon surgery. Through this the synovial sheath is opened proximal to the A_1 pulley and the errant tendon retrieved. A core suture is placed in this proximal tendon end. The suture ends are cut equally long and sufficient to reach beyond the window in which the work is to be done. A piece of silicone tubing is selected from a range of nasogastric feeding tubes of

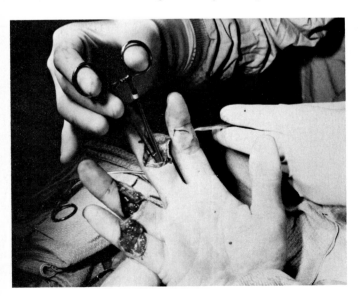

Figure 101–7. The wrist is flexed and the hand supported. The grasp on the hemostat is here shown, it being the most sensitive that can be achieved with this instrument.

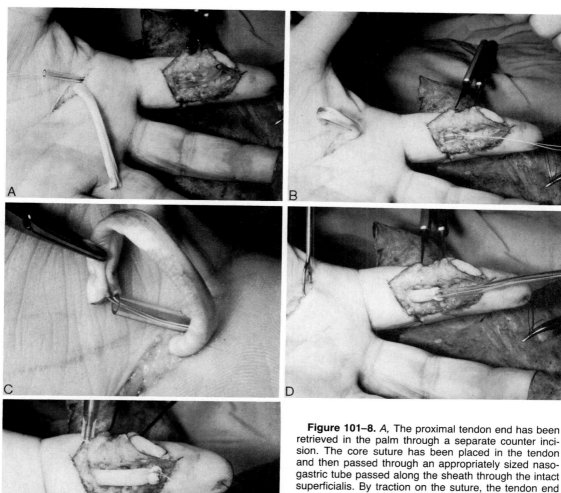

Figure 101–8. *A,* The proximal tendon end has been retrieved in the palm through a separate counter incision. The core suture has been placed in the tendon and then passed through an appropriately sized nasogastric tube passed along the sheath through the intact superficialis. By traction on the suture, the tendon end is abutted against the nasogastric tube in *B* and *C. D,* Grasping the tube and the contained suture and irrigating proximally, the tendon is drawn easily into the proximal interphalangeal window. Since the repair has to be done in the distal interphalangeal window, the tendon is pulled out to length and transfixed with a needle in *E.*

Illustration continued on following page

appropriate caliber to fit snugly into the canal: 8 to 14 gauge is usually suitable. The end is taper cut and is passed from one window to the next. The end of the tubing close to the tendon is now cut squarely and the suture passed along the tube, employing a needleholder to advance the suture. This will pass with ease, but only if both the tubing and the suture are as dry as possible. The suture is pulled out of the far end of the tube until the tendon end abuts firmly against the near end of the tubing. Using the same needleholder, the far end of the tubing con-

taining the tendon suture is grasped firmly, the proximal end is irrigated and inspected to ensure that there is no impediment to progress, and the tendon is drawn through into the distal window.

This technique is especially useful in passing a profundus tendon through an intact superficialis, for the tubing laid on the chiasm of Camper and advanced proximally always passes through the right path in the superficialis.

Because the needle has been removed before the suture is passed through the tubing,

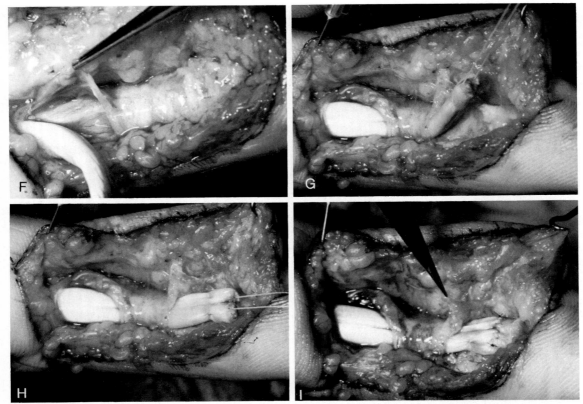

Figure 101–8 *Continued F,* The L-shaped cut in the proximal interphalangeal window is held open with forceps and the tendon is passed through into the distal window *(G). H,* The tendon is now positioned overlying the distal stump and the repair can satisfactorily be completed *(I).*

the core suture in these circumstances comes finally to resemble the Tajima technique, with two separate sutures in the two ends and two knots buried in the repair.

Of necessity in most cases the tendon end has been grasped by a hemostat or similar instrument in the process of retrieving it, thereby inflicting unwanted injury on the epitenon. To avoid further damage, it is important not to reposition the instrument or for any other reason to release the tendon, otherwise it may be lost into the sheath. Instead, the tendon should be drawn gradually and gently out to the required length, approximately 5 mm beyond the cut distal end, the position of which can be seen or is certainly known (Fig. 101–9). In situations in which the proximal tendon must be advanced beyond its normal length to pass beneath a pulley (see below), it should be transfixed at that excess length. This requires stronger traction and may require preliminary transfixion before the required length is

delivered, to obtain a more secure hold on the tendon. This maneuver may result in some flexion of joints proximal to the point of transfixion, which flexion can be controlled by a lead hand. The tendon should be transfixed proximally to retain it in the selected relationship. Straight, cutting needles for this purpose have the disadvantage of potential damage to the tendon, while round-bodied needles are difficult to drive through the tendon. A suitable compromise is a hypodermic needle, 23 gauge, the cutting bevel being oriented in the coronal plane so as to be parallel to the tendon fibers and thereby be less likely to injure them. The hypodermic has the added advantage that it cannot possibly be overlooked later, even in the most complex injury. The needle should be passed through as immobile a structure as can be found adjacent to the tendon. In the digit an annular pulley is ideal. In so doing, the surgeon must ensure first that there is sufficient tendon (in excess of 1 cm) between the cut

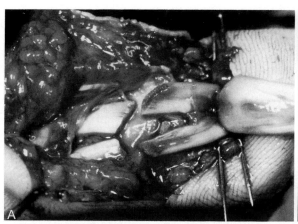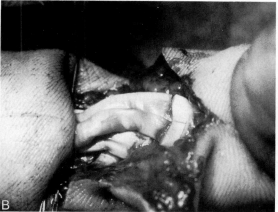

Figure 101–9. Tendon abutment. In *A* the tendons are *unsatisfactorily* abutted. There is a gap of some 5 mm between the tendon ends, which is unacceptable for tendon repair. *B,* The abutment shown in this illustration of the profundus tendon is acceptable and is mandatory in all flexor tendon repairs.

end and the point of transfixion to permit free rotation during placement of the peripheral suture, and second that the needle does not transfix either neurovascular bundle.

Whichever is first retrieved in a digit, the flexor digitorum superficialis or the flexor digitorum profundus, the other usually follows it by a variable distance. Both can be transfixed to the proper length at the same time, but there is some merit in transfixing and repairing the deep tendon before fully retrieving the second. This improves exposure and avoids unnecessary handling and drying of the more superficial tendon. In the digit distal to the midpoint of the proximal phalanx, the deep tendon is the superficialis, the superficial one the profundus. Thus, if the profundus is first retrieved it is drawn out until the other tendon emerges. The superficialis is grasped, drawn out to length, and transfixed. Before the profundus is released, the hand should be placed at neutral and the weight of the hemostat on the tendon supported in order to check the amount of profundus retraction. If any doubt exists, there is little harm in transfixing it temporarily in a somewhat retracted but accessible position. Finally, when flexion of distal joints is necessary to permit adequate exposure of the distal tendon end, this can also be maintained by use of a transfixion needle through a distal pulley. Suturing can now begin.

By inspecting the amount of distal tendon that can be delivered into the selected window, the surgeon now must make a decision regarding the technique of repair.

1. If 1 cm or more of distal tendon is exposed in the window or can be brought into it by joint manipulation, the repair is straightforward and is described below.

2. If the tendon lies under the annular pulley distal to the window, but can be brought into it by the 5 mm required to place the superficial running suture (hereinafter referred to as the peripheral suture), the initial step of the repair should be conducted by carefully opening the next retinacular portion distally. The distal tendon is then delivered into that second window, taking care to protect any vincular structures. The deep suture (henceforward called the core suture) is passed first beneath the intervening annular pulley, inserted into the distal end as described below, and then returned beneath the pulley with the distal end. This is not simple. It is a maneuver most often undertaken at the region of the middle phalanx and A_4 pulley. Taking it again in sequence, but in more detail, the retraction of the distal tendon end under the annular pulley is best done by means of a closed fine hemostat passed proximally beneath the pulley alongside the tendon until it is proximal to the short vinculum. The hemostat is then turned transversely beneath the tendon and lifted against its undersurface. This usually delivers the tendon into the distal wound. If it fails, proximal retraction on the distal edge of the annular pulley with a skin hook may achieve it. In the rare situation when that also fails, the short vinculum of the flexor digitorum profundus can be coagulated, giv-

ing greater mobility to the tendon stump. The core suture is now placed in the distal end in the standard manner described below, after the needle is first passed beneath the annular pulley from the proximal to the distal window (Fig. 101–10). This is best done with the needle reversed, i.e., with the suture end leading, thereby avoiding the sharp end snagging on the pulley, the periosteum, or the vinculum. After the core suture is placed, the needle is returned in the same manner and along the same course, thereby reducing the chance of the suture passing on either side of

any strands of tissue that might then arrest proximal passage of the tendon, the next step to be undertaken. In this maneuver the tendon *must not be pulled* beneath the pulley by means of the deep suture. Such traction serves only to bunch the tendon, preventing its passage and, if continued, causing disruption of the fibers at the tendon end. Such disruption makes the second, peripheral tendon suture ineffective. Instead, the tendon should be eased proximally through the pulley. This is greatly facilitated if the distal window has been opened with an L-shaped

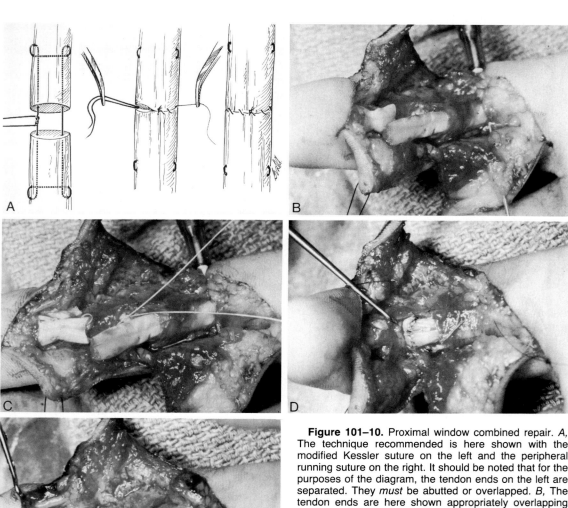

Figure 101–10. Proximal window combined repair. *A,* The technique recommended is here shown with the modified Kessler suture on the left and the peripheral running suture on the right. It should be noted that for the purposes of the diagram, the tendon ends on the left are separated. They *must* be abutted or overlapped. *B,* The tendon ends are here shown appropriately overlapping outside the A₄ pulley. *C,* The suture has been passed beneath the A₄ pulley into the distal window where the core suture has been inserted in the distal stump. *D,* The tendon is then drawn through into the proximal interphalangeal window beneath the A₄ pulley, employing an L-shaped funnel cut. The repair is completed with a peripheral running 6-0 nylon suture. *E,* The retinacular window is then closed with running monofilament nylon.

incision as described above, for the major portion of the tendon end can be laid into the funnel so created in the sheath, and the surgeon need only guide that segment which protrudes from the L incision safely beneath the pulley. The tendon end should first be drawn up to the edge of the pulley, but not forced against it, by traction applied to the core suture by the surgeon's nondominant hand. Continuing to apply that gentle traction, the surgeon should now ease all aspects of the periphery of the tendon beneath the pulley edge, using a fine periosteal elevator. If necessary this step can be eased by the assistant holding the pulley in its normal relationship perpendicular to bone, using two skin hooks. Tears or contusions of the epitenon on the free tendon end are disastrous to the subsequent peripheral suture and *must not be inflicted* (Fig. 101–11). Patience and care are therefore required. On completion of this difficult task, the surgeon proceeds with a standard repair as described below.

3. If the distal tendon cannot be delivered into the proximal window for the 5 mm required to perform the peripheral suture despite passive joint flexion, the repair must be performed in the next distal window. That window should be opened as previously described, and the proximal tendon end advanced beneath the intervening pulley (see Fig. 101–8). This may require previous placement of one-half of the core suture to aid in advancement, which is achieved in a manner similar to that detailed in the last paragraph.

Several different configurations of core suture have been described (Ketchum, 1985).

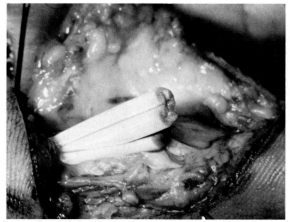

Figure 101–11. Epitenon. This tendon end demonstrates undamaged epitenon, which must be preserved if a satisfactory peripheral running suture is to be performed.

The two main groups are (1) those that crisscross diagonally across the tendon, the Bunnell suture, and its modifications; and (2) those in which the suture runs parallel to the fibers, the Mason (1940) and Kessler (1973) sutures and their modifications. Urbaniak, Cahill, and Mortenson (1975) showed that the former group tended to strangulate the tendon ends, producing a significant reduction in tensile strength as compared with the Kessler type of suture five days after repair. For this reason the author uses a modification of the Kessler suture, which approximates very closely to the suture described by Kirchmayer in 1917.

When one tendon end is to be passed beneath a pulley after placement of one-half of the core suture, clearly that end must be sutured first; otherwise, it is of no consequence which end is chosen. The outer aspect of the tendon—the epitenon—must never be handled, for it will either split, making the later peripheral suture unsatisfactory, or suffer damage that predisposes to adhesions (Hansson, Lundborg, and Rydevik, 1980). Instead, the tendon end should be grasped firmly with the heavier of the pair of toothed dissecting forceps in the hand set. The security of this grasp should be tested by applying a little gentle traction to the tendon end, for it must resist the pressures applied during the passage of the needle.

Several suture materials have been used for the core suture (Ketchum, 1985), of which the braided man-made fibers are probably the most reliable, using the 4-0 gauge for the average adult tendon and scaling down accordingly in flexor tendon repairs in children. The choice of needle is up to the surgeon, either straight or curved. The only important aspect of using the needle in the tendon is that, whether curved or straight, the advancing tip of the needle should always be parallel to the tendon fibers in making the first pass. The needle should not be inserted exactly into the center of the tendon, for it has been shown that the blood supply to the tendon runs primarily on its deep dorsal surface (Caplan, Hunter, and Marklin, 1975). With this in mind, the core suture is inserted into the more superficial half of the tendon as far as possible. Placing the core suture requires three passes of the needle in each of the cut ends.

1. Holding the tendon end with the toothed forceps, the tip of the needle is inserted into one superficial-lateral quadrant of the tendon

end. The needle is advanced parallel to the fibers for approximately 1 cm and then driven out through the anterolateral surface of the tendon at 11 o'clock. Particular caution should be observed in driving the needle through the epitenon to ensure that the back end of the curved needle does not impinge on the epitenon at the cut end of the tendon, thereby disrupting it and spoiling it for subsequent peripheral suture. The suture should then be drawn through the tendon until the last centimeter of a 10 cm length of suture protrudes from the tendon end. This passage is always simple with monofilament suture, and for this reason some surgeons prefer it. If a braided suture is employed, it should be passed through the fat of the finger on a number of occasions before being used on the tendon, in order to ensure its smooth movement. Despite this precaution, the surgeon using braided suture should watch the passage of the suture through the tendon closely for any tendency for the braided suture to gather tendinous material in its substance.

2. The second transverse pass of the core suture should be made in a different plane from that of the initial pass. Pennington (1979a) showed in a rather novel manner that this plane within the tendon should be superficial to that of the initial longitudinal pass of the core suture. In this way the suture locks on the tendon fibers in a manner in which it does not if the transverse pass is placed deep to the longitudinal. Apart from being superficial to the longitudinal one, this transverse pass should lie somewhat closer to the tendon end than the point from which the longitudinal suture had emerged by some 1 to 2 mm. The tendon should still be held by the forceps as described above, and supported laterally against the phalanx, the sheath, or the ring finger of the hand holding the forceps. The needle is inserted into the tendon further lateral than the point from which it emerged, closer to the tendon end by 1 to 2 mm and aimed so that it passes superficial to the first pass of the suture (enters at 10 and emerges at 2 o'clock). The loop in the suture on this, the first of the tendon ends to be sutured, can be drawn tight.

3. The next longitudinal pass is exactly parallel to and at the same depth as the first longitudinal pass emerging from the tendon end in the other lateral superficial quadrant (enters at 1 o'clock and passes deep to the transverse pass) (Fig. 101–12). Once again the loop can be tightened down. Where the

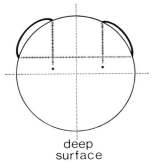

deep
surface

Figure 101–12. Core suture. The relationship of the three passes of a core suture in a tendon end is demonstrated. The longitudinal suture, which is represented as a dot just above the horizontal midtendinous line, is seen running deep to the transverse suture. The longitudinal pass emerges from the tendon at 11 and 1 o'clock respectively, while the transverse suture is at 2 and 10 o'clock.

passage of the core suture in one tendon end preceded a manipulation of that tendon end with respect to the fibrous flexor sheath (see above), that manipulation should now be undertaken. After it is completed, or if no such manipulation is necessary, the relationship between the two tendon ends should be checked to ensure that no gap has developed between them. If all is still well, the other cut end of the tendon is grasped in a similar fashion and the suture passed in a manner identical to that described above, with the exception that the loops of the suture, of which there are two lying 1 cm from the tendon end, are left long until all passes of the suture have been made. The suture can now be tightened down with a needleholder and a skin hook, taking care to abut the two tendon ends as this is done. The skin hook is used to hold the second loop while the needleholder tightens down the first loop so as to approximate the tendon ends. Approximation is the appropriate degree of contact between the tendon ends. Any bunching or "concertina" effect should be avoided. At this juncture it can be appreciated why it was so important to hold the two tendon ends overlapping or abutting on one another with the use of the transfixion needles, for the tendon ends should *not* be pulled together by the core suture (see Fig. 101–9). If it were so employed, inevitable bunching would result. It would also be extremely difficult to have balanced tension in the two longitudinal limbs of the Kessler suture. The knot is now tied to lie between the cut tendon ends. If a braided suture is being employed, only one hitch should be made in the first throw of the

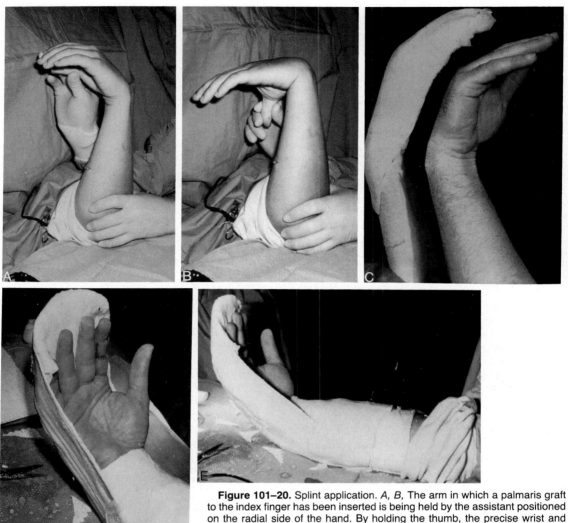

Figure 101–20. Splint application. *A, B,* The arm in which a palmaris graft to the index finger has been inserted is being held by the assistant positioned on the radial side of the hand. By holding the thumb, the precise wrist and metacarpophalangeal joint posture can be established by the surgeon who applies the cast from the ulnar aspect. *C,* The dorsal hood is constructed to have 20 degrees less than full wrist flexion and 45 to 60 degrees of metacarpophalangeal joint flexion. *D, E,* The dorsal splint is held in place with circumferential dressings.

Illustration continued on following page

zation employing rubber band flexion (Young and Harmon, 1960; Lister and associates, 1977). In the survey referred to above, 22.2 per cent of all surgeons used the Duran technique, and 59.2 per cent the rubber band (Strickland, 1985d). In both a dorsal block splint is used; the Duran method incorporates Velcro straps to hold the fingers at all times, apart from two or three sessions per day of passive motion of the digital joints. In the other technique the rubber band is applied to the involved finger alone. Previously all fingers were so held, but consideration of the

anatomy of the flexor digitorum profundus showed this to be incorrect. Since all tendons of the flexor digitorum profundus have a common origin, free extension of uninvolved fingers reduces tension on one cut tendon held by traction and probably also encourages its frequent extension.

The splint is constructed in the operating room on completion of repair. The position is best obtained and maintained by resting the elbow on the hand table with the forearm vertical (Fig. 101–20A). An assistant sitting at the shoulder holds the thumb (in finger

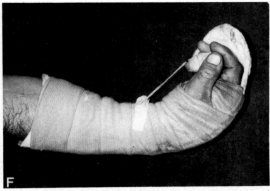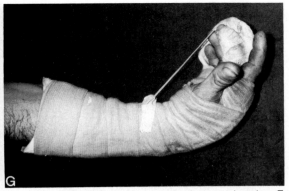

Figure 101–20 *Continued F, G,* The finger is held into flexion by a rubber band attached to the forearm dressing. Full extension against the splint should be possible and should be done repeatedly.

repairs). The surgeon sitting at the axilla positions the hand for the assistant to maintain, and applies the splint entirely from the ulnar side. The wrist is first flexed fully (Fig. 101–20B) then backed off by 20 degrees. A dorsal slab of 4 inch plaster is then applied, extending from the upper forearm to just beyond the fingertips. The slab is held in place with an open weave bandage around the forearm and wrist. The maximal extension position of the fingers is then ensured by holding the fingers against the plaster on their dorsal aspect while it sets. The metacarpophalangeal joints should be flexed 45 to 60 degrees and both interphalangeal joints should be fully extended. While the splint sets, an ulnar buttress is added to strengthen the cantilevered extension block (Fig. 101–20C). This ulnar buttress gains significance in flexor pollicis longus lacerations, since the best line of pull for the rubber band is gained by attaching it to a hole through that buttress. In such flexor pollicis longus injuries, the dorsal wrist and metacarpophalangeal block should be as above, but the finger block can be omitted beyond the proximal phalanx. A thumb extension block must be added with both metacarpophalangeal and interphalangeal joints at 0 degrees.

The rubber band is attached to the digit at the time of surgery. This is done by passing a 4-0 monofilament nylon through the fingernail twice and knotting it to create a double loop in which a rubber band is hitched (Fig. 101–20D). This band must be short and strong enough and its point of attachment proximal enough to flex the digit fully toward the wrist; it must be long and elastic enough and must attach sufficiently far distally to permit the patient to extend the finger fully

and frequently (Fig. 101–20E,F,G). For adults a No. 18 rubber band is usually correct, for children a No. 16.

The rubber bands are attached to the forearm bandage with a safety pin. This step is omitted until later consultation in patients unable to understand an explanation of its significance.

In some cases the above splintage is changed (see Table 101–1).

In children under 6 years of age, the splint is quite different. It is a long arm cast in which the elbow is flexed to 90 degrees, the wrist is flexed fully, the metacarpophalangeal joints are flexed by 90 degrees, and the interphalangeal joints are fully extended. The anterior surfaces of the fingers are left free, the dorsal hood being continued from the fingertip to join the cast on the upper arm. In children over 6 years the standard splint is fitted but the rubber band is not attached proximally.

The proximal attachment of the rubber band flexes the injured digit. By making that attachment, the surgeon potentially inflicts

Table 101–1. Factors Causing Modification in the Standard Flexor Repair Splint

Associated Factor	Modification
Direct nerve or vessel repair	Flex extension block by amount determined at repair to be safe
Palmar plate repair	Flex block by 20 degrees at involved joint
Fracture, extensor tendon, replantation	Omit rubber band; early active and passive motion
Intoxicated, retarded, or unconscious patients; children 6–9 years	Omit proximal rubber band attachment until review at day 1 or 2
Young children 0–6 years	Omit rubber band, special splint

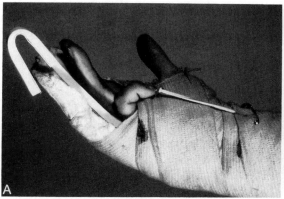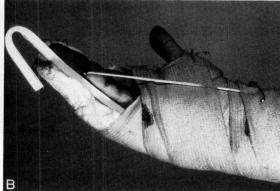

Figure 101–21. *A, B,* Metacarpophalangeal block. This patient has sustained a laceration of the flexor tendons in the region of the carpal tunnel, which had to be opened. The wrist was therefore splinted at neutral. It was found on follow-up that the small finger was not extending satisfactorily, and therefore a block to be applied to the proximal phalanx was constructed out of aluminum foam splint.

on the patient the worst complication of primary flexor tendon repair—a flexion contracture. Two conclusions should be drawn: (1) the band should not be attached proximally in those who cannot understand or whose cooperation is at all doubtful; and (2) it is important to understand the personal responsibility for supervision of postoperative therapy that the surgeon accepts by using the rubber band. All patients should be seen by the surgeon within one or two days of surgery. The splint should be checked and any inadvertent block to full interphalangeal extension (Fig. 101–21) overcome by rebuilding it, or by providing a block to the dorsal aspect of the proximal phalanx to act as a fulcrum around which full extension can be achieved. Patients with rubber band traction in place should be observed and encouraged to repeat their exercises many times a day.

A danger in follow-up is a long lapse between appointments. The patient may appear to be doing well at five days and is given an appointment for two weeks later; he therefore is absent during the two weeks when scar forms. He should be seen by the operating surgeon twice weekly, if only for encouragement. If the patient misses an appointment he should be called the same day and chided to meet the surgeon the next day—anywhere! Faced with such attention and determination, most patients get the message that this is an important time in their lives.

The next critical decision is when to remove the splint and the rubber band. At an office visit three to four weeks after repair or reconstruction, the band is released and the active range of motion is checked. If this is good the only risk is rupture: the splint is removed, but the rubber band is attached to the wrist for a further three to four weeks (Fig. 101–22). If the band is discarded at this

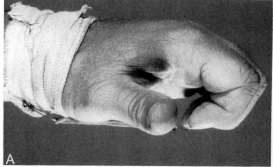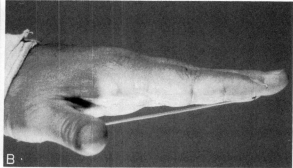

Figure 101–22. Four weeks after surgery. This patient was found to have good active flexion following repair of both tendons over the proximal phalanx in the index finger. On removal of the dorsal splint, therefore, the rubber band was once again attached to a bandage around the wrist, allowing him to continue exercise *(A, B)*. The final result is shown in Figure 101–31.

time there is a great danger of rupture. If active motion is poor, the band is discarded and the patient attends therapy daily, because the dangers now are adhesion, flexion contracture, and poor range of motion. In either circumstance the patient is given a new set of instructions: no lifting of anything until eight weeks after the injury.

If after eight weeks there is a persistent flexion contracture, dynamic splintage can be employed without risk of tendon rupture. The splint should flex the wrist, and block the metacarpophalangeal joint at 30 degrees with a No. 18 rubber band extending the finger. In severe contractures, static overnight splints such as the joint jack may be tried after eight weeks, but the prospects in such cases are bleak.

Before leaving the first responsible encounter after repair, the patient should be told how to contact the surgeon. Should rupture occur, he usually knows it, for he will report a "pop" during some unauthorized activity. The proper management of such a rupture is immediate exploration and repeat repair, from which results are usually good.

SECONDARY RECONSTRUCTION

Many factors determine whether tendon reconstruction will succeed in restoring function to an impaired digit, and therefore whether it should even be attempted.

Age. While it is generally recognized that healing and rehabilitation potential decreases with advancing years, the adverse aspect of infancy is not so widely known. Children under 8 years of age—sometimes younger, sometimes older—handle pain by sustained immobility of the part, in a pattern seen universally in other species. Other species do well, but they have not undergone tendon surgery! Evidence is cited elsewhere in this text of the merits of mobilization following repair, graft, and tenolysis. In the young, such mobilization cannot be achieved.

Occupation. The demands of an occupation for manipulative skills influence the patient's awareness of hand function and his commitment to efforts to restore that function. The demands of a strict schedule may unreasonably restrict the time available for reconstruction. The musician with a tendon laceration is the role model for one who will do well; in practice, such a patient is rare, but the characterization is accurate.

Initial Injury. Injuring agents produce typical wounds. Thus, the knife differs from the table saw, the lawnmower, and the punch press in the extent of tissue damage it can cause. The more extensive the tissue damage, the more widespread is the subsequent scar. The quantity of the scar is in turn inversely proportional to the range of motion that can reasonably be expected after all primary and reconstructive surgery is completed. A sharp laceration, dividing only the profundus tendon, is clearly the most propitious injury. The nerve damage, fractures, joint involvement, and devascularization associated with more severe trauma all reduce the reconstructive potential of the digit.

Initial Care. As the patient tells of his primary care, the surgeon can form a fairly accurate impression of its quality. High quality primary care will have done most to assist him in his task, by thorough debridement of contaminated and avascular tissue, rigid fixation of the skeleton, provision of good skin cover, and repair of significant blood vessels. Subsequent care will have included physical therapy directed at maintaining joint motion.

Previous Operations. All previous surgical procedures on the involved part, whether or not for the presenting complaint, will have resulted in scar that to a large degree is cumulative. This is particularly true if many different incisions have been employed. If those operative procedures included tendon surgery, whether primary repair or subsequent graft, the prognosis should be very guarded.

Examination of the involved limb should include all structures, including those remote from the injury, since their impairment may seriously influence the outcome of surgery. Also, in this litigious age, only a thorough and recorded preoperative examination protects the surgeon from ill-founded postoperative accusations of iatrogenic disability.

PHYSICAL EXAMINATION

Skin. Soft, mobile skin is essential for digital motion, and therefore for success in operations on the tendons that produce that motion. The skin should be inspected while it is handled and massaged. Scars, grafts, and flaps should be noted: their presence indicates inevitable interference with the blood supply. The severity of that interference is indicated by the lack of mobility detected by massage. Skin that is poorly supplied will be fixed—an ominous finding. If the scars are still red, the surgeon is wise if he adheres to conservative management until they fade and soften. Once the scars are quiescent, he must assess whether the skin cover can be improved by replacement in the form of a regional flap.

Blood Supply. While handling the digit the examiner detects any differences in temperature between it and adjacent, uninjured fingers. The digital Allen test should be performed and the findings confirmed by Doppler examination. If one digital artery is absent, supply may be adequate, but incisions should be planned on that side of the finger to maximize flow to the skin flaps. Where both are absent, the chances of preoperative ischemia and postoperative scarring are very high. The results of surgery will be poor and plans should be made in that knowledge. Digital arterial reconstruction is possible, but is rarely practical together with the other procedures indicated. When it is elected to try to improve the blood supply, reversed vein grafts taken from the anterior aspect of the forearm or arterial grafts from the posterior interosseous artery are used.

Sensation. Dry, smooth skin will probably be insensate. This can be confirmed by the static and moving two-point discrimination tests. If sensibility is seriously impaired, the results of tendon surgery are known to be poor. Reconstruction of the digital nerves requires grafts, commonly taken from either the lateral or the medial (author's preference) cutaneous nerves of the forearm (see Chap. 109).

Bone. An intact skeleton is one of the prerequisites for successful tendon surgery. Radiographs should be studied for evidence of fracture, malunion, or nonunion. If nonunion is suspected, the region should be stressed in an attempt to elicit tenderness, the sure clinical sign of persistent lack of union. Firm union is an essential requirement for tendon surgery, so appropriate steps should be taken at preliminary surgery to ensure its presence. Malunion may be a direct cause of tendon entrapment by impalement, but also may be a more subtle origin of poor digital function. Apart from its presence indicating an area of periosteal loss to which the tendon may be adherent, certain angulations seriously affect the biomechanics of the finger and preclude successful tendon surgery. One example, commonly encountered, is the apex-palmar angulation of the proximal phalanx. If permitted to heal unreduced, a flexion contracture of the proximal interphalangeal joint is almost inevitable, with an apparent loss of full flexion of the metacarpophalangeal joint. In fact, the latter flexes fully, but the malunion angulates the phalanx into extension. The flexion of the proximal interphalangeal joint comes about through the change in forces acting on that joint, and is analogous to the Z-deformity observed in rheumatoid patients. This deformity denies any chance of successful tendon surgery. Correction of this and other malunions is essential before the tendons are approached.

Joint. It is self-evident that little is gained from working on a tendon so that it may motor a joint that is, however, too irretrievably damaged to permit that motion. In examining the joint, the surgeon should measure the range of motion from full passive extension to full passive flexion. In so doing, he should assess the congruity and integrity of the surfaces of the joint. Impairment is revealed as grinding, grating, or other evidence of irregularity. Precisely taken true anteroposterior and lateral views of the joints should be studied for irregularities and for loss of joint space, which indicates loss of cartilage. Where the joint surfaces are good but motion is still restricted, this may be due to any one of several of the structures around the joint. If flexion is restricted—an extension contracture—the dorsal skin may be scarred, the extensor tendon adherent, or the dorsal capsule contracted; on the palmar surface, adhesion of the flexor tendon may be preventing free proximal movement and thereby blocking flexion. If extension is incomplete—a flexion contracture—this similarly may be due to skin, fascia, tendon sheath, or flexor tendon on the palmar surface or the extensor tendon dorsally. Within the joint itself, the true collateral ligament of the proximal interphalangeal joint is taut in all positions and therefore is not involved in contractures. The palmar plate, however, may become shortened, preventing extension, or adherent, blocking flexion. Pure tendon adhesions can easily be detected, for passive motion exceeds active on the *same* side of the joint as the adhesion, but equals it on the opposite side. In other words, a pure flexor tendon adhesion has greater passive than active flexion, but equal passive and active extension.

Problems of joint contracture and their management are dealt with in Chapter 105.

When any suspicion persists with regard to the bones or joints of the involved digit, such as doubtful union or irregular articular surfaces, polytomography may clarify the issue.

Having evaluated and in some instances attended to the skeleton, the skin envelope, and the blood and nerve supply, the examiner can concentrate on that which moves the digit, the musculotendinous apparatus.

Extensor. Complex injuries may involve both surfaces of the digit. Extensor tendon disorders may adversely affect flexor function. Adhesion of the extensors is revealed on examination by the presence of passive extension greater than that which can be achieved actively, provided only that flexor adhesions and joint contracture have not clouded the issue. The extensor adhesions preclude active extension, thereby impeding therapy after flexor surgery and predisposing to flexor tendon adhesions and joint contracture. In addition, such adhesions prevent full flexion. They clearly must be removed. Since tendon surgery on both aspects of the digit is depressingly unsuccessful, extensor tenolysis must be performed as a prelude, with a vigorous therapy program thereafter, necessary because the wounded flexor can take little or no part in the process.

Flexor. Finally, to the heart of the matter. This obtuse, even coy, approach to examination has good reason. Experience has shown that when one goes directly to the main problem, other, often significant findings are missed.

If the flexor tendon has been cut at some time past and not repaired, then little is to be learned beyond that detailed above. In most instances of early rupture, the situation is similar. Such a digit commonly has a full passive range of motion (Fig. 101–23). This, of course, is a much preferable situation to the unsuccessful, adherent tendon repair that leaves a fixed, flexed finger. Here lay the major merit in declaring the flexor sheath a "no man's land" (Bunnell, 1948; Manske, Gelberman, and Lesker, 1985). When the injury is to the flexor digitorum profundus alone in Zone I, careful palpation over the palmar aspect of the middle phalanx may detect the cut proximal end of the tendon, held out to length by persistent vincular attachments. In such cases, however long it is since the time of injury, direct repair may still be possible. When this is not so and direct repair cannot be effected, a decision must be made regarding the best way to control the distal interphalangeal joint. In making that decision, it should be remembered that Littler (1977)

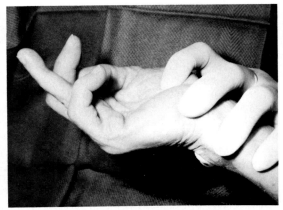

Figure 101–23. Tendon rupture. Shortly after primary repair, this patient reported that she felt a "pop" in the finger. The surgeon elected to take no further action, and here at six weeks following injury it can be seen that she had a fully extended digit that showed full passive flexion. Subsequent grafting was successful.

showed that the active flexion of the distal interphalangeal joint contributes only 3 per cent of the total arc of motion of the digit at all three joints, and only 15 per cent of the "extrinsic" arc of motion of the interphalangeal joints. The intact superficialis produces at the proximal interphalangeal joint, by contrast, 20 per cent of the total arc and 85 per cent of the extrinsic arc. Should one hazard that proximal interphalangeal motion by passing a tendon graft around or through the intact superficialis? Or should one simply stabilize the distal interphalangeal joint by tenodesis if a stump of tendon remains, or by arthrodesis if it does not? At one time, the author favored the latter view unequivocally. However, in 1982 McClinton, Curtis, and Wilgis reported the results of 100 such procedures, with an average distal interphalangeal range of motion of 48 degrees. These authors adjudged 13 per cent as failures, in which loss of proximal interphalangeal motion exceeded 20 degrees and distal interphalangeal motion was less than 20 degrees. Still a dilemma persists. Should we risk a 13 per cent failure rate in attempting to gain 3 per cent of an arc of motion? As a compromise, we should heed the advice of Stark and associates (1977a) who recommended the procedure only in selected young people. This is especially appropriate in avulsion injuries in those with open epiphyses, because arthrodesis without damage to the growth plate is difficult. In the supple hands of such young people, hyperextension of the distal interphalangeal joint with possible pseudo-bouton-

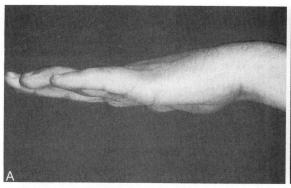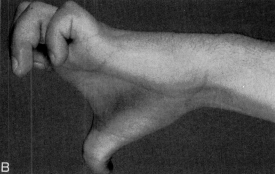

Figure 101–24. Following an avulsion of the profundus tendon that was neglected for some months, it was elected to undertake arthrodesis of the distal interphalangeal joint. The resulting extension and interphalangeal flexion is shown in *A* and *B,* respectively.

nière deformity will result from neglect. In all others, arthrodesis or tenodesis is still preferred (Fig. 101–24).

In all other instances of an unrepaired injury, once the full passive range of motion has been confirmed, it suffices merely to determine the source of the tendon graft (see below).

When previous repair or reconstruction has been performed, several problems may beset the patient.

Flexion Contracture. The causes of this most common complication of flexor tendon surgery have been discussed above—injury to other structures, poor patient selection, excessive sheath excision leading to adhesions or bowstringing, an ill-designed splint, or poorly supervised therapy. If no active motion exists, the course of the tendon should be palpated during attempts at flexion, to try to ensure its integrity. Tension beneath the skin suggests an intact tendon, although such tension may be transmitted through scar. The severity of the contracture should be determined by measuring the extension deficit, i.e., the sum in degrees at each joint of the failure to achieve a straight finger. The joints involved are noted, because the adhesion will lie distal to the most distal joint retaining a normal range. The active and passive flexion should be recorded; the latter often exceeds the former. In most flexion contractures, it is not possible to distinguish between tendon adhesions alone and adhesions combined with joint contracture.

Bowstringing. This results almost solely from excessive incision of the retinacular system, very rarely from rupture of an intact pulley. The effect is to increase the moment arm of the tendon at the joints it crosses. This causes more powerful flexion of the joint(s), but also a need for more tendon excursion to achieve full flexion. This excursion is not available. Bowstringing therefore results in incomplete flexion *and* extension, the latter sometimes causing a flexion contracture of the most involved joint. Its presence is confirmed by asking the patient to flex the digit against resistance, while the examiner palpates the tendon.

TENOLYSIS OR EXPLORATION

Since the surgeon often does not know what procedure will be required, as discussed above, the attempted tenolysis may simply be the exploratory prelude to more complex procedures (i.e., delayed repair, graft, silicone rod, pulley reconstruction, or distal interphalangeal joint arthrodesis). Tenolysis may be performed after primary tendon repair or after one- or two-stage tendon graft. Some authors state that tenolysis is indicated mainly where the passive range exceeds the active and all joint contractures have been overcome (Strickland, 1985b). Such a patient would certainly be ideal, but is also rare. All too frequently the candidate has a severe contracture that cannot be overcome by therapy. Passive flexion may often exceed active but is a secondary bonus. The contracture is the problem.

The timing of tenolysis has been studied extensively, recommendations varying from 12 weeks (Wray, Moucharafieh, and Weeks, 1978) to nine months (Rank, Wakefield, and Hueston, 1973). In fact, an absolute time does not exist. The procedure is performed when all associated injuries have been treated effectively (see above), when maximal benefit from therapy has been achieved, and when the skin of the involved digit is soft and mobile.

Although the surgeon may have to proceed with graft or pulley reconstruction requiring later supplemental regional or general anesthesia, the merits of local anesthesia for tenolysis are so cogent as to dictate its use in all patients capable of cooperating. Such merits include the ability of the patient to participate in the tenolysis by active motion of the part when requested, and second, the golden opportunity to show the patient the result of the procedure while pain does not restrict it. If he has seen full motion, his motivation to achieve that range in postoperative therapy is immeasurably enhanced (Schneider and Mackin, 1984). Digital or wrist block can be employed. The latter requires that the surgeon block the metacarpophalangeal joints in a little flexion when testing or demonstrating extension, otherwise the intrinsic paralysis causes clawing with poor active proximal interphalangeal extension. Bupivacaine 0.5 per cent is used, the 12 hour duration of anesthesia providing pain relief during the early postoperative therapy that is an essential feature of tenolysis. Some surgeons leave an indwelling catheter alongside the appropriate nerve to permit supplementary anesthesia for several days. The author reserves that technique for second tenolyses.

With supplemental analgesia and tranquilization in the form of fentanyl-droperidol or diazepam, the patient can often tolerate an upper arm tourniquet for 30 minutes or more. If more time is required, a secondary pediatric tourniquet around the mid-forearm can provide it. The secondary tourniquet also overcomes the problem of paralysis of extrinsic tendons that occurs after 20 to 30 minutes of ischemia and negates patient participation.

The digit is opened from tip to palm through the incisions discussed above. Such extensive exposure may seem excessive, but experience shows that it is invariably necessary, and starting the procedure with full display of the sheath saves time limited by the use of local anesthesia. The entire sheath should be preserved, working through retinacular windows, both for reasons discussed above (Fig. 101–25). The two tendons should first be mobilized fully at the proximal interphalangeal window. Often the two cannot be distinguished from each other. The profundus should then be dissected distally where it is the sole tendon, and the two dissected as far

proximally as they are distinct structures. The superficialis and profundus should then be dissected one from the other in the palm out as far as the A$_1$ pulley. Tenolysis then proceeds from both directions toward the point of fusion and adhesion. Traction on the tendons away from the bed and each other reveals the correct plane, which is then pursued by dissection with a standard knife or Beaver blade (McDonough and Stern, 1983) (Fig. 101–25). Traction on the tendon is *never* applied with forceps, otherwise the damage caused to the surface would surely result in adhesions. Instead, a right-angled retractor or a soft rubber catheter should be placed around the tendon(s). Pulleys, which should never be divided, are retracted with a hook or right-angled retractor and the plane of dissection followed beneath them. Once this has been pursued as far as possible, the dissection must go to the next window, the pulley being retracted in the other direction. If a valid channel can be opened at any point below the pulley from one window to the next, a rubber catheter or a retractor can be passed from one to the other and put around one or other tendon. This tendon can then be drawn from one window to the other beneath the pulley, permitting further separation of the two tendons from the pulley and bed, and from each other. At the point of primary repair, revealed by the presence of suture material, the tendon should be inspected for the presence of scar. This is seen as an area of gray between the more yellow tendinous material, and is usually that area of the tenolyzed tendon of the smallest diameter. If this area is too narrow, it is likely to rupture; if too long, it is likely to flex the digit incompletely (see below). In separating the superficialis and profundus, once all local dissection is apparently completed, one should be secured distally and the other proximally, and traction applied in opposite directions. The tendon held should then be exchanged and the traction repeated in opposite directions. This often separates long and undetected intertendinous adhesions. A point will be reached at which the surgeon believes that the tenolysis may be complete. Three steps are taken in turn to prove this. The tendon is drawn as far distally as possible from beneath a pulley and marked with ink at the edge of the pulley. By then drawing it proximally, the surgeon can observe whether or not that mark emerges beneath the pulley, indicating clearance at least on that surface.

geon's forearm. When it reaches the upper third of the calf, the sharp stripper is substituted for the dull. With a levering motion on the stripper while pulling on the tendon, it is detached through the muscle belly.

Extensor Digitorum Longus of Second, Third, and Fourth Toes. The extensor digitorum longus and the extensor digitorum brevis both act on only four toes, the former on the four lateral toes, while the latter only rarely sends a slip to the fifth. Grafts may therefore be taken only from the central three. A feature of the extensor digitorum longus is that there are many intertendinous connections on the dorsum of the foot. Thus, while grafts can be taken with a stripper, it may be difficult. Also, because of these connections, the grafts obtained are less smooth than others. For this reason the author tries not to use the extensor digitorum longus graft unless the recipient bed has been previously prepared by use of a silicone rod. When the grafts are taken from all three toes, as described below, the interconnections may be left intact. If so, it is important in inserting the grafts to attach the common proximal end first, or there is imbalance between the tension of the grafts to the three digits.

Harvest. Through longitudinal incisions over the proximal phalanx of each of the second, third, and fourth toes, the extensor hood is exposed. The tendons of the extensor digitorum longus and brevis are dissected, the latter lying lateral to the former. Further transverse incisions are made over the dorsum of the foot, some 3 inches apart over the line of the extensor digitorum longus, which is detected by repeatedly flexing and extending the toes. Using the same guide, the tendons are isolated at each wound, the most proximal of which is above the extensor retinaculum on the anterior surface of the leg. The extensor digitorum longus is now divided in each of the wounds over the toes. Three hemostats are passed into the toe wounds along the tendon from the wound next proximal, and the tendons are grasped and withdrawn in retrograde fashion. This maneuver is repeated, progressing proximally one wound at a time.

When more than one graft is required, it is perfectly permissible (Farmer, Farkas, and Herbert, 1983) to split one of the thicker grafts longitudinally. This is done with three hemostats, holding respectively the conjoined end and the two ends resulting from a small knife cut in the other end. The hemostats are pulled away from one another at angles of 120 degrees while the knife is advanced from one tendon end to the other, splitting the fibers.

TECHNIQUE

The distal attachment is prepared first, by dissecting the insertion of the flexor digitorum profundus off the underlying palmar plate of the distal interphalangeal joint. Continuing in that plane with a small rigid knife, such as a No. 67 Beaver blade, the proximal portion of the insertion is lifted from the distal phalanx, exposing bare bone. At this point the choice lies between going through, around, or along the bone. The first two carry some risk of damage to the nail bed; the author therefore follows the third course. Two 20 gauge needles are passed through the pulp of the finger some 3 to 4 mm from the free edge of the nail plate and 5 mm apart, parallel to one another and aiming proximally, in such a way that the needles slide along the anterior surface of the distal phalanx to emerge side by side beneath the flexor digitorum profundus insertion just where the bone has been exposed. For the moment they are left there.

In the palmar wound the superficialis tendon is dissected, pulled out to length, and, if not required as a graft or motor (see below), cut off and discarded. The profundus tendon is located best by its position and by dissecting in the lumbrical, which should be left attached. If, as in most cases, the injury has been distal to the lumbrical, the profundus will have undergone little or no myostatic contraction. In any event the end of the tendon, once dissected clear, should be firmly grasped with a tissue forceps or a heavy suture. The portion grasped is later discarded. Longitudinal distraction should now be applied to the proposed motor to the graft for a timed three minutes, during which time little or nothing may happen. In other instances, however, the distraction initially achieved may gradually increase. This comes about because tissues distorted by injury commonly demonstrate what is known in engineering as "creep." This is the phenomenon whereby deformation under constant load increases with the passage of time. If this is not done, it is impossible to select the tension appropriate for any graft, since the extent of "creep" that occurs *after* grafting is variable and unpredictable. On completion of the period of distraction, the total excursion that can be achieved from the relaxed to the fully distracted position should be measured. Potential total active excursion varies according to the configuration of the muscle belly, but as a general rule it is twice the passive excursion measured on the operating table.

The graft is now taken from its bed where it has been left, prepared for transfer (see p. 4551). If a rod is to be replaced, the suture placed in the graft is now stitched into the rod, which is then drawn through and out of the distal window. If no rod is in the bed, the graft must be passed beneath the retained segments of the sheath. This may be difficult if the intact segments are long or if the graft is of a wide diameter, approximating to the caliber of the tendon sheath. In such a situation, passage of the graft can be facilitated by placing in the tendon sheath a pediatric nasogastric feeding tube of appropriate size. After the needle has been removed the suture in the end of the graft can be passed along the tubing, which should be kept dry for that purpose. The suture, once through, is drawn through until the tendon graft abuts against the tubing. Grasping both the suture and the tubing at the distal end, the surgeon can easily bring the graft into position.

The two ends of suture in the graft are now passed through the 20 gauge needles previously placed through the pulp of the finger. The needles are removed and the graft is drawn up tightly beneath the flexor digitorum profundus insertion by traction on the sutures, which are then tied over a dental roll. The distal repair is completed with one or two figure-of-eight sutures through the graft and the distal stump, taking care not to cut the pull-out suture through the pulp in the process. The distal repair is now tested by applying traction to the proximal end of the graft and allowing the finger to flex fully. This demonstrates first that the repair is secure, and second that the graft is capable of producing motion equal to the passive range. If the distal interphalangeal joint does not flex fully, the distal repair is abutting against the A_4 pulley; it should be modified. The A_4 pulley of course should not be incised to achieve this. The excursion of the tendon necessary to produce full flexion of the finger should be measured. If this is more than the estimated total active excursion of the motor (see above), it is possible that the pulleys are incompetent or insufficient. This can be tested by placing temporary bands of umbilical tape

around the finger and repeating the test. If this confirms the need by reducing the excursion necessary to produce full flexion, additional pulleys should be constructed. If pulley deficiency is not the problem, the excursion in the selected motor is inadequate. The surgeon must then decide whether to accept that limitation or to seek another motor. This most commonly is the superficialis of the injured digit. If for some reason this is not available, the superficialis of an adjacent intact finger can be transferred.

The proximal tenorrhaphy should now be performed (Fig. 101–27). An end to end juncture can be undertaken if the motor and graft are of comparable diameter, but this is rarely the case, and in any event such a join is less strong than a weave, which is therefore preferred (Pulvertaft, 1956). Using the grasp already established on the end of the motor tendon, it is drawn distally until it is rendered tense. A tendon-weaving forceps is then passed through the motor tendon some 5 mm from the grasping forceps, and the proximal end of the graft is placed in the weaver and then drawn through the motor tendon. An estimate of tension is then made and the first stitch is placed in the weave. This, and all subsequent stitches, start in the slot of the motor created by the weaving forceps, passing through the graft, the other side of the slot, over and back through all three tendon layers. Finally the stitch is passed through the final side of the slot to be tied, thereby leaving the knot within the slot. The tension can now be assessed. Provided the motor has been loaded as described above, the correct tension is that which brings the digit into a proper cascade with the other unaffected fingers. This is best observed by removing all instruments from the hand and flexing and extending the wrist while observing that cascade. Motion in the digit under repair should be exactly coordinated with those adjacent throughout the full range. If the tension is incorrect, adjustment is simply made. A mark is made with a pen on the graft adjacent to the motor on that side of the motor toward which the graft must be moved to correct the tension. This mark acts as a point of reference. The single suture placed earlier is then removed, adjustment made, a new suture placed, and the process repeated until tension is deemed to be correct. A second suture is then placed in similar fashion on the opposite side of the graft in the same slot. The weave is repeated through two further slots, each

102

Ray A. Elliott, Jr.

Extensor Tendon Repair

A minor interest, perhaps even a lack of respect for, extensor tendon injuries was quite evident in the early training, publications, and scientific programs devoted to surgery of the hand. Although the volume of published concern for flexor tendon and neurovascular injuries continues to outweigh that for extensor tendon injuries, it is gratifying to see an increasing number of thoughtful contributions related to the extensor mechanism. Unfortunately, there is still a tendency to consider the emergency room presentation of an extensor tendon injury as a fitting challenge for the neophyte. Unlike the usual flexor tendon injury in which the retracted ends must be sought some distance from the wound, extensor tendon ends seen within the wound may appear to present an opportunity for a "simple surgical experience of the first order." However, for the unwary, that is where the fun stops. The proper diagnosis and treatment of injury to the extensor mechanism is serious business, owing in part to the delicate nature and balance of the mechanism (Tubiana and Valentin, 1964a,b). The unique presentation and requirements of treatment at the various levels of encounter can serve to organize discussion.

GENERAL CONSIDERATIONS

Before delving into the details of anatomy, function, pathologic physiology, and treatment related to specific structures and levels of injury, it is well to review the considerations common to most extensor injuries.

The Injury

The open wounds most frequently associated with loss of continuity of the extensor mechanism are laceration, crush, avulsion, and deep abrasion. Their relative frequency varies with the level of injury. Avulsion of the extensor tendon from its insertion onto the middle or distal phalanx is often a closed injury. The type of wound and level of injury give the trained hand surgeon useful information regarding the possible underlying defect.

Priority. All injuries should have a priority of treatment. In the hand the highest priority is given to vascular insufficiency, loss of cover, and an unstable fracture. Most flexor tendon and nerve injuries also have a priority higher than extensor tendons in cases in which the repairs are incompatible. However, prompt repair of an injury to the extensor mechanism is valuable when feasible (Mason, 1936); subtle imbalance can quickly lead to fixed deformity.

Lacerations. A tendon injury in a clean wound made by a sharp instrument carries the best prognosis for an uncomplicated restoration of function (Fig. 102–1). Most lacerations can be made surgically clean by irri-

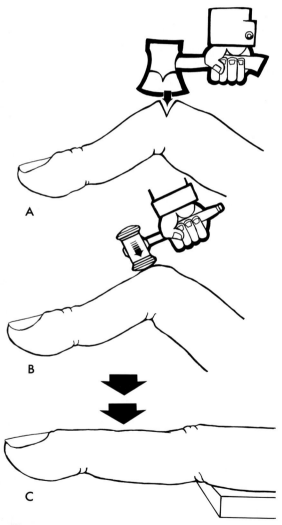

Figure 102–1. Common types of injury to extensor tendons. *A,* Lacerations are most frequent. *B,* Crush can cause immediate or delayed rupture. *C,* Forced flexion of an actively extended joint may avulse tendon insertion with or without associated fracture.

gation and debridement of nonviable tissue. However, if there is any question about viability of the cover or residual contamination, it is better to delay the tendon repair. In the author's experience, a repair within 10 to 14 days carries the same prognosis as an earlier repair. Highly contaminated wounds, such as a human bite, require aggressive wound treatment and delayed tendon repair. If conditions are proper, exploration will obviate the delayed rupture sometimes seen with undiagnosed partial division.

Crush Injuries. Associated fractures are common in this group of tendon injuries. The healing tendon may adhere to the fracture site, but with precise bone reduction, accurate tendon repair, and internal fixation, simultaneous repair is usually feasible. Interposition of soft tissue between the healing bone and tendon may be helpful, but synthetic sheeting has proved disappointing. In a closed injury with tendon crush or partial division, there is always the possibility of a delayed rupture at 10 to 14 days when the healing fibers soften. Exploration or precautionary splinting is always indicated if tendon damage is suspected (see Fig. 102–11).

Avulsion Wounds. Incomplete avulsion injuries of the dorsal cover present unique problems in management. For example, a beveled wound may harbor a tendon injury in the deeper portion beneath an intact cover. The classic ring finger degloving may avulse the tendon from the distal phalanx, but seldom damages the remaining extensor mechanism per se, because the separation occurs above the deep fascia. However, flaps that depend on retrograde venous drainage and arterial nutrition demand careful management to avoid progressive necrosis and secondary tendon involvement (Elliott, Hoehn, and Stayman, 1979).

Complete avulsion injuries require replacement of the missing structures. When cover and tendon are avulsed, the reconstructed cover must have a subcutaneous stratum to facilitate gliding of tendons (Weeks, 1967). Free skin grafts can be used over paratenon, but they will not survive on extensive bare tendon. Biologic dressings afford the best protection for denuded tendons if definitive repair of the cover must be delayed for hours or days (Elliott and Hoehn, 1973); electrolyte dressings are not an effective alternative. When a joint and tendon are seriously damaged at the same level, arthrodesis is often the best choice (see Fig. 102–21).

Deep Abrasion. This injury is more common on the dorsal surface of the hand and fingers. The extensor mechanism is vulnerable beneath the thin cover. The principles of treatment are the same as for the complex avulsion injuries discussed above.

Other Types of Wound. Thermal burns of the thin dorsal cover of the hand and fingers can be very damaging to the underlying extensor mechanism. Early removal of the burned cover and prompt resurfacing with skin grafts may prevent progressive damage and tendon involvement (see Chap. 129). Electrical burns often cause more extensive deep damage that requires amputation or complex reconstruction (see Chap. 132).

The mangled hand is certain to have severe associated injuries. Because of the priorities noted above, extensor tendon repairs are often delayed in favor of more acute concerns.

The Golden Period. Early teaching defined a six-hour postinjury "golden period" for tendon repair in a surgically clean wound (Bunnell, 1944). Today, this period can be extended considerably. Closure of the wound and the use of antibiotics allow delay of the tendon repair for up to 10 to 14 days after injury if necessary (Carter and Mersheimer, 1966). Delay of the primary repair is a good option if the surgical environment and technique can be improved by the delay. Biologic dressings provide a dependable protection for exposed tendons if wound closure must be delayed for a few hours or days.

Closed Tendon Avulsion. Avulsion of an extensor tendon from its bony insertion on the distal or middle phalanx usually occurs as the result of forceful flexion of an actively extended joint; most recreational injuries have a history of a strike on the tip of the outstretched digit. Treated early, this type of injury may respond to simple splinting of the involved interphalangeal (IP) joint. An associated avulsion of a small fragment of bone can often be ignored; treatment of a major avulsion involving the articular surface is more complex. The treatment options vary with the level of injury.

Extensor Tendon Peculiarities

Paratenon. The extensor mechanism is extrasynovial except at the wrist level, where synovial sheaths facilitate free gliding of tendons beneath the dorsal carpal ligament (Tubiana, 1968). Distal to these sheaths, the tendons on the dorsum of the hand are surrounded by paratenon. This delicate, transparent, vascular layer of deep fascia supplies a segmental circulation to the tendons via their deep surface (Smith, 1968). The vascular leash is a short, effective tether compared with a synovial mesentery, and thus gliding is rather limited (Zbrodowski, Gajisin, and Grodecki, 1980). The vascularity of paratenon and the proliferation of unsatisfied extra synovial tendon ends both contribute to the dense, adhesive scar seen after some neglected or poorly managed extensor injuries (Redfern, Curtis, and Wilgis, 1982). On the positive side, tendons divided in paratenon do not retract very far and their retrieval is relatively easy.

Tendon Plus Scar. A good quality tendon repair is important for another reason. If a scar-filled gap between tendon ends is more than a few millimeters in length, the tendon unit plus scar may be too long to move the more distal joints into full extension. This problem is best prevented by accurate tendon approximation and proper splinting to prevent stretching of the fresh scar. Although good spontaneous improvement has been seen with contracture of the maturing scar, this is not common; early and prolonged splinting is much more certain. Some older deformities respond to prolonged splinting alone, but the most dependable results are seen after tendon-scar shortening and splinting in combination (Elliott, 1970).

Early Motion. Active motion during the first two weeks after repair may increase the bulk of tendon healing, lengthen the interposed scar, or even break the union (Bunnell, 1964). However, early guarded active motion may benefit selected injuries proximal to the metacarpophalangeal (MP) joint (Dargan, 1969; Merritt, 1986). Injuries treated by splinting alone require a full period of immobilization without periodic "testing." As a rule, extensor tendon repairs are splinted longer than flexor tendon healing repairs in order to prevent injury to the repair by the more powerful flexors.

Tendon Characteristics. Although extensor action is weaker, and active excursion is less than that of the flexors, the extensor mechanism is able to accommodate the full range of motion of the flexors. The distal shift of the extensor expansion of the fingers during digital flexion is an example of this accommodation (Rosenthal, 1984). A cross section of the extensor tendons of the forearm and at the wrist is similar to that of the flexor tendons (Kilgore and Graham, 1977). Overlying the metacarpals, they become thinner and flatter, and expose a broader surface area to injury. Beyond the metacarpophalangeal level, exposure to injury is even greater as the delicate extensor mechanism expands to wrap the dorsum and sides of the proximal and middle phalanges, protected only by a thin cover of skin and fascia.

Patient Factors

Acute Injuries. The details of a social and work history often become secondary when the planned treatment can promptly restore the extensor mechanism and return good function to the hand. However, there are subtle treatment variations that depend on the age, health, occupation, and wishes of the patient. After weighing all factors, a qualified hand surgeon should discuss the options and recommend one preferred treatment.

Established Deformities. Recommendations for the correction of established deformities may vary greatly. For example, an awkward deformity that interferes with work may motivate repair, whereas the same deformity in a sedentary person may be of less concern. Discomfort, clumsiness, and poor appearance are common motivations for reconstruction. The patient's occupation and recreation may mandate precise needs. Even more than with acute injuries, the options must be discussed with and the choice guided by an experienced surgeon.

Age. Young patients should be encouraged to seek the greatest possible function. Informed olders patient may elect some compromise of function in return for a timely, less complicated rehabilitation. A combination of satisfactory function and reasonable appearance is a standard goal for any age group.

Treatment Conditions and Technique

The Surgeon. The surgeon who accepts a patient for the treatment of an extensor tendon injury should have experience or expert guidance. Truly good results do not come easily. Knowledge of anatomy, pathologic physiology, treatment options, and follow-up care are essential. Probably the function of more hands has been saved by an informed and judicious decision to close the skin, prescribe antibiotic coverage, and delay the tendon repair than by a decision to operate without experience or guidance.

Environment and Preparation. Wound explorations and open tendon repairs should be carried out in a bloodless field, preferably in an operating room environment. Proper wound preparation sets the stage for an uncomplicated course. Thorough wound irrigation and conservative debridement of all nonviable tissue should be a surgical habit. If tendon repair must be delayed, skin closure and interim splinting should be considered.

Anesthesia. Local infiltration anesthesia is used most often on the hand. General anesthesia or nerve block is reserved for extensive and complex wounds, and for treatment of uncooperative or very young patients. Vasoconstrictors are never used. Repairs in the forearm and at the wrist level are easier under general anesthesia or nerve block in order to gain muscle relaxation; the author prefers the efficiency of general anesthesia whenever feasible.

Exposure. The traumatic wound is often extended to facilitate accurate diagnosis and repair. Undulating and zigzag longitudinal incisions are preferred; short transverse incisions give the poorest exposure. On the hand and wrist the author usually incorporates the traumatic wound and tries to cross the joints transversely. Straight-line longitudinal incisions are used on the forearm where linear contracture is less frequent. Remember that any incision may occasionally hypertrophy; fortunately, most soften and fade with time when well placed.

A bloodless field aids exposure, and a digital or arm tourniquet is routine. The latter is readily tolerated by most adults for up to 45 minutes, and periodic release extends that time. Elevation of the extremity, manual exsanguination, and a tourniquet pressure of 250 mm Hg for adults is the author's preference.

Tendon Retrieval. Meticulous handling of tissues is fundamental in hand surgery. It has a special significance in tendon surgery when scar formation at each contact point has been well documented (Potenza, 1964). With tendons freshly severed in the finger, extension of the next most distal joint beyond the level of injury brings the tendon ends together. On the dorsum of the hand and with injuries in the synovial sheaths at the wrist, retrieval usually requires extension of both the wrist and metacarpophalangeal joints. A combination of wrist extension and milking of the forearm muscles is used for selected injuries above the wrist, along with increased surgical exposure. Transcutaneous, fine, hypodermic needle fixation of tendons divided in their sheath facilitates a tension-free repair, but joint positioning alone is sufficient for injuries in paratenon.

ANATOMY AND FUNCTION

Dorsal Skin

The dorsal cover of the hand consists of skin and layers of superficial and deep fascia. The skin is noticeably thinner, softer, and more pliable than on the palm. Missing are the fibrous septa, callus, and fat padding that fix and protect the palmar structures. The redundant dorsal skin seen with joint extension becomes taut and thinned with flexion. Thus, the relatively superficial extensor mechanism is susceptible to injury, particularly over the metacarpophalangeal and interphalangeal joints made prominent by finger flexion.

Superficial Fascia

The superficial layer of dorsal fascia has a delicate, fatty component that contains large lymphatic and venous channels, and a relatively insignificant arterial supply. A deeper membranous portion is loosely attached to the deep fascia by areolar tissue (Rosenthal, 1984). It is this areolar plane that balloons with traumatic and inflammatory edema, and leaves the deep fascia and extensor mechanism intact in the classic degloving injury.

Deep Fascia

The deep fascia of the dorsal forearm condenses at the wrist to become the dorsal carpal ligament. Vertical septa from the deep surface of the ligament to the radius and ulna define a series of fibro-osseous canals through which the extrinsic tendons pass en route to their insertions on the hand. At this level the tendons are enclosed in sheaths of synovium.

Distal to the termination of the synovial sheaths, the deep fascia splits to envelop the extensor tendons in a peritendinous fascia known as paratenon. The clinical significance of paratenon is discussed under Extensor Tendon Peculiarities above.

Wrist Extension

The dedicated extensors of the hand at the wrist are the extensor carpi radialis longus (ECRL) and brevis (ECRB) and the extensor carpi ulnaris (ECU). The two radial extensors have muscle origins on the medial side, and the ulnar extensor on the lateral side, of the elbow and forearm. All three become tendinous in the distal half of the forearm. The ECRL and ECRB tendons pass through the second dorsal compartment to insert on the dorsal base of the second and third metacarpals, respectively. The ECU tendon passes through the sixth compartment to insert on the base of the fifth metacarpal (Kaplan, 1965).

Although their principal function is wrist extension, as synergistic muscles for flexion of the digits they also stabilize the wrist and conserve the flexion forces for action on the digits. The ECRL and ECU tendons, acting with their corresponding wrist flexors, also abduct and adduct the wrist. The ECRB is the purist wrist extensor because of its more central insertion; therefore, preservation of this tendon often has a priority in reconstruction.

Extension of the wrist is a secondary function for the extensors of the fingers and thumb. Their efficiency as digital extensors is enhanced by synergistic wrist flexion. The synergistic action of tendons inserting on the hand is particularly important when tendon transfers are planned (Bunnell, 1964) (see Chap. 114).

Extrinsic Finger Extension

Extensor Digitorum Communis. Extension of the fingers is produced by a combination of extrinsic and intrinsic muscle action (Harris and Rutledge, 1972). The principal extensor of the fingers at the metacarpophalangeal joint is the extensor digitorum communis (EDC). It has an origin at the elbow and in the forearm and becomes tendinous in the distal forearm, giving rise to three or four tendons that pass together through the fourth dorsal compartment. The EDC tendon to the little finger may arise at the proximal metacarpal level from the ulnar side of the EDC tendon to the ring finger. The EDC tendons to the index, middle, and ring fingers are more constant (Schenck, 1964). A variety of intertendinous connections (juncturae tendinum) over the distal portion of the metacarpals limits the independent action of the EDC on the middle, ring, and little fingers and may limit independent EDC extension of the index finger (Fig. 102–2). The tendons of the EDC continue over the proximal phalanxes in the extensor expansion. Authors argue about the presence and nature of a formal attachment of EDC tendons to the capsule of the metacarpophalangeal joint or to the base of the proximal phalanx, but this is a moot point, because the EDC tendons never *function* as if there is a significant insertion at this level (Harris and Rutledge, 1972).

Extensor Indicis Proprius. Independent extension of the metacarpophalangeal joint of the index finger is the primary function of the extensor indicis proprius (EIP) tendon. The EIP muscle arises on the ulnar side of the dorsal forearm, and the tendon passes through the fourth dorsal compartment at the wrist deep to and along the ulnar side of the EDC to the index finger, to insert into the extensor expansion. The EIP contributes to ulnar deviation of the finger, but the ability to point is a more significant function.

Extensor Digiti Quinti Minimus. Independent metacarpophalangeal extension of the little finger is supplied by the extensor digiti quinti minimus (EDQM) muscle, whose origin resembles that of the EDC to which it is occasionally fused (Schenck, 1964). The tendon travels alone through the fifth dorsal compartment and is ulnar to the EDC to the little finger, en route to its insertion into the extensor expansion. The EDQM frequently splits into two tendons, the ulnar one remaining independent, and the radial one joined to the EDC tendon to the ring finger. Independent extension of the little finger is often weak and of little importance.

Intrinsic Finger Extension

The interosseous and lumbrical muscles are the principal extensors of the interphalangeal joints of the fingers (Littler, 1967). They take their origin from adjacent metacarpal bones and from the profundus tendons, respectively. The first dorsal interosseous muscle is the most vulnerable to injury. The other inter-

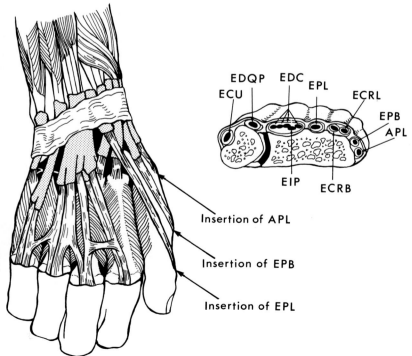

Insertion of APL

Insertion of EPB

Insertion of EPL

EDQP EDC EPL
ECU   ECRL
                        EPB
                        APL

EIP ECRB

Figure 102–2. Functional anatomy of extensor tendons on the wrist, hand, and thumb. Dedicated extensors of the hand at the wrist are the extensor carpi radialis (ECRL) and brevis (ECRB) and extensor carpi ulnaris (ECU). Metacarpophalangeal joints of fingers are extended by the extensor digitorum and proprius tendons of the index (EIP) and little (EDQP) fingers. Variable intertendinous connections over the distal metacarpals limit independent extensor digitorum communis (EDC) action. The abductor pollicis longus (APL) assists thumb extension by stabilizing the first metacarpal. The extensor pollicis longus (EPL) and brevis (EPB) extend the metacarpophalangeal and interphalangeal joints; only the EPL can hyperextend the distal phalanx. Six fibro-osseous compartments formed by the dorsal carpal ligament attachments to bone determine where the tendons enter the hand.

osseous muscles and the lumbrical muscles lie deeper and are better protected by the metacarpals. The intrinsic tendons are more vulnerable after they merge on the dorsum of the middle phalanx.

Extensor Apparatus of Fingers

The complex anatomy and function of the extensor mechanism in the fingers have been detailed and debated by numerous authors. At and beyond the metacarpophalangeal joint, extension forces are transmitted by a fascinating array of fibers held together by a delicate elastic membrane (Schultz, Furlong, and Storace, 1981). This apparatus, also known as the extensor expansion or the extensor hood, covers the dorsum and portions of the sides of the proximal and middle phalanges, and has anatomic or functional insertions into the base of both of these phalanges

(Fig. 102–3). It has a tendon system to transmit tension and produce motion, and a retinacular system to stabilize the tendon system (Rosenthal, 1984). A working knowledge of the anatomy and physiology of this apparatus is important to any surgeon treating hand injuries.

Anatomy of Tendon System. The sagittal bands are vertically oriented fibers of the apparatus that cover the capsule and collateral ligaments of the metacarpophalangeal joint, and separate them from the intrinsic muscles (Harris and Rutledge, 1972). During extension, these bands lie as a hood over the metacarpophalangeal joint; during flexion they are distal to the joint axis.

The central band of the tendon system is a continuation of the EDC tendon. Although there may be some proximal attachments (Tubiana and Valentin 1964a,b), most of the central tendon fibers end in the distal part of the proximal interphalangeal (PIP) joint cap-

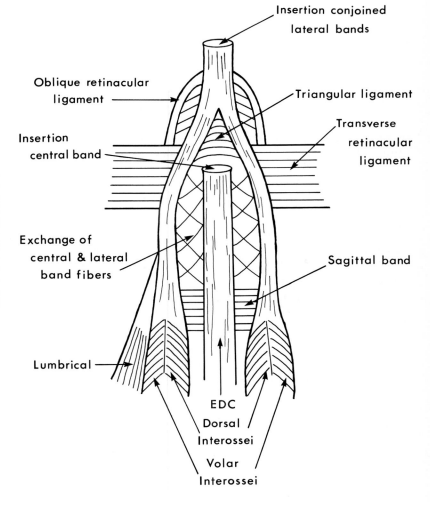

Figure 102–3. Functional anatomy of finger extension. The extensor digitorum communis (EDC) extends the metacarpophalangeal joints; when the latter is fixed it can extend the proximal interphalangeal joints. The interossei and lumbricals are principal interphalangeal joint extensors. The tendon system, stabilized by a retinacular system, exchanges fibers in a delicate elastic membrane of extensor expansion.

Insertion conjoined lateral bands

Oblique retinacular ligament

Triangular ligament

Transverse retinacular ligament

Insertion central band

Exchange of central & lateral band fibers

Sagittal band

Lumbrical

EDC
Dorsal Interossei
Volar Interossei

sule with a bone insertion on the base of the middle phalanx (Hauck, 1923). Some fibers of the EDC are exchanged with each of the lateral bands (Haines, 1951).

Distal to the sagittal bands, the intrinsic muscles contribute proximal vertical and distal oblique fibers to the sides of the central tendon. The lateral bands are predominantly tendinous extensions of the oblique fibers of the intrinsics, with contributions from the EDC (Smith, 1974). Distal to the proximal interphalangeal joint they first are separated by a portion of the apparatus known as the triangular ligament, and then merge to form a conjoined tendon and a terminal tendon. The latter blends with the capsule of the distal joint and inserts on the base of the distal phalanx.

Anatomy of Retinacular System. The principal components of the retinacular system are the transverse and oblique fibers described by Landsmeer (1963), who called them "ligaments." After arising from the proximal phalanx and flexor tendon sheath in the volar compartment, transverse fibers of the system pass through a window in Cleland's ligament volar to the axis of the proximal interphalangeal joint, to insert on the lateral bands dorsal to the axis and on the triangular ligament that separates them at this level (Milford, 1968). The deeper and more tendinous oblique fibers have a broad insertion on the side of the lateral bands from the level of the proximal interphalangeal joint to at least the distal third of the middle phalanx (Tubiana and Valentin, 1964a,b). One author believes there is also an insertion into the base of the distal phalanx as well. The author's experience with the treatment of the boutonnière deformity would exclude any functional significance of such an attachment, if indeed it exists.

Physiology. The published motion (Hauck, 1923; Stack, 1962; Zancolli, 1968; Evans and Burkhalter, 1986) and electromyographic (Backhouse and Catton, 1954) studies of the extensor mechanism are excellent. Evaluation and treatment of finger deformities caused by division or contracture of the extensor apparatus are facilitated by basic knowledge about the dynamics of the mechanism.

The primary function of the EDC tendon is extension of the proximal phalanx at the metacarpophalangeal joint, but with this joint in extension or flexion and further active extension blocked, the EDC can also extend the middle and distal phalanges (Zancolli, 1968). The EDC is unable to extend the two distal phalanges against normal flexor tone if the metacarpophalangeal joint is allowed to hyperextend.

Normally the extensor hood over the metacarpophalangeal joint level is free to slide proximally with MP extension and distally with MP flexion. With the hood in the distal position, the interossei contribute to flexion of the metacarpophalangeal joint through their vertical fibers, and have little or no effect on the proximal and distal interphalangeal joints. With the hood in the proximal position and the metacarpophalangeal joints stabilized in extension, the interossei can act through the oblique fibers and lateral bands to extend the middle and distal phalanges (Littler, 1967).

The lumbrical muscles, like the interossei, provide flexion of the metacarpophalangeal joint through vertical fibers. In contrast, however, they are effective extensors of the middle and distal phalanges regardless of the position of the metacarpophalangeal joint. If the latter is held in flexion by action of the intrinsic muscles, the EDC tendon is able to exert an effective extension force across the proximal and distal interphalangeal joints (Bunnell, 1964).

The two lateral bands, which normally lay quite dorsal to the axis of motion of the extended proximal interphalangeal joint, shift volarward with PIP flexion. This lateral band shift permits flexion of the distal interphalangeal joint during active flexion of the proximal interphalangeal joint (Smith, 1974). However, the intact triangular ligament limits the extent of the shift and prevents the lateral bands from dropping below the axis of motion to become flexors of the proximal interphalangeal joint.

Thumb Extension

The extensor pollicis longus (EPL) tendon transverses the wrist in the third fibroosseous compartment, and from this radial dorsal approach is an effective adductor and supinator of the first ray. This tendon also extends the metacarpophalangeal joint and can hyperextend the interphalangeal joint.

The extensor pollicis brevis (EPB) enters the hand via the first dorsal wrist compartment along with the abductor pollicis longus (APL), the important stabilizer of the first metacarpal base. The EPB extends the carpometacarpal and metacarpophalangeal joints and has a bone insertion on the base of the proximal phalanx. Frequently its action is extended to the distal phalanx as well (Kaplan, 1965).

The extensor anatomy at the thumb metacarpophalangeal joint level resembles the anatomy at the proximal interphalangeal joint level of the fingers. The adductor pollicis and abductor pollicis tendons contribute to a dorsal expansion, which has transverse fibers that act like the transverse retinacular ligaments of the fingers (Milford, 1968). This expansion stabilizes the EPB and EPL tendons and exchanges their extension forces. Thus, the intrinsics of the thumb are able to extend (but not hyperextend) the interphalangeal joint, and fibers of the dorsal apparatus transmit energy from the EPL tendon to extend the metacarpophalangeal joint (Rosenthal, 1984).

INJURIES AT SPECIFIC LEVELS

It is important to classify injuries to the extensor mechanism by the level of injury; each level has its own peculiar deformity and treatment (Elliott, 1970). Although the extensor mechanism can be injured anywhere between origin and insertion, the injuries at joint levels are the most frequently discussed and debated.

Voluminous conflicting literature on any

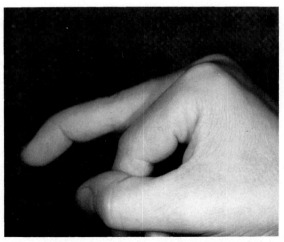

Figure 102–4. Classic mallet deformity. The distal phalanx is flexed. The patient is unable to extend the distal interphalangeal joint actively, even with active proximal interphalangeal joint extension.

subject tends to stand as a monument to the confusion of student and teacher alike. There is no better example than the literary attention given to extensor tendon injuries at the interphalangeal joint levels. The author's mission to uncomplicate the potentially complicated yields a basic message: "Restore the anatomy, and be patient in the rehabilitation."

Division of the extensor mechanism over the interphalangeal joint usually involves the joint, because of the intimate fusion of the tendon and joint capsule at these levels (Bunnell, 1944). At the metacarpophalangeal and wrist levels, there is a distinct separation of tendon and joint capsule that permits independent injury and repair.

Distal Interphalangeal Joint Level

The Deformity (Mallet Finger). Complete division of the terminal tendon beyond the insertion of the oblique retinacular ligaments results in a deformity known as mallet finger (Fig. 102–4).

Classically the distal phalanx is flexed at the distal interphalangeal joint and cannot be extended actively, even with active extension of the proximal interphalangeal joint. The addition of proximal interphalangeal hyperextension and metacarpophalangeal flexion seen in patients with a relaxed volar plate mimics the swan-neck deformity noted with volar plate rupture. The latter results in a hyperextension deformity at the proximal interphalangeal level, which leads to a secondary flexion deformity at the metacarpophalangeal and distal interphalangeal joints.

A primary flexion or hyperextension deformity at any joint level of the hand or wrist results in a tendon imbalance that tends to create the opposite deformity in the alternate remaining uninjured joints (Thompson, Littler, and Upton, 1978).

Open Injuries. With an open wound and preservation of at least a cuff of distal tendon, the severed tendon ends are approximated with interrupted sutures of 5–0 nylon or a continuous pull-out suture of 4–0 monofilament wire (Fig. 102–5). The author prefers a separate closure of the skin, rather than a simultaneous tendon and skin approximation as advocated by Doyle (1982). The tendon ends are brought together for the repair by

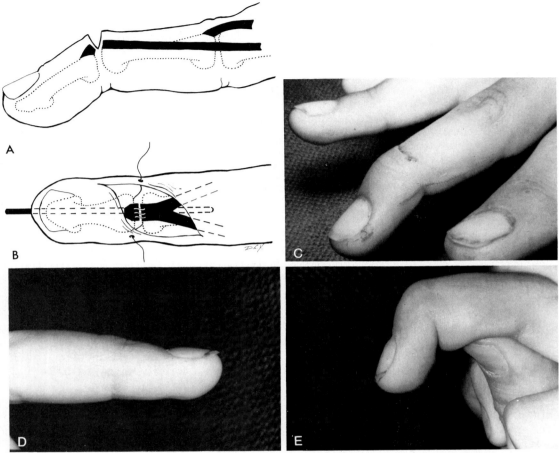

Figure 102–5. Acute mallet deformity. *A,* Open wound. *B,* Tendon repair. The distal interphalangeal joint is fixed in full extension. *C,* Fresh laceration. *D,* Postoperative extension at two months. *E,* Postoperative flexion.

positioning the distal interphalangeal joint in extension or hyperextension. A degree of hyperextension is preferred during postoperative splinting, but persistent blanching of the dorsal skin must be avoided (Rayan and Mullins, 1987); there is already a deficient blood supply in the tendon at this level.

Division of the terminal tendon is treated with splinting alone if a wound is grossly contaminated, if there are higher priority injuries, and when the tendon has been avulsed from bone. For the last-named injury, a pull-out wire suture tied over a distal button is an alternative repair technique (Nichols, 1960).

Closed Injuries. The only routine indication for opening an acute closed deformity is an associated major articular fracture (Stark, Boyes, and Wilson, 1962). Accurate reduction

and direct wiring of the avulsed fragment restores the articular surface and the normal insertion of the adherent tendon. Hyperextension of the distal phalanx disturbs the reduction by forcing the bone fragment out of the joint. Therefore, splinting alone is seldom feasible; after open reduction and fixation the distal interphalangeal joint is held in extension, or mild flexion, but not hyperextension (Lange and Engber, 1983).

In all other closed tendon injuries, including those with a minute bone avulsion, immobilization of the distal interphalangeal joint in hyperextension is the treatment of choice, but again dorsal skin blanch is avoided (Fig. 102–6). The tendon is often frayed by this type of injury and unable to hold sutures. Splinting avoids the more complex procedures required to suture tendon, particularly to bone. Splinting alone produces

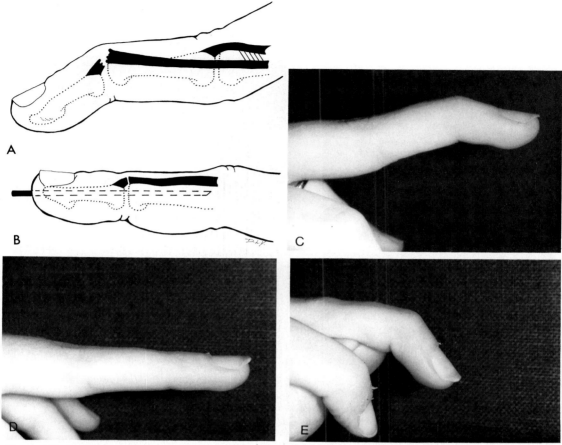

Figure 102–6. Acute mallet deformity. *A,* Closed injury. *B,* The distal interphalangeal joint is pinned in full extension. *C,* Fresh avulsion injury with mild proximal interphalangeal recurvation. *D,* Extension at three months. *E,* Flexion at three months.

the best results in most closed injuries at this level, and there may be fewer complications (Stern and Kastrup, 1988).

Established Deformity. Untreated deformities develop a significant length of scar between the tendon ends because of the unopposed flexion of the distal phalanx. Immature scar usually contracts in response to prolonged continuous splinting, and thus a trial with splinting is justified even a few months after the injury (Kaplan, 1959; McFarlane and Hampole, 1973). A dentist colleague refused a splint and obtained full extension after six months, allegedly without any treatment. That fortunate result must be considered a rarity; most untreated patients develop a significant deformity.

When more than 1 or 2 mm of scar bridges the traumatic gap, the tendon-scar unit may be too long to extend the distal phalanx fully. Prolonged splinting may improve deformities more than one month old, but some compromise of the result is expected. After the scar is mature, the length of the tendon-scar unit probably will not be changed by splinting alone. At this point the scar actually may look and function like tendon.

Clumsiness and catching on a pocket are common complaints in patients with less than 165 degrees of active distal interphalangeal extension. Surgical correction can benefit these patients (Fig. 102–7). Excising the extra length of the tendon-scar unit and prolonged postoperative splinting has produced good results (Elliott, 1965, 1970). The tendon or mature scar is freed from the distal joint and transected just proximal to the joint. The proximal segment is elevated from the middle phalanx until gentle traction gives some gliding. Gentle traction on the distal segment must extend the distal interphalangeal joint. After the latter is fixed in hyperextension

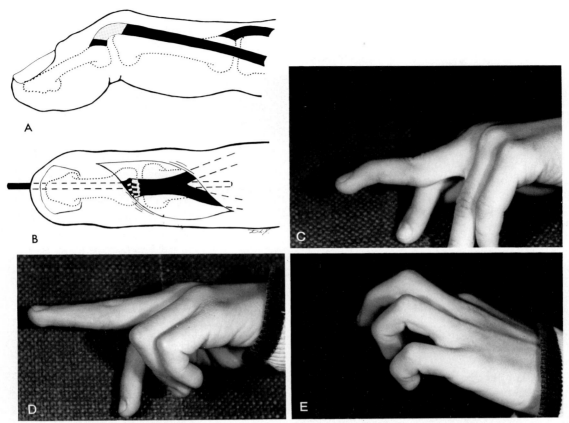

Figure 102–7. Established mallet deformity. *A,* Scar plus tendon is too long for distal interphalangeal extension. *B,* Excision of excess length, repair, and the distal interphalangeal joint fixed in full extension. *C,* Addition of proximal interphalangeal hyperextension and matacarpophalangeal flexion to classic mallet deformity mimics swan-neck deformity secondary to proximal interphalangeal volar plate rupture. *D,* Deformity corrected by restoring distal interphalangeal extension. *E,* Active flexion three months postoperatively. (From Elliott, R. A.: Injuries to the extensor mechanism of the hand. Orthop. Clin. North Am., *1*:355, 1970.)

with a C-wire introduced through the distal pulp, firm traction is applied to the end of the proximal segment as the excess length is serially resected and interrupted sutures of 5–0 nylon are placed. With this technique, all the potential crush from the traction maneuver is discarded and maximal tension is established. The average resected length is only 1 or 2 mm.

Verdan (1966) lysed the mature scar and resected a segment of tendon over the middle phalanx somewhat more proximal to the joint. He noted that the mature scar behaved like tendon, and the anastomosis was away from the distal interphalangeal joint. The alternative turn-key maneuver of Verdan (1966) plicated the intact tendon to shorten it, but this approach produces palpable bulk and excessive shortening of the tendon-scar unit, and therefore is not recommended.

Associated Proximal Interphalangeal (Swan-Neck) Deformity. The hyperextension of the proximal interphalangeal joint and flexion of the metacarpophalangeal joint resulting from the flexion deformity of the distal interphalangeal joint is dependent on a combined laxity of the proximal interphalangeal volar plate and imbalance of the extensor tendon system (see Figs. 102–6*C* and 102–7*C*). This deformity, known as swan-neck deformity, classically results from a rupture of the volar plate and secondary flexion of the adjacent joints.

When secondary to a mallet finger, proximal interphalangeal hyperextension is corrected by restoring at least 165 degrees of extension at the distal interphalangeal joint. This tendon imbalance does not respond to proximal interphalangeal splinting alone. It can also be corrected, however, by lengthen-

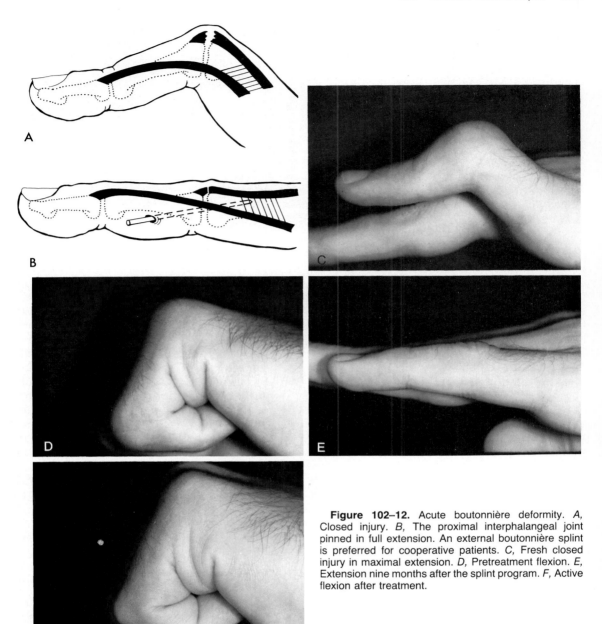

Figure 102–12. Acute boutonnière deformity. *A,* Closed injury. *B,* The proximal interphalangeal joint pinned in full extension. An external boutonnière splint is preferred for cooperative patients. *C,* Fresh closed injury in maximal extension. *D,* Pretreatment flexion. *E,* Extension nine months after the splint program. *F,* Active flexion after treatment.

stored, an excellent range of active motion should be obtainable for most patients. Prolonged splinting or section of the conjoined tendon may improve function, but the best reported results (Elliott, 1971) used an anatomic repair and prolonged splinting in combination (Fig. 102–14). Long-standing deformities may require weeks or months of directive and dynamic splinting to gain full passive motion. The results improve if a maximal range of passive motion is obtained

preoperatively; the postoperative range of active motion seldom exceeds the preoperative passive motion (see Fig. 102–13*B*).

The author still favors the anatomic repair that he presented to the American Society for Surgery of the Hand in 1965 (Figs. 102–15 to 102–17). An undulating incision is used to expose the extensor mechanism over the proximal one-third of the middle phalanx and the distal one-half of the proximal phalanx. The lateral bands are defined and freed from

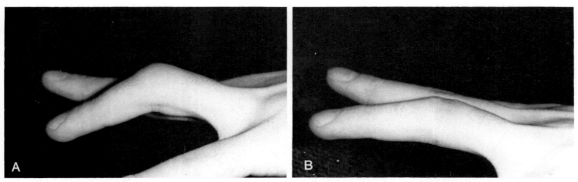

Figure 102–13. Boutonnière deformity with proximal interphalangeal dislocation. *A,* Preoperative active extension after 12 weeks of splinting. *B,* Postoperative active extension matched preoperative passive extension.

the contracted fibers of the transverse retinacular ligaments. Next, the tendon and scar overlying the proximal interphalangeal joint is dissected from the capsule of the joint and divided proximal to the joint. This obviates the need for a tendon-bone reconstruction in all cases. Proximally the scar and central band are reflected in the areolar plane until free tendon excursion is evident. The proximal interphalangeal joint is then fixed in 180 degrees of extension with a transarticular wire, and the central band and scar are advanced with firm traction as the excess length is serially amputated and a repair is accomplished with interrupted 5–0 nylon sutures. The triangular ligament is repaired with two sutures, and the central band and scar are trimmed to accommodate the lateral bands

in their normal dorsilateral position. Approximation of the lateral bands over the proximal interphalangeal joint (Mason, 1930; Kaplan, 1936) prevents normal flexion and may result in rupture of the repair or a tendon imbalance (Fig. 102–18). Unfortunately, this is a common error.

After the anatomic repair, if the distal interphalangeal joint cannot be flexed passively, a release of the oblique retinacular ligaments may be indicated. The author has never needed this release, but Zancolli (1968) described it as a routine requirement in his practice. We both use an anatomic reconstruction, but perhaps there is a subtle difference in our repairs.

Deformities with Impaired Passive Motion. Unless full passive extension of the

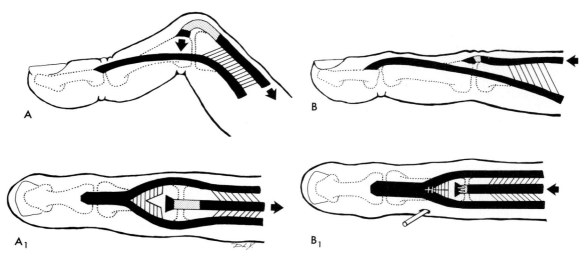

Figure 102–14. Established mobile boutonnière deformity. *A,* Preoperative deformity with retracted central band plus a scar too long for *full active* proximal interphalangeal extension, tear of triangular ligament, and volar displacement of lateral bands below the axis of the joint. *B,* Excision of excess length, anatomic repair, and the proximal interphalangeal joint fixed in full extension.

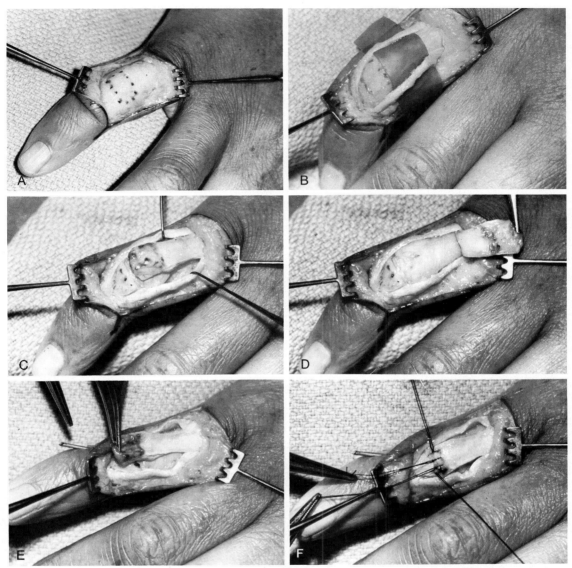

Figure 102–15. Anatomic repair of established, mobile boutonnière deformity. *A,* Exposure through an undulating incision. The scar is outlined over the proximal interphalangeal joint. *B,* Lateral bands are sharply defined and separated from the transverse retinacular ligaments. *C,* Scar transected, leaving a cuff of tissue on the middle phalanx for repair of central band insertion. *D,* Scar and tendon elevated in the areolar plane deep to the vascular leash. *E,* Middle proximal interphalanggeal joint pinned in full extension. Traction on the scar advances the central band and relaxes the lateral bands. *F,* Excess length serially excised and scar to car anastomosis completed.

Illustration continued on following page

proximal interphalangeal joint is obtained before the extensor tendon reconstruction, restoration of a full range of active motion is unlikely (see Fig. 102–13). Preoperative splinting or surgical release of contracted volar structures improves some results. When proximal interphalangeal flexion is fixed, relief of the associated distal interphalangeal hyperextension usually improves comfort and function. Fusion in a functional position may be the best treatment for acute flexion deformities of the proximal interphalangeal joint, particularly those with joint destruction (see Fig. 102–21).

The anatomic repair described above for mobile deformities restores active motion, which seldom exceeds the preoperative passive motion. Tenotomy of the conjoined ten-

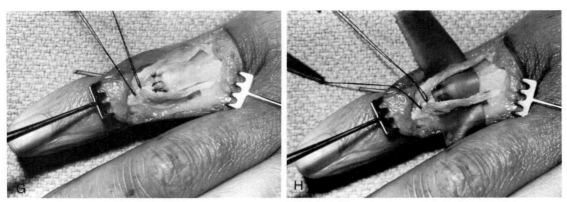

Figure 102–15 *Continued. G,* Lateral bands repositioned by approximation in triangular ligament area. *H,* Note the anatomic position of the lateral bands. (From Elliott, R. A.:Boutonnière deformity. *In* Cramer, L. M., and Chase, R. A. (Eds.): Symposium on the Hand. St. Louis, C. V. Mosby Company, 1971.)

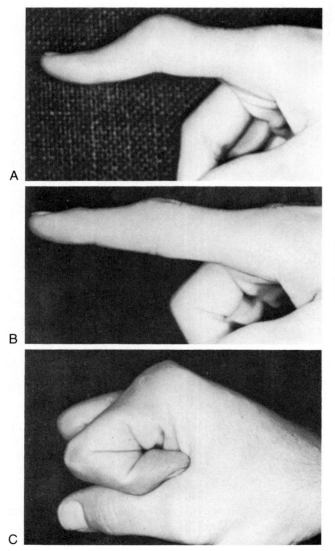

Figure 102–16. Established boutonnière deformity. *A,* Mobile preoperative deformity in a 19 year old male. *B,* Postoperative active extension. *C,* Postoperative (untrapped) active flexion. (From Elliott, R. A.: Boutonnière deformity. *In* Cramer, L. M., and Chase, R. A. (Eds.): Symposium on the Hand. St. Louis, C. V. Mosby Company, 1971.)

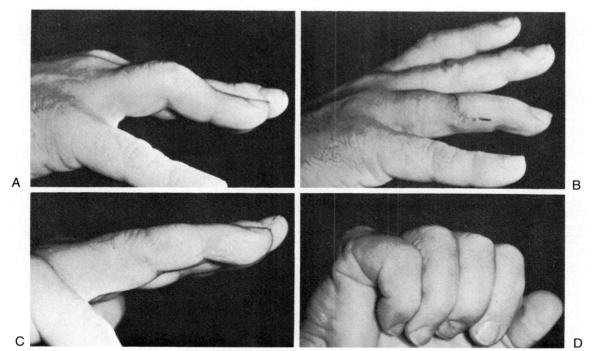

Figure 102–17. Established boutonnière deformity. *A,* Mobile deformity recurrent in a 51 year old male eight months after repair, an inadequate two week splinting period, and early aggressive therapy "because of his age." *B,* Two weeks after secondary anatomic repair. The proximal interphalangeal joint is pinned and the lateral bands are relaxed. *C,* Postoperative active extension at four months. *D,* Postoperative active flexion. (From Elliott, R. A.: Injuries to the extensor mechanisms of the hand. Orthop. Clin. North Am., 1:335, 1970.

don just distal to the triangular ligament (Fig. 102–19) relieves distal interphalangeal hyperextension and improves the extensor tendon balance and active extension at the proximal interphalangeal joint (Dolphin, 1965). A tenotomy beyond the insertion of the oblique retinacular ligaments results in a mallet deformity. Fusion of the proximal interphalangeal joint is not difficult and failure is rare. The ulnar two fingers require more flexion than the radial two, to satisfy the needs of most patients.

Splinting Techniques. Splinting is recommended for the treatment of acute closed injuries (Elliott, 1971), for the trial treatment of some older injuries (Chase, 1971), and for the preoperative correction of flexion contractures (Elliott, 1973). The directive splint preferred by the author counters the firm pressure of a strap pressure on the dorsum of the proximal interphalangeal joint, and distal interphalangeal flexion is not restricted. Following a design credited to John Micks, the Christensen Orthopedic Supply Company*

originally manufactured these splints with a web strap and buckle fastener. At the author's suggestion, a Velcro fastener was substituted for ease of patient application (Fig. 102–20). Moleskin is added to both end plates to prevent slipping and absorb moisture.

The occasional fixed flexion contracture that requires a greater corrective pressure is treated with the "Joint Jack" splint of Watson and Ritland.† As soon as acute flexion is overcome, the COSCO splint is substituted in order to exercise the distal interphalangeal joint.

Dynamic splinting is reserved for patients with a full range of passive motion who are prone to joint stiffness. These "substituting" splints are not strong enough, however, to overcome true contractures.

The transarticular wire used to stabilize the proximal interphalangeal joint with open repairs facilitates wound care. An external gutter splint is used for one week after re-

---

*COSCO, 986 Artesia Blvd, Hermosa, CA 90254.

†Joint Jack Company, 198 Millstone Road, Glastonbury, CT 06033.

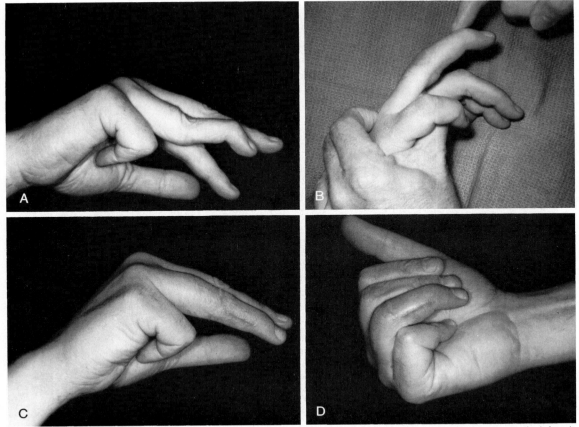

Figure 102–18. Treatment failure. *A,* The surgeon converted boutonnière deformity to a severe swan-neck deformity by central band advancement and approximation of lateral bands over the proximal interphalangeal joint. *B,* Intrinsic positive deformity demonstrated by passive metacarpophalangeal extension and pressure on the dorsum of the middle phalanx. *C,* Rebalancing obtained with dissection and separation of the lateral bands and step lengthening of the central band. *D,* Active flexion eight weeks after surgery.

moval of the wire to permit healing of the articular perforations.

A Velcro strap is used to regain flexion during later rehabilitation. This "directive" splint is never used before eight weeks, and seldom before three months, after extensor reconstruction in order to avoid stretching the repair scar.

Immobilization Period. All acute injuries and all late repairs are ideally splinted for seven weeks. Rigid proximal interphalangeal joint fixation and active flexion of the distal interphalangeal joint is the program during the first six weeks. Internal fixation is always followed by at least one full week of external splinting. A night splint is used during the final week.

After splinting is discontinued, active extension exercise of the proximal interphalangeal joint and active distal interphalangeal flexion is encouraged. After eight weeks an active and passive exercise program is introduced. The time frame for maximal recovery is six to nine months. For patients over 50 years of age, the entire splinting program is shortened by one week. Failure to maintain proximal interphalangeal extension is an indication to continue the splinting until the maximal result is obtained.

After release of contractures of scar or tendon, active and passive motion exercises are started within hours or days. After a fusion, manual support of the joint permits early exercise of the other joints.

Treatment of Failures. Patients in whom there are symptomatic splinting failures should be offered surgical treatment. Symptomatic failures after tendon surgery at the proximal interphalangeal level may benefit if the conjoined tendon is sectioned over the

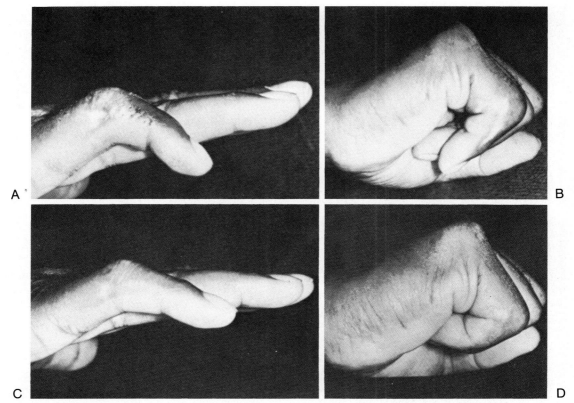

Figure 102–19. Established boutonnière deformity with limited proximal interphalangeal mobility and limited distal interphalangeal joint flexion in a 57 year old laborer. *A,* Maximal active and passive extension after six weeks of directive splinting. *B,* Preoperative flexion. *C,* Active and passive extension after conjoined lateral band tenotomy. *D,* Postoperative proximal and distal interphalangeal flexion. (From Elliott, R. A.: Injuries to the extensor mechanism of the hand. Orthop. Clin. North Am., *1*:335, 1970.)

proximal portion of the middle phalanx (see Fig. 102–19). This relieves the tension on the terminal tendon and improves the balance of the entire extensor mechanism; improved flexion of the distal interphalangeal joint and extension of the proximal interphalangeal joint usually result. Fusion of the proximal interphalangeal joint can also improve function in selected patients (Fig. 102–21).

Proximal Phalanx Level

The Deformity. An injury over the proximal phalanx may involve the central tendon, the intrinsic expansion, or both. The central tendon is vulnerable in its dorsal location; the intrinsic tendons are protected on the sides of the digit, except on the radial and ulnar sides of the index and little fingers, respectively. Division of the central tendon over the distal portion of the phalanx results in a boutonnière deformity, but unilateral division of an intrinsic tendon does not usually demonstrate a gross deformity and therefore may go undetected without specific testing of the involved intrinsic. Scar adherence

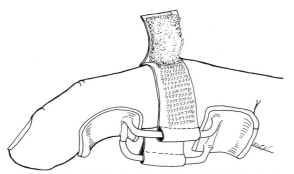

Figure 102–20. Boutonnière splint (COSCO). Padded rigid plastic splint with adjustable Velcro fastener. This directing splint is used for immobilization when the proximal interphalangeal joint has been fully extended. The splint design permits both metacarpophalangeal and distal interphalangeal flexion.

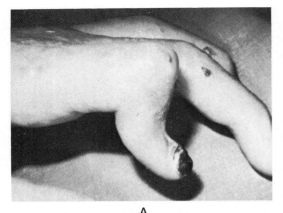

A

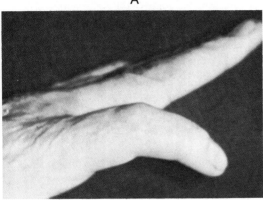

B

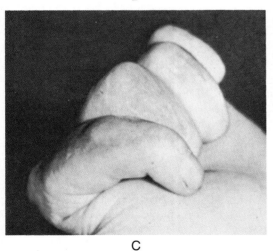

C

Figure 102–21. Fixed boutonnière deformity in a young adult. *A,* Burn destruction of the central band at the proximal interphalangeal level with distal interphalangeal joint tenodesis. *B,* Extension after proximal interphalangeal fusion and conjoined lateral band tenotomy. *C,* Postoperative function with active flexion of metacarpophalangeal and distal interphalangeal joints. (From Elliott, R. A.: Injuries to the extensor mechanism of the hand. Orthop. Clin. North Am., *1*:335, 1970.)

to the immovable deep structures blocks active and passive flexion and active extension of the proximal interphalangeal joint, while preserving full passive extension (Rosenthal, 1984).

Treatment. Most injuries at this level are open wounds. Anatomic repair with interrupted 5–0 nylon sutures is ideal for the clean wound. Splinting alone is reserved for the highly contaminated wound. Although the type of splinting is the same as for injuries at the proximal interphalangeal joint level, injuries over the proximal phalanx require only four weeks of immobilization.

Metacarpophalangeal Joint Level

The Deformity. Division of the central tendon at the level of the metacarpophalangeal joint causes an extensor lag, and diminishes active extension of the proximal phalanx of the middle or ring finger against resistance. Loss of extension may not be as evident on the index or little finger unless the adjacent proper tendon is also divided.

Treatment. Highly contaminated human tooth injuries are common at this level. Primary tendon repair is contraindicated in such wounds and the prognosis is compromised by the infection, articular destruction, and scar, despite aggressive management. In clean wounds the joint capsule and extensor tendon are repaired separately. The flat structures are repaired with interrupted 5–0 nylon sutures; a Bunnell pull-out wire suture with a distal button is an option for the common extensor repair. Four weeks of immobilization with the wrist and metacarpophalangeal joints in extension is usual, but Dargan (1969) obtained his best results with active motion after only two weeks. Merritt splints the wrist in extension and the involved metacarpophalangeal joint in dynamic hyperextension and encourages full motion of all other joints (Merritt, 1986). His patients have not required hand therapy after the splint is discontinued. Wolock, Moore, and Weiland (1987) protect fresh repairs on the dorsum of the hand with a retention stitch woven into the tendon proximal to the repair and a distal button, but their splinting is prolonged and involves the interphalangeal joints. It is important that the proximal and distal interphalangeal joints always remain free; splinting them in full extension along with the metacarpophalangeal and wrist joints can cause unnecessary discomfort from tension on the flexors.

Metacarpal Level

The Deformity. Division of an extensor tendon over the midmetacarpal might be expected to mimic the deformities seen at the metacarpophalangeal joint level. In fact, the liberal intertendinous connections of the extensor digitorum communis serve to transfer extension forces between the digits and lessen the deformity (Fig. 102–22). An associated injury to the intertendinous connections may therefore increase the deformity. A pure intertendinous division may go unnoticed. At this level, scar adherence to the underlying fascia produces a tenodesis that can prevent simultaneous flexion at the metacarpophalangeal and interphalangeal joints. Initiating flexion at one joint draws the other joints into extension (Rosenthal, 1984).

Treatment. It is well to repair all divided structures, even the intertendinous bands, because unsatisfied tendon ends proliferate rapidly in paratenon, and scarring can be severe. The flat tendons on the dorsum of the hand distal to the tendon sheaths are repaired and splinted in the same way as injuries at the metacarpophalangeal joint level.

A tendon repair near the dorsal carpal ligament may not glide beneath the ligament with full wrist extension. The author does not hesitate to section a portion of the ligament in this event.

Thumb Joint Levels

The Deformities (Fig. 102–23). Division of the extensor pollicis longus (EPL) tendon at the interphalangeal joint results in a mallet deformity similar to that seen at the distal interphalangeal level of the fingers. With division of the EPL over the proximal phalanx, if the extensor expansion is intact, intrinsic extension is possible at the IP level, but not hyperextension.

Injuries at or proximal to the metacarpophalangeal joint vary in their behavior. If only the extensor pollicis brevis (EPB) is severed, the deformity may be minimal, or may resemble the boutonnière deformity seen at the proximal interphalangeal level of the fingers. With the weakened metacarpophalangeal extension, and the relative strength of unopposed flexion, tension on the EPL increases and interphalangeal hyperextension completes the deformity. The boutonnière deformity can also result from severe disruption of the extensor expansion and volar migration of the EPL below the joint axis (Rosenthal, 1984). The displaced EPL then acts as a metacarpophalangeal flexor, and hyperextension of the distal phalanx results from the increased tension on the distal EPL fibers. Division of the EPL causes a mild flexion deformity of the metacarpophalangeal

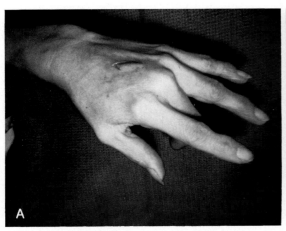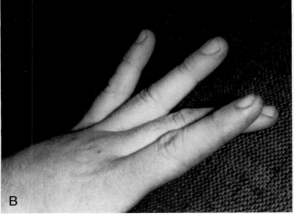

Figure 102–22. Division of the extensor digitorum communis tendon of the middle finger over the metacarpus. *A,* Deformity with division including, or distal to, the intertendinous connections. *B,* Partial metacarpophalangeal joint extension through preserved intertendinous connection(s) from adjacent intact EDC tendon(s).

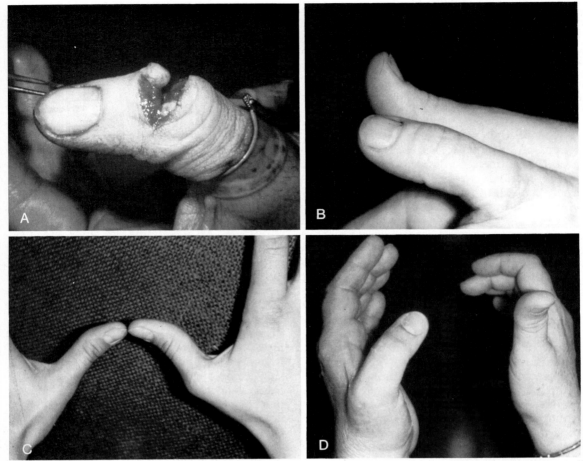

Figure 102–23. Common thumb deformities. *A,* Division of the extensor pollicis longus tendon at the interphalangeal joint results in a mallet-type deformity. *B,* With division of the EPL tendon over the proximal phalanx and an intact extensor expansion, intrinsic and occasionally extensor pollicis brevis extension is possible at the interphalangeal level, but not hyperextension. *C,* Isolated division of the EPB tendon at the metacarpophalangeal level as in this patient, or severe disruption of the extensor expansion and displacement of the EPL tendon below the axis of the metacarpophalangeal joint, will cause a boutonnière deformity. *D,* On the left hand both the EPL and EPB tendons are severed proximally to the metacarpophalangeal joint. Active extension is lost at the interphalangeal and metacarpophalangeal joints. (From Elliott, R. A.: Injuries to the extensor mechanism of the hand. Orthop. Clin. North Am., *1*:335, 1970.)

and interphalangeal joints, and complete loss of interphalangeal hyperextension. When both the EPL and EPB tendons are severed, there is a marked flexion deformity at both thumb joints.

Treatment. The principles, repair techniques, and splinting are essentially the same as for the fingers. Tendons lacerated on the thumb are always repaired separately, and only the involved joint requires splinting. More proximal injuries need extension of the wrist as well. EPL repairs can be relaxed further with adduction and supination of the first ray. Wrist immobilization is continued for four weeks, and thumb joints are fixed for five weeks.

Figure 102–24. Step-cut lengthening for tendons and ligaments. *A,* Design of the incisions for division. *B,* The lengthening repair.

Injuries at Other Levels

Division of extensor tendons at or near the wrist presents no difficulty in diagnosis, but tendon retrieval and repair is complicated by the dorsal carpal ligament. If better exposure is needed, or if the repair tends to hang up on the proximal or distal border of the ligament, the latter can be partially divided without hesitation. With complete division of the ligament, however, tendons may bowstring with dorsiflexion of the wrist. Although this is not a serious functional or cosmetic deformity, it can be avoided by a step-cut division and a lengthening repair of the ligament (Fig. 102–24). Extensor tendons at the wrist and in the forearm resemble the flexor tendons, in contrast to the relatively flat tendons on the dorsum of the hand and digits. The buried suture techniques described for flexor tendons (see Chap. 101) are preferable at these levels of injury.

REFERENCES

Backhouse, K. M., and Catton, W. T.: An experimental study of the functions of the lumbrical muscles in the human hand. J. Anat., 88:133, 1954.

Bingham, D. L., and Jack, E. A.: Buttonholed extensor expansion. Br. Med. J., 2:701, 1937.

Bunnell, S.: Surgery of the Hand. 1st Ed. Philadelphia, J. B. Lippincott Company, 1944.

Bunnell, S.: Intrinsic muscles of fingers. In Bunnell, S. (Ed.): Surgery of the Hand. 4th Ed. (revised by Boyes, J. H.). Philadelphia, J. B. Lippincott Company, 1964.

Campbell, C.: Personal communication, 1965.

Carducci, A. T.: Potential boutonnière deformity: its recognition and treatment. Orthop. Rev., 10:121, 1981.

Carter, S. J., and Mersheimer, W. L.: Deferred primary tendon repair: results in 27 cases. Ann. Surg., 164:913, 1966.

Cascells, S. W., and Strange, T. B.: Intermedullary wire fixation of mallet finger. J. Bone Joint Surg., 39A:521, 1957.

Chase, R. A.: Boutonnière deformity (discussion). In Cramer, L. M., and Chase, R. A. (Eds.): Symposium on the Hand. St. Louis, C. V. Mosby Company, 1971.

Curtis, R. M., Reid, R. L., and Provost, J. M.: A staged technique for the repair of the traumatic boutonnière deformity. J. Hand Surg., 8:167, 1983.

Dargan, E. L.: Management of extensor tendon injuries of the hand. Surg. Gynecol. Obstet., 128:1269, 1969.

Dolphin, J. A.: The extensor tenotomy for chronic boutonnière deformity of the finger. J. Bone Joint Surg., 47A:161, 1965.

Doyle, J. R.: Extensor tendons—acute injuries. In Green, D. P. (Ed.): Operative Hand Surgery. New York, Churchill Livingstone, 1982, pp. 1441–1464.

Elliott, R. A.: Extensor tendon injuries at the interphalangeal joint levels. Presented to American Society for Surgery of the Hand, Chicago, 1965.

Elliott, R. A.: Injuries to the extensor mechanism of the hand. Orthop. Clin. North Am., 1:335, 1970.

Elliott, R. A.: boutonnière deformity. In Cramer, L. M., and Chase, R. A. (Eds.): Symposium on the Hand. St. Louis, C. V. Mosby Company, 1971.

Elliott, R. A.: Splints for mallet and boutonnière deformities. Plast. Reconstr. Surg., 52:282, 1973.

Elliott, R. A., and Hoehn, J. G.: Use of porcine skin for wound dressings. Plast. Reconstr. Surg., 52:401, 1973.

Elliott, R. A., Hoehn, J. G., and Stayman, J. W.: Management of the viable soft tissue cover in degloving injuries. Hand, 2:69, 1979.

Evans, R. B., and Burkhalter, W. E.: A study of the dynamic anatomy of extensor tendons and implications for treatment. J. Hand Surg., 11A:774, 1986.

Fowler, S. B.: Extensor apparatus of the digits. J. Bone Joint Surg., 31B:477, 1949.

Goldner, J. L.: Deformities of the hand incidental to pathological changes of the extensor and intrinsic muscle mechanisms. J. Bone Surg., 35A:115, 1953.

Grundberg, A. B., and Reagan, D. S.: Central slip tenotomy for chronic mallet finger deformity. J. Hand Surg., 12A:547, 1987.

Haines, R. W.: The extensor apparatus of the finger. J. Anat., 85:251, 1951.

Harris, C., and Rutledge, G.: The functional anatomy of the extensor mechanism of the finger. J. Bone Joint Surg., 54A:713, 1972.

Hauck, G.: Die Ruptur der Dorsalaponeurose am ersten: Interphalangealgelenk, zugleich ein Beitrag zur Anatomie und Physiologic der Dorsalaponeurose, Arch. Klin. Chir., 123:197, 1923.

Kaplan, E. B.: Extensor deformities of proximal interphalangeal joints of fingers. J. Bone Joint Surg., 18:781, 1936.

Kaplan, E. B.: Anatomy, injuries and treatment of extensor apparatus of the hand and digits. Clin. Orthop., 13:24, 1959.

Kaplan, E. B.: Functional and Surgical Anatomy of the Hand. 2nd Ed. Philadelphia, J. B. Lippincott Company, 1965.

Kilgore, E. S., and Graham, W. P.: The Hand, Surgical and Nonsurgical Management. Philadelphia, Lea & Febiger, 1977.

Landsmeer, J. M.: The coordination of finger joint motions. J. Bone Joint Surg., 45A:1654, 1963.

Lange, R. H., and Engber, W. D.: Hyperextension mallet finger. Orthopedics, 6:1426, 1983.

Littler, J. W.: The finger extensor mechanism. Surg. Clin. North Am., 47:415, 1967.

Lucas, G. L.: Fowler central slip tenotomy for old mallet deformity. Plast. Reconstr. Surg., 80:94, 1987.

Mason, M. L.: Rupture of tendons of the hand. Surg. Gynecol. Obstet., 50:611, 1930.

Mason, M. L.: Immediate and delayed tendon repair. Surg. Gynecol. Obstet., 62:449, 1936.

McFarlane, R. M., and Hampole, M. K.: Treatment of extensor tendon injuries of the hand. Can. J. Surg., 16:366, 1973.

Merritt, W. H.: Complications of hand surgery. In Greenfield, L. J. (Ed.): Complications in Surgery and Trauma. Philadelphia, J. B. Lippincott Company, 1984, p. 852.

Merritt, W. H.: Immediate active motion following extensor tendon repair. Am. Soc. Surg. of Hand Correspondence Newsletter, No. 45, 1986.

Milford, L. W., Jr.: Retaining Ligaments of the Digits of the Hand. Philadelphia, W. B. Saunders Company, 1968.

Nichols, H. M.: Manual of Hand Injuries. 2nd Ed. Chicago, Year Book Medical Publishers, 1960, p. 181.

Potenza, A.: Prevention of adhesions to healing flexor tendons. J.A.M.A., *187*:181, 1964.

Pratt, D. R.: Internal splint for closed and open treatment of injuries of the extensor tendon at the distal joint of the finger. J. Bone Joint Surg., *34A*:785, 1952.

Rayan, G. G., and Mullins, P. T.: Skin necrosis complicating hyperextension of mallet finger. J. Hand Surg., *12*:548, 1987.

Redfern, A. B., Curtis, R. M., and Wilgis, E. F.: Experience with peritendinous fibrosis of the dorsum of the hand. J. Hand Surg., 7:380, 1982.

Rosenthal, E. A.: The extensor tendons. *In* Hunter, J. M., et al. (Eds.): Rehabilitation of the Hand. St. Louis, C. V. Mosby Company, 1984.

Schenck, R. R.: Variations of extensor tendons of the fingers. J. Bone Joint Surg., *46A*:103, 1964.

Schultz, R. J., Furlong, J., and Storace, A.: Detailed anatomy of the extensor mechanism at the proximal aspect of the finger. J. Hand Surg., *6*:493, 1981.

Smith, J. W.: Tendon injuries. *In* Grabb, W. C., and Smith, J. W. (Eds.): Plastic Surgery. Boston, Little, Brown & Company, 1968.

Smith, R. J.: Balance and kinetics of the fingers under normal and pathological conditions. Clin. Orthop., *92*:104, 1974.

Spinner, M., and Choi, B. Y.: Anterior dislocation of the proximal interphalangeal joint, a cause of rupture of the central slip of the extensor mechanism. J. Bone Joint Surg., *54A*:1329, 1970.

Stack, H. G.: Muscle functions in the fingers. J. Bone Joint Surg., *44B*:899, 1962.

Stack, H. G.: Mallet finger. Lancet, *2*:1303, 1968.

Stark, H.: Troublesome fractures and dislocations of the hand. AAOS Inst. Course Lect., *19*:130, 1970.

Stark, H., Boyes, J., and Wilson, J.: Mallet finger. J. Bone Joint Surg., *44A*:1061, 1962.

Stern, P. J., and Kastrup, J. J.: Complications and prognosis of treatment of mallet finger. J. Hand Surg., *13A*:333, 1988.

Thompson, H. S., Littler, J. W., and Upton, J.: The spiral oblique retinacular ligament (SORL). J. Hand Surg., *3*:482, 1978.

Tubiana, R.: Surgical repair of the extensor apparatus of the fingers. Surg. Clin. North Am., *48*:1021, 1968.

Tubiana, R., and Valentin, P.: The anatomy of the extensor apparatus of the fingers. Surg. Clin. North Am., *44*:897, 1964a.

Tubiana, R., and Valentin, P.: The physiology of the extension of the fingers., Surg. Clin. North Am., *44*:907, 1964b.

Verdan, C. E.: Repair of tendons. *In* Flynn, J. E. (Ed.): Hand Surgery, Baltimore, Williams & Wilkins Company, 1966.

Weeks, P. M.: The chronic boutonnière deformity: a method of repair. Plast. Reconstr. Surg., *40*:248, 1967.

Wolock, B. S., Moore, R. J., and Weiland, A. J.: Extensor tendon repair: a reconstructive technique. Orthopedics, *10*:1387, 1987.

Zancolli, E. A.: Structural and Dynamic Basis of Hand Surgery. 2nd Ed. Philadelphia, J. B. Lippincott Company, 1968.

Zbrodowski, A., Gajisin, S., and Grodecki, J.: Vascularization and anatomical model of the mesotendons of the extensor digitorum and extensor indicis muscles. J. Anat., *130*:697, 1980.

103

R. Christie Wray, Jr.

Fractures and Joint Injuries of the Hand

GENERAL PATIENT EVALUATION

The initial approach to all patients with a hand injury should be directed at obtaining as much a history of possible life-threatening associated injuries and systemic diseases as a history about the injury itself. The mechanism of injury is a valuable guide to the likelihood of associated injuries. Patients with injuries from industrial accidents, home accidents, sports, or simple fights are unlikely to have significant associated injuries. In contradistinction, those whose hands are injured by high speed automobile accidents, high velocity gunshot wounds, or deliberate beatings are much more likely to have associated injuries. The most common life-threatening associated injuries involve intracranial, intrathoracic, or intra-abdominal organs. Cardiovascular disease, particularly a recent myocardial infarction or unstable angina, and uncontrolled diabetes might alter the usual treatment of fractures and dislocations. Even for minor injuries, one should obtain a history of the patient's general health, drug allergies, current medications, and previous hospitalizations.

The physical examination can be confined to the injured part in patients with minor injuries. The usual complete history and physical examination is necessary for those requiring a regional or inhalation anesthetic. General examination of the injured hand should include a demonstration of the active (but not passive) range of motion just to the point of producing mild pain. The patient should not move the hand beyond his pain tolerance until radiographs are obtained. Light touch sensibility should be tested in the tips of all digits. Median nerve motor function in the hand should be demonstrated by palmar abduction of the thumb. Ulnar nerve function should be demonstrated by abduction of the little and index fingers. Abnormal findings on these screening tests are an indication for more complex testing. Specific physical examination techniques for various parts of the hand are described in the section concerning each specific bone or joint.

Survey radiographs (the entire hand), and radiographs for the wrist and specific area (scaphoid, finger, ray) may all be used at various times. The patient's localization of pain and the physician's localization of tenderness aid in the determination of the area to be studied radiographically. If one cannot localize the injury, survey radiographs should be taken and followed by localized films if needed. Radiographs must be obtained in at least two planes, preferably 90 degrees apart. A recurring error is evaluation and treatment based on either a single radiograph (generally an anteroposterior) or an anteroposterior and a 10 degree oblique. Determination of the presence or absence of fractures or dislocations and the degree of displacement can be tragically mistaken when insufficient radiographs are obtained. The author is aware of at least three malpractice cases based primarily on insufficient radiographs of injured hands. Indications for specific radiographs are discussed under the sections on individual bones and joints.

General care of the injured is beyond the scope of this chapter, but for those with open wounds the guidelines for tetanus prophylaxis of the Communicable Disease Center are recommended (Table 103–1).

The frequency of injuries of individual bones and joints have varied depending on the reporting source. The referral patterns of an individual surgeon or group of surgeons may produce skew in the frequency of various injuries. In general, however, distal phalangeal fractures are the most common (about 50 per cent) followed by metacarpal (30 per cent), proximal phalangeal (about 15 per cent), and middle phalangeal (about 5 per cent) (Dobyns and associates, 1982). Injuries involving the distal interphalangeal (DIP) joint are common (about 18 per cent). However, proximal interphalangeal (PIP) joint injuries are even more common (about 55 per cent). Injuries involving the metacarpophalangeal (MP) joint are second in frequency (about 21 per cent). The carpometacarpal (CMC) joints are the least often injured (about 6 per cent).

The frequency of various etiologies of hand injuries varies, as does the frequency of individual bones and joints injured. This variance is likewise dependent on the referral patterns of individual physicians (Wray, Young, and Holtman, 1984). In general, industrial accidents are the most common and athletic injuries the second most common causes of fractures and joint injuries in the hand. Accidents at home, motor vehicle accidents, and gunshot wounds are less common.

GENERAL PRINCIPLES OF TREATMENT

Almost invariably, treatment of fractures and joint injuries involves one of four types: closed reduction external fixation (CREF), closed reduction internal fixation (CRIF), open reduction internal fixation (ORIF), or open reduction external fixation (OREF). Some fractures require little or no reduction and little external fixation. For classification this "treatment" can be listed as CREF. Rarely, no treatment of any kind is rendered. The reason for not treating the fracture or dislocation is almost always related to associated diseases or injuries abrogating the delivery of the usual care. The frequency with which ORIF, OREF, CRIF, and CREF are used varies with the practice and referral patterns of individual surgeons. If all emergency room visits are considered, CREF is certainly the most common treatment. In the author's referral practice in the Division of Plastic Surgery at the University of Rochester and at Washington University, ORIF is the most common treatment (Weeks, 1981).

Certain general principles of treatment are useful; specific treatment regimens are given in the following sections under the individual bones and joints. Early active motion is the cornerstone of treatment for most fractures and some joint injuries in the hand. Prolonged immobilization usually causes joint stiffness and is almost always detrimental to hand function. The definition of "prolonged" is difficult owing to the multiplicity of factors involved in producing joint stiffness. How-

Table 103–1. Tetanus Prophylaxis

Previously Adsorbed Toxoid Doses	Clean Minor Wounds		Other Wounds	
	Tetanus-Diphtheria Toxoid	*Tetanus Immune Globulin*	*Tetanus-Diphtheria Toxoid*	*Tetanus-Immune Globulin*
Unknown or <3	Yes	No	Yes	Yes
≥3	Yes if >10 yrs since last dose	No	Yes if >55 yrs since last dose	No

Modified from Morbidity and Mortality Weekly Report, *34*:426, 1985.

ever, two factors are most important in determining whether an individual will develop joint stiffness after a hand injury. The degree of joint stiffness after a given injury is directly related to the patient's age. Permanent joint stiffness following an injury is extremely rare in infants and young children. Joint stiffness is uncommon in the teenager and becomes increasingly common as the patient ages. Past the age of 50, some degree of permanent joint stiffness is almost invariable after a severe hand injury with displaced fractures, ligamentous injuries, and associated injuries to nerves, tendon, or skin. Joint stiffness is frequently severe in patients over the age of 50 and is the determinant of hand function. The second important factor is the severity of the injury, which can be estimated by obtaining an accurate history, observing the degree of displacement and/or dislocation of the bone or joint, and noting the presence of associated injuries to other structures in the hand or body (Dobyns and associates, 1982).

Treatment usually involves early rest and elevation of the injured part followed by very early active range of motion exercises of the uninvolved joints and early motion of the involved joints. Any immobilization that prevents joint motion should be removed as early as possible. Rarely the immobilization is continued longer than six weeks; it usually is discontinued after four weeks. At times, short-term stability may have to be sacrificed to allow joint motion. Immobilization between periods of exercises is frequently used to allow early active motion. When the fracture is clinically stable in the cooperative patient, uninhibited active range of motion not against resistance is encouraged. The period of immobilization and active motion not against resistance ranges from one to eight weeks. Final restoration of maximal range of motion, however, may require many months. During this time, the patient is encouraged to utilize the hand maximally, and dynamic splinting may be used. The ultimate goal is, of course, a normal range of motion.

Equipment. Although numerous external and internal fixation devices have been described for fractures of the hand, a select few are sufficient for the vast majority of fractures and joint injuries (Weeks, 1981; Dobyns and associates, 1982). External fixation is most commonly accomplished with the stack splint (Fig. 103–1) or plaster. Internal fixation is usually with Kirschner wires (K-wires) or

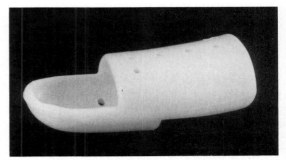

Figure 103–1. Stack splint. Similar models are available from various companies.

wire suture material; ASIF (Swiss Association for the study of Internal Fixation) screws and plates are occasionally useful. Nitrogen powered drills (from the Zimmer, Stryker, or 3M companies) are the current standard for the insertion of K-wires. Previously, the only available battery powered drills had insufficient power; newer drills such as Dyonics have mostly overcome this deficit. The K-wires generally used are 0.035, 0.045, or 0.062 inch in diameter; occasionally 0.028 inch wires are useful.

Anesthesia. The choice of anesthetic is dictated by the duration of the anticipated procedure (Weeks and Wray, 1978; Weeks, 1981). Inhalation (general) anesthesia or skillfully administered axillary block anesthesia should be selected for procedures expected to last two or more hours. Inhalation anesthesia is more appropriate in the extremely anxious patient. Not infrequently, tourniquet pain limits the use of axillary block anesthesia to less than two hours. The infiltration of local anesthesia directly into the skin beneath the tourniquet reduces the incidence of tourniquet pain. For procedures up to about 1½ hours in length, intravenous regional anesthesia (Bier block) is quite effective and is quickly and simply administered by the surgeon. Double tourniquets are placed about the arm. A butterfly needle or angiocath is inserted into a peripheral vein. The limb is then exsanguinated using a Martin bandage, and the distal tourniquet is inflated first. The proximal tourniquet is then inflated and the distal tourniquet deflated. The Martin bandage is unwrapped and 0.5 per cent lidocaine without epinephrine at a dose of 3 mg per kg is injected intravenously. This results in the anesthetic diffusing under the area of the most distal tourniquet. The intravenous access route is removed. The proximal tourniquet is left inflated until tourniquet pain dictates that the distal tourniquet be inflated. Following inflation of the distal tourniquet, the proximal one is deflated.

FRACTURES WITHOUT JOINT INJURY

Carpal Bones

SCAPHOID

Acute, subacute and non-united scaphoid fractures are the most common pure fractures involving the carpals. Indeed, scaphoid fractures are over three times as common as all other carpal fractures combined (Dobyns and Linscheid, 1975). These fractures usually result from a fall on the outstretched hand with the wrist in dorsiflexion and radial deviation. In most of the injuries the pain is not severe and the tenderness may be more diffuse than localized. Radiographs, including special views for the scaphoid (pronation and ulnar deviation), are necessary for the diagnosis (Fig. 103–2). If initial radiographs fail to

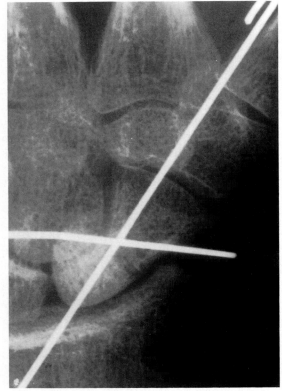

Figure 103–2. Open reduction internal fixation of an open fracture of the scaphoid. Anteroposterior radiograph.

demonstrate the fracture, a short-arm thumb spica cast is applied for two weeks. After two weeks, the cast is removed and radiographs are repeated. If the clinical impression of scaphoid fracture persists but the radiographic results are again normal, the cycle of temporary casting followed by more radiographs is repeated. Early indications are that computed tomography (CT) scans may demonstrate the fracture when the usual radiographs are normal or nondiagnostic. The CT scans are probably going to replace conventional and trispiral tomograms. The most important determinants for prognosis are stability and displacement. Subclassifications into location (proximal, middle, distal thirds, and tuberosity) also aid in making an accurate prognosis. Displaced fractures show some "movement" in radiographs taken in different planes. Stable fractures can be treated with a thumb spica cast. Controversy exists over whether the cast should be above or below elbow. The author believes an above elbow cast should be used for two weeks and then changed to a below elbow cast. Immobilization is continued until there is radiographic evidence of healing. The unstable fracture requires a long-arm thumb spica cast until there is radiographic evidence of healing. If adequate immobilization of the displacement cannot be obtained, open reduction and internal fixation, generally with a K-wire or occasionally with a screw, is indicated (Maudley and Chen, 1972; Linscheid and associates, 1972; Herbert, 1974; Eddeland and associates, 1975). The approach for ORIF is as described below for the Russe technique of bone grafting.

The treatment of established scaphoid nonunion remains somewhat controversial (Eddeland and associates, 1975). If the fracture is stable and there is no evidence of collapse or arthritis, no treatment may be needed in the *elderly* patient. In younger patients, the author considers that bone grafting is the treatment of choice. For larger fractures the Russe (1960) technique is utilized. Bone grafting using the technique of Matti (Trojan, 1974) is the treatment of choice for a small proximal third fracture.

In the Russe technique an incision about 6 cm long and centered on the tip of the radial styloid is made parallel to the radial border of the flexor carpi radialis. The joint capsule is opened. The fracture is identified and reduced into anatomic alignment if possible. If the reduction is stable, no fixation is needed.

Chap. 91). For a single metacarpal fracture, a 5 cm long longitudinal incision centered over the fracture is used. For multiple fractures either transverse or S-shaped incisions are chosen. K-wires are usually adequate for fixation. Although other techniques produce greater rigidity, non-union of an adequately reduced fracture immobilized with K-wires is exceedingly rare. Generally, the author uses crossed K-wires or transverse K-wires into an adjacent metacarpal. For very unstable oblique or spiral metacarpal fractures, open reduction and screw fixation can be used. Occasionally, plates can be used on unstable transverse metacarpal fractures (Fig. 103–7). The semilongitudinal K-wire introduced through the site of the collateral ligament at the metacarpophalangeal joint is also helpful in unstable fractures. In general, K-wires can be left exposed and bent at the skin surface to avoid interval migration. After the fracture has healed, the wires are removed without the need for anesthesia in most patients.

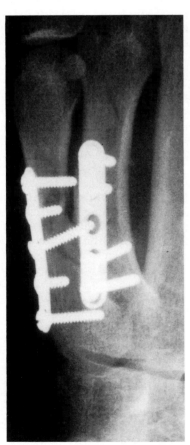

Figure 103–7. After open reduction internal fixation with ASIF plates of the patient in Figure 106–6. Oblique radiograph.

MALUNION OR NON-UNION

The most commonly treated metacarpal malunion results from malrotation of the fracture. Generally, a transverse osteotomy through the proximal end of the metacarpal is used for correction. Again, any of three types of anesthesia may be employed. A longitudinal incision centered over the metacarpal and equal to its length is used. A line is drawn on the bone with marking solution parallel to the long axis prior to the osteotomy. Transverse osteotomy through the thin cortical portion of the midshaft should be avoided, but occasionally distal osteotomies are satisfactory. The bone distal to the osteotomy is rotated until the fingers are parallel *while flexed.* A step-off in the line drawn on the metacarpal confirms the change in longitudinal alignment. The osteotomy site is held with crossed and/or transverse K-wires. For the rare persistent angulatory malunion a dorsal closure osteotomy and fixation with K-wires is used.

Proximal Phalanx

All types of fractures (transverse, spiral, comminuted) occur in the proximal phalanx. Transverse fractures through the "neck" just proximal to the distal end are quite common (Fig. 103–8). These and more proximal transverse fractures can be treated by closed reduction and external fixation by a short arm cast or a ulnar gutter splint that immobilizes the metacarpophalangeal and proximal interphalangeal joints and leaves the distal interphalangeal joint free to move. The metacarpophalangeal joint is immobilized in 90 degrees of flexion and the proximal interphalangeal joint in extension. For those fractures that are originally undisplaced, displacement during the course of cast treatment is unlikely (Wright, 1968). However, for those that have a major displacement originally, redisplacement during external (cast) fixation is quite probable. Thus, radiographs to evaluate the adequacy of reduction should be taken immediately after reduction and again one week after injury. If closed reduction is possible but the reduction is not stable, internal fixation with K-wires is recommended (Weeks, 1981). These are best inserted with the metacarpophalangeal joint flexed 90 degrees. The proximal "shoulder" of the proximal phalanx is palpated just distal to the metacarpocarpal head. A K-wire is inserted

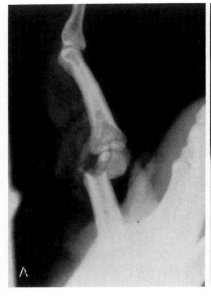 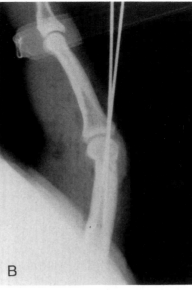

Figure 103–8. *A,* Fracture of the neck (distal end) of the proximal phalanx. Open lateral radiograph. *B,* After open reduction internal fixation of the fracture. Lateral radiograph.

with a power drill angled diagonally across the phalanx (Fig. 103–9). This method of fixation is best for transverse fractures located throughout the length of the phalanx and is occasionally useful for oblique fractures. One should be particularly cautious about proximal telescoping of any oblique fracture treated with external fixation. Oblique fractures that are unstable can be held with transverse K-wires. At times these can be inserted percutaneously with an image intensifier, but usually ORIF is necessary.

Fractures that are unstable or unreducible require ORIF. Both dorsal and midlateral incisions have been recommended. The author finds the dorsal incision the length of the phalanx most satisfactory. The extensor mechanism can be incised longitudinally and repaired, or at times reflected by incision lateral to the most dense fibers. Internal fixation is usually most easily achieved with K-wires. The author prefers retrograde pinning by first inserting the K-wires through at the site of fracture and then out through the lateral wall of the proximal fragment, preferably in the midaxial line. The fracture is then reduced and the K-wires are driven back across the fracture. Various experimental studies have indicated that either plates or looped wires are more stable than simple crossed K-wires. However, repeat displacement following crossed K-wire fixation is extremely rare. For very unstable fractures, direct interosseous wiring can be combined with K-wire fixation. K-wire fixation also is generally satisfactory in the oblique fractures that require open reduction. Two ASIF screws placed across both fracture fragments also provide satisfactory fixation.

Middle Phalanx

The mechanism of injury and physical and radiographic findings are similar to those described for fractures of the metacarpal (see above). If these fractures are stable and nondisplaced, external fixation is used. A short-arm volar plaster splint with an aluminum extension for the finger is satisfactory. The metacarpophalangeal joint is held in 90 degrees of flexion and the proximal and distal interphalangeal joints in almost full extension. Splinting is generally maintained for three to four weeks and then the finger is treated with "buddy taping" without splinting. Motion against resistance is not allowed for an additional two weeks.

Open fractures generally are both unstable and significantly displaced. One or, at most, two attempts at closed reduction and either external or internal fixation (K-wires being inserted with an image intensifier) is justified. However, if CREF or CRIF is not successful, ORIF should be used (Kilbourne, 1968; Weeks, 1981). Generally, the fracture is approached through the laceration or an extension of the laceration. If no laceration

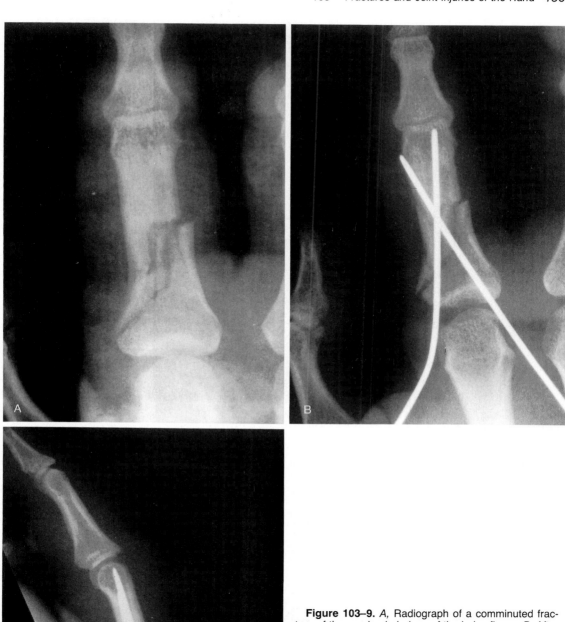

Figure 103–9. *A,* Radiograph of a comminuted fracture of the proximal phalanx of the index finger. *B,* After closed reduction internal fixation with Kirschner wires. Posteroanterior radiograph. *C,* Lateral radiograph.

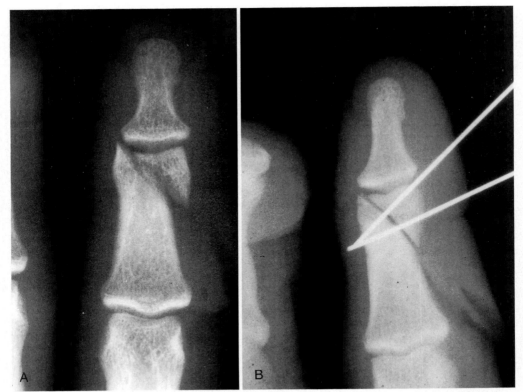

Figure 103–10. *A*, Fracture of the middle phalanx. Open posteroanterior radiograph. *B*, After open reduction internal fixation with Kirschner wires. Posteroanterior radiograph.

is present, a dorsal skin incision the length of the phalanx is made. The extensor mechanism is elevated along the radial or ulnar border without an incision through the extensor mechanism. Generally, the fractures are pinned with K-wires placed in the retrograde fashion as described above for the proximal phalanx (Fig. 103–10). If smaller diameter (0.035 inch) K-wires are used, they frequently remain within the medullary cavity. However, if larger wires (0.045 inch) are used, they can be made to exit through both cortices. Screw fixation is almost never employed owing to the mass of the screw and its impingement on the extensor mechanism. The additional stabilizing force obtained with a interrosseous wire must be weighed against the fact that the wire is usually in contact with the extensor mechanism. In general, crossed K-wires lend sufficient stability.

Distal Phalanx

If the distal interphalangeal joint is not involved by the fracture, the patients can generally be treated quite simply by an external splint. The Stack splint (Fig. 103–1) generally is easily applied and well tolerated. Occasional epiphyseal separations require reduction but usually are stable when reduced. Epiphyseal separations may present as a mallet deformity. The mallet appearance is due to the flexor profundus attaching to the distal fragment and the extensor mechanism to the

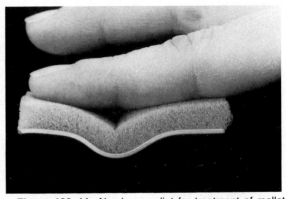

Figure 103–11. Aluminum splint for treatment of mallet finger, shown without tape for clarity.

proximal fragment. Closed reduction is performed after digital block anesthesia. If the nail has been displaced, it is replaced under the nail fold for increased stability. If the patient is too small for the smallest Stack splints, a bent aluminum splint is used to immobilize the distal interphalangeal joint (Fig. 103–11). A small K-wire may even be needed to immobilize the distal interphalangeal joint and hold the fracture in a reduced position. Non-union is not rare after distal phalangeal fractures, but is rarely symptomatic.

DISLOCATIONS, SUBLUXATIONS, AND FRACTURES WITH JOINT INJURY (See Chap. 104)

Carpal Bones

Most carpal dislocations and fracture-dislocations are the result of acute hyperextension (dorsiflexion) injuries (Taleisnik, 1978). The majority of the injuries are closed and occur after a fall or vehicular accidents. Motorcycle operators and passengers seem to be particularly prone to these injuries. The more rare open injuries are frequently industrial accidents from rapidly rotating shafts, wheels, or drums whose axis of rotation is at right angles to the forearm. As the carpals are of near-equal strength, fracture-dislocations occur with similar frequency. As the dorsal flexion continues, the lunate may be retained in position and the remaining carpal bones dislocate about it, causing a dorsal perilunate dislocation (Table 103–2). The scaphoid may or may not undergo rotary subluxation. With the dislocating force concentrated more on the ulnar radial side, a transscaphoid perilunate fracture-dislocation may result (Fig. 103–12). With the stress on the radial side of the wrist and into hyperextension, the fracture may occur further proximal through the radial styloid, again producing a dorsal perilunate fracture-dislocation (Table 103–2). The volar perilunate or dorsal lunate dislocations are much less common. Complete dislocation of the scaphoid is less common but well described. Virtually any pattern of fracture and/or dislocation of the carpal bones can occur and have been

Table 103–2. Carpal Dislocations and Fracture-Dislocations

Dorsal perilunate—volar lunate dislocation
 Isolated rotatory subluxation of scaphoid
 Transradial dorsal perilunate—volar lunate fracture-dislocation

Dorsal trans-scaphoid perilunate fracture-dislocation
 Dorsal trans-scaphoid transradial perilunate fracture-dislocation

Volar perilunate—dorsal lunate dislocation

Unusual dislocations and fracture-dislocations

reported but are classified under "unusual fracture-dislocations" owing to their rarity. Table 103–2 lists the injuries in order of decreasing frequency.

The usual patient with a closed dislocation or fracture-dislocation has surprisingly few symptoms (Green, 1982). The wrist is held in a near-neutral position in the flexion-extension and radioulnar axes. Pain develops if the patient attempts to move the wrist. Pain and limitation of motion are the usual findings, but are not dramatic. Palpation directly over the carpals elicits tenderness, but again this is not dramatic. Function of the median nerve should be carefully evaluated. The presence of normal median nerve function initially followed by loss of function is an indication for open decompression of the median nerve at the wrist. If the patient initially has some median nerve impairment, observation may be safe; however, if symptoms progress, decompression is indicated.

The anteroposterior radiograph may show only subtle changes, but a lunate that appears triangular is an indication of lunate dislocation. The lateral radiographs are usually diagnostic and should be taken with the wrist in neutral position. An oblique radiograph is a helpful addition but of itself is usually nondiagnostic. A "wrist instability series" consisting of posteroanterior views with the hand in radial and ulnar deviation and lateral views in dorsiflexion, volar flexion, and fist compression are useful in determining the effects of old injuries but are not the subject of this chapter. Radiographs taken after traction has been applied may clarify the exact nature and extent of the injury. Both anterior, posterior, and lateral radiographs should be taken.

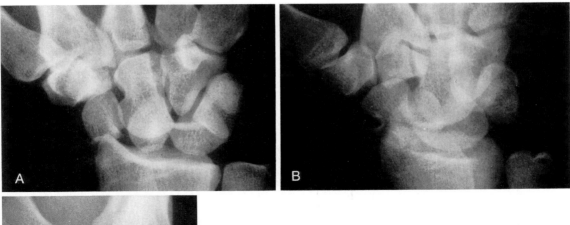

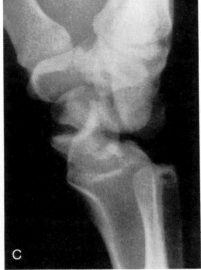

Figure 103–12. *A,* Transscaphoid perilunate fracture-dislocation. Antero-posterior radiograph. *B,* Oblique radiograph. *C,* The lunate remains in the lunate fossa of the radius. Lateral radiograph.

DORSAL PERILUNATE—VOLAR LUNATE DISLOCATIONS

Dorsal perilunate or volar lunate disloca-tions can usually be treated by closed reduc-tion (Figs. 103–13, 103–14) (Watson-Jones, 1943; Green, 1982). Inhalation, brachial block, or intravenous regional anesthesia is obtained. The fingers are placed in finger-traps and 10 to 15 lbs of weight is placed on a sling about the arm. The elbow is flexed to 90 degrees and the weight is left in place for five to ten minutes. The fingertraps are then removed while the surgeon continues longi-tudinal traction with his hand. Generally a right-handed surgeon maintains the traction with the left hand. The patient's hand is dorsiflexed while the right thumb stabilizes the lunate on the volar aspect of the wrist.

Gradual palmar flexion of the hand while the longitudinal traction is maintained usually results in reduction of the dislocation. If the injury has preceded treatment by several days, open reduction may be required. The dislocation is immobilized in a short-arm thumb spica cast with the wrist neutral. Post-reduction radiographs are necessary to en-sure the adequacy of reduction, the certainty of lunate and capitate alignment, and the lack of scaphoid rotation. Radiographs should be taken at weekly intervals for the first three weeks. In general, six to eight weeks of im-mobilization are sufficient. After immobili-zation is discontinued, cautious resumption of activities and gradually increase of dorsi-flexion and volar flexion loads leads to strengthening of the ligaments.

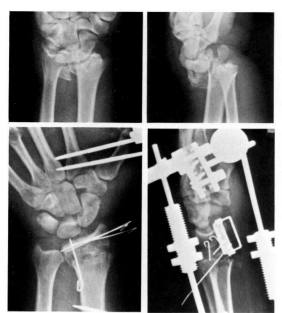

Figure 104–16. Radiograph showing a comminuted distal radial fracture above, and the combined use of an external fixator and Kirschner wires for a comminuted distal radial fracture below.

final wrist motion than is seen following stabilization with an external fixation device.

Elderly Patients. If the patient's activity level and general health are consistent with the need for a "normal wrist," a similar pro-

tocol is followed as with a younger individual attempting to achieve and maintain an anatomic reduction. If, however, the patient is physiologically or chronologically elderly, a closed reduction is employed to restore length and volar tilt as much as possible, and a short arm cast is employed for six weeks. Following removal of the cast, a removable splint is applied that the patient can be weaned from over a subsequent two to three weeks. The distal radial fracture that results from this type of care frequently shows considerable radial shortening, but the complaints of ulnar wrist pain in this age group tend to be minimal. If the patient has discomfort about the distal ulna after fracture healing, a distal ulnar resection or recession is employed (Darrach, 1912a, b, 1913; Milch, 1963; Darrow and associates, 1985).

RADIAL STYLOID FRACTURES

Once known as a chauffeur's fracture, the radial styloid fracture is significant not only because it is intra-articular, but because the major extrinsic ligaments of the wrist arise from the radial styloid.

Treatment. Small avulsion fractures are treated with a short arm cast in 15 degrees of radial deviation and 15 degrees of palmar flexion for six weeks. Large avulsions are treated with open reduction and internal fix-

Figure 104–17. Plating of an uncomminuted distal radial fracture through a dorsal approach.

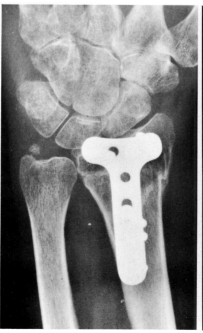
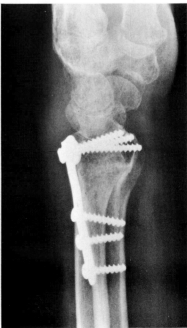

ation of the radial styloid fracture, followed by plaster immobilization until union is achieved (Fig. 104–18). Anatomic restoration of the bony architecture restores the normal relationships of the radiocapitate and radiotriquetral ligaments. Six weeks of plaster immobilization after fixation of the fracture result in both bony and ligamentous healing.

LUNATE LOAD FRACTURES

A fall on the outstretched upper extremity may cause a compression fracture of the lunate fossa of the radius as the lunate itself is driven back into the radius (Fig. 104–19). Tomography is frequently necessary to reveal the joint incongruity that results from this fracture. Although the severity of the original injury may result in chondrolysis and secondary degenerative joint disease no matter what treatment is undertaken, the author prefers an open reduction of the wrist with an elevation of the depressed fragment and fixation with Kirschner wires, followed by iliac crest bone grafting of the bony defect. The pins are removed at six weeks and plaster immobili-

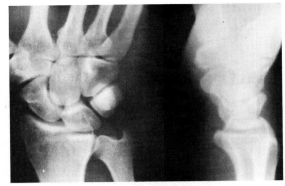

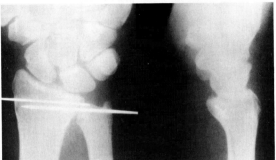

Figure 104–19. A lunate load fracture is pictured above on an AP and lateral film. Below, the depressed fracture has been elevated, stabilized with Kirschner wires, and the bony defect left after elevating the lunate fossa, bone grafted.

zation is carried out for an additional two to four weeks.

Distal Ulna

DISTAL ULNAR FRACTURES

Most distal ulnar fractures are styloid fractures that occur in association with distal radial fractures, and are relatively insignificant (Reeves, 1966; Bowers, 1982). These need no special treatment. Although many do not heal, this seldom leads to long-term problems (Fig. 104–20). If the nonunited ulnar styloid fragments are symptomatic, the fragment can be easily removed (Reeves, 1966). Occasionally, however, one sees a larger ulnar styloid fragment associated with an unstable distal ulna. In this instance, the TFCC insertion into the distal ulna remains on the avulsed fragment, thus leaving the residual ulna unsupported.

Treatment. Screw fixation of ulnar styloid fragments associated with an unstable distal ulna is extremely difficult. The author prefers a tension band wiring technique (Fig. 104–

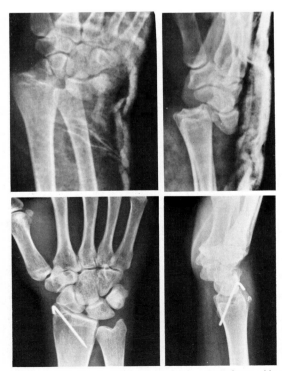

Figure 104–18. A dislocated wrist is seen along with a large avulsion of the radial styloid. Reduction of the carpus and hand was achieved when the radial styloid was reduced *(below).*

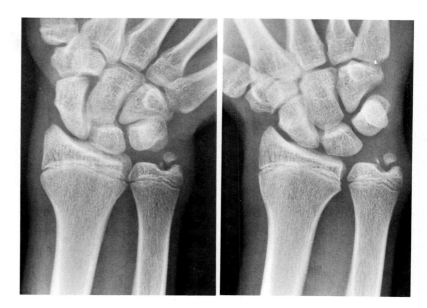

Figure 104–20. Nonunion of an ulnar styloid fracture that is asymptomatic. There is no evidence of wrist instability.

21). However, because of the paucity of soft tissue about the distal ulna, the fixation device must frequently be removed after bony union.

Ulnar head fractures are rare. They are usually the result of a direct blow to the wrist, generally in young adults. If the fracture fragment is small, involving very little of the articular surface, the bony fragment can be removed. However, if the fragment is large, every attempt should be made to restore the ulnar head congruency by internally stabilizing the fracture with either a Kirschner wire or a small interfragmentary screw. Distal ulnar resections in young people should be avoided if at all possible.

SUBLUXATION AND DISLOCATION

Subluxation or dislocation of the distal ulna is frequently not appreciated acutely, since radiography is notoriously inaccurate in evaluating the distal radioulnar joint (Milch, 1942; Dameron, 1972; Hamlin, 1977). A single cut CT scan, however, at the level of Lister's tubercle, is virtually diagnostic for distal radioulnar joint incongruity (Fig. 104–22) (Mino, Palmer, and Levinsohn, 1983). Subluxation or dislocation of this joint can be successfully treated with simple immobilization in a long arm cast for six weeks if the injury is seen acutely (Darrach, 1912b; Bowers, 1982).

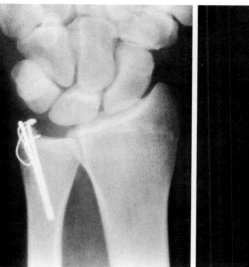
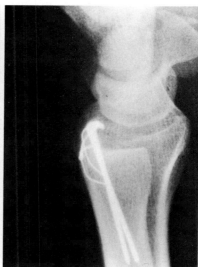

Figure 104–21. Tension band wiring of an ulnar styloid fracture. Stabilization of the fracture restored stability to the distal radioulnar joint.

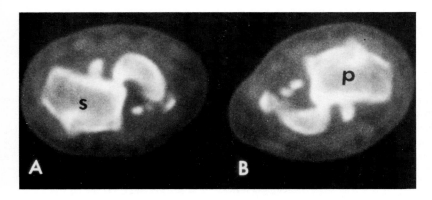

Figure 104–22. A CT scan of the distal radioulnar joint, showing palmar fracture dislocation of the distal ulna in *(A)* supination (s) and *(B)* pronation (p).

The position of immobilization is full supination for a dorsal dislocation and full pronation for a palmar dislocation. Untreated or unrecognized injuries to the distal radioulnar joint may lead to a very disabling problem that is difficult to treat: chronic distal ulnar instability.

Treatment. For chronic subluxation or dislocation of the distal radioulnar joint, the author prefers to reattach the ulnar styloid process or to reattach the avulsed or stretched out TFCC (Rose-Innes, 1960; Heiple, Freehafer, and Van't Hof, 1962; Albert, Wohl, and Rechtman, 1963; Dameron, 1972; Alexander, 1977; Blatt and Ashworth, 1979; af Ekenstam, 1984; Darrow and associates, 1985). The capsule is tightly reinforced over the ligamentous repair, and the arm is immobilized in supination for six weeks for a dorsal incongruity and in pronation for six weeks for a palmar incongruity. If it is not possible to achieve a stable reduction at the time of surgery, a Lauenstein procedure, as repopularized by Taleisnik, is preferred (Fig. 104–23) (Carroll and Inbriglia, 1979; Bowers, 1982).

Carpal Fractures and Dislocations

The seven major carpal bones, excluding the pisiform, are arranged into two horizontal rows, with the scaphoid acting as the connecting link between the two. The proximal carpal row is the "interculated segment" in a link system that is stabilized by (1) the bony architecture of the carpal bones and (2) the extrinsic and intrinsic carpal ligaments. Carpal fractures and dislocations are the products of many factors, including (1) the geo-

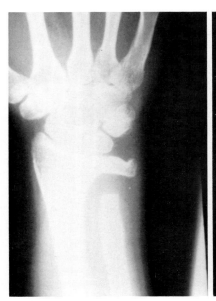
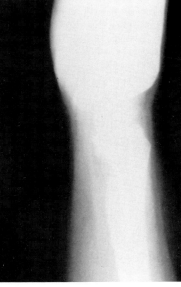

Figure 104–23. Fusion of the ulnar head to the distal radius with a bony cuff proximally has again become a popular treatment of chronic distal radioulnar joint dislocation.

metric configuration of the articulation; (2) the attachment and relative strength and elasticity of the ligaments and capsule; (3) force considerations, including points of application, magnitude, rate of loading, and direction; and (4) the status of the skeleton in terms of demineralization.

The perilunar area of the wrist has been termed the "vulnerable zone" by Johnson and Mayfield, since this is where most fracture dislocations of the wrist occur (Fig. 104–24) (Mayfield, Johnson, and Kilcoyne, 1976, 1980; Mayfield, 1980; Johnson, 1980). These carpal fractures and dislocations are the result of a hyperextension hypersupination injury to the wrist. As force is applied to the palm, the scaphoid hyperextends and either fractures or ruptures the scapholunate interosseous ligament. With further load, the lunate extends and the head of the capitate fractures and/or dislocates. With progression to the ulnar side of the lunate, the triquetrum in a similar fashion fractures and/or dislocates. When all the perilunar carpals fracture with dislocation, it is called a "greater arc injury." When all the perilunar carpals dislocate without fracture, it is called a full perilunar dislocation or "lesser arc injury." Any combination of greater or lesser arc injuries may occur. All fractures and dislocations of the carpus should not be thought of in terms of an isolated fracture or dislocation, but in terms of the fractured bone, the injured ligament, and the resultant loss of normal carpal relationships and the consequent instability patterns that may develop.

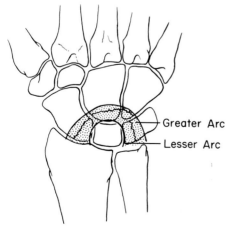

Figure 104–24. Dislocations taking place about the lunate are lesser arc injuries. Fracture dislocations taking place about the lunate through adjacent carpal bones are termed greater arc injuries.

CARPAL FRACTURES

Fracture of Scaphoid

In every case of closed injury to the wrist with no obvious deformity, one must assume the presence of a scaphoid fracture until (there is) radiological proof of the contrary.

BOYES, 1970

The scaphoid is second only to the distal radius in incidence of fracture about the wrist (Desault, 1805; Bentzon and Randlov-Madsen, 1946; Cooney, 1980b; Verdan and Narakas, 1968). Scaphoid fractures have been reported in all age groups, but usually occur in young male adults and generally involve the waist of the scaphoid (Eddeland and associates, 1975; Greene, Hadied, and LaMont, 1984). The mechanism of injury is a fall on the outstretched upper extremity, the impact load producing a hyperextension supination injury to the wrist (Weber and Chao, 1978; Weber, 1980). The location of the scaphoid fracture and the fracture stability dictate, to some extent, the treatment program (Cooney, 1980b). Approximately 70 per cent of scaphoid fractures occur in the middle third of the scaphoid, 20 per cent in the distal third, and 10 per cent in the proximal third (Cooney, 1980b).

Acute Scaphoid Fractures

Historically, scaphoid fractures have had a relatively high incidence of nonunion (Ruby, Stinson, and Belsky, 1985). This can be attributed to two factors: (1) the precarious blood supply of the proximal pole of the scaphoid and (2) the fact that many fractures are not radiographed acutely and therefore are missed (Taleisnik and Kelly, 1966; Gelberman and Menon, 1980; Leslie and Dickson, 1981; Gelberman and associates, 1983). One must therefore develop a high index of suspicion for scaphoid fractures. If a fracture is suspected, the wrist should be immobilized in a long arm thumb spica cast (even if radiographic results appear normal) for two weeks, and then x-rayed again (Archambault, 1980).

Approximately 10 per cent of all scaphoid fractures are displaced and unstable when first seen. In these instances, the blood supply to the proximal pole has usually been disrupted (Gelberman and associates, 1983). Open reduction and internal fixation is generally needed to restore anatomic alignment of these fractures (Adams, 1928). If treated

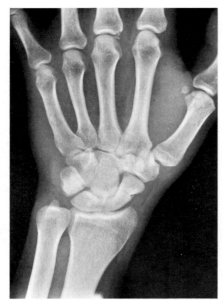

Figure 104–25. An undisplaced scaphoid fracture is best treated with plaster immobilization.

with immobilization without an anatomic reduction, these fractures may proceed to nonunion and progressive carpal collapse.

Treatment

Nonoperative. Undisplaced scaphoid fractures should be treated in plaster until there is radiographic (tomographic) evidence of union (Fig. 104–25) (Archambault, 1980). The author prefers a long arm thumb spica cast for eight weeks followed by a short arm

thumb spica (Goldman, Lipscomb, and Taylor, 1969). The length of immobilization needed to effect union varies considerably, depending on the location of the fracture and the promptness of initiation of immobilization after the fracture. A scaphoid fracture that does not heal with six months of immobilization should be considered a nonunion.

Operative. Unstable scaphoid fractures (Fig. 104–26) are best treated with open reduction and internal fixation with K-wires or a Herbert screw (Fig. 104–27) (Maudsley and Chen, 1972; Sprague and associates, 1985).

Scaphoid Nonunions

Asymptomatic scaphoid nonunions are frequently seen. Most of these go on to develop symptoms of post-traumatic arthritis with time (Fig. 104–28) (Mazet and Hohl, 1961). The goals of treatment for a scaphoid nonunion should be twofold: union and restoration of normal carpal alignment (Fisk, 1970; Cooney, Linscheid, and Dobyns, 1979; Boeckstyns and Busch, 1984; Green, 1985). If the patient is young and active, the author recommends treatment for an asymptomatic scaphoid nonunion (Cooney, 1980b). Treatment for a symptomatic nonunion is always advisable when there is associated carpal collapse.

Treatment. For a stable scaphoid nonunion without collapse, the author prefers a Russe bone grafting approach, utilizing iliac

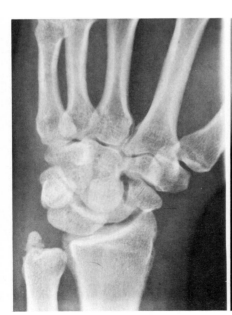
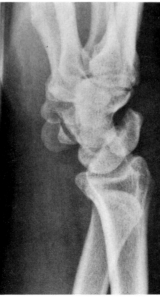

Figure 104–26. An unstable displaced scaphoid fracture with carpal malrotation.

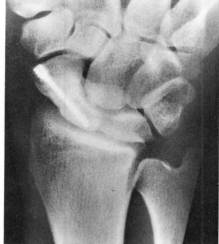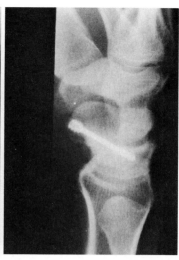

Figure 104–27. An unstable scaphoid fracture has been reduced and stabilized (Herbert screw), thereby correcting associated carpal malalignment.

crest bone (Murray, 1934; Russe, 1960; Dooley, 1968; Green, 1985). Internal fixation is not routinely used. The patient is immobilized postoperatively in a long arm thumb spica for eight weeks, followed by a short arm cast until union is observed by tomography.

For an unstable nonunion with associated collapse, the author prefers a Russe approach, but in this instance, utilized internal fixation (Murray, 1934; Matti, 1937; Russe, 1960; Green, 1985). The iliac crest bone is fixed in place with two Kirschner wires inserted parallel to one another and parallel to the longitudinal axis of the scaphoid.

Electrical stimulation is presently popular for the treatment of scaphoid nonunions (Bora, Osterman, and Brighton, 1981; Beckenbaugh, 1985). The author prefers to utilize this method in two circumstances: (1) when conventional bone grafting has failed or (2) when surgery is not feasible because of a patient's philosophy or physical condition.

Other surgical procedures to treat scaphoid nonunions, such as radiostyloidectomy, proxial row carpectomy, limited wrist fusion, or pan wrist fusion, should be viewed as salvage procedures and reserved for the treatment of localized degenerative joint disease, secondary to scaphoid nonunions (Andrews, 1932; Agner, 1963; Axelsson, 1971).

Proximal Pole Fractures

If the proximal fragment is relatively large, the author still prefers conventional bone grafting via the volar Russe approach. If union fails to occur or the fragment is very small, the fragment is excised through a dorsal approach and soft tissue is inserted. If carpal collapse begins to occur at a later date as a result of excision of the proximal pole, a limited wrist fusion is performed as a salvage procedure.

Fractures of Lunate

Acute fractures of the lunate are rare (Adams, 1925). Most lead to avascular necrosis despite treatment, and are then dealt with as Kienböck's disease. Nevertheless, all acute fractures of the lunate should be immobilized

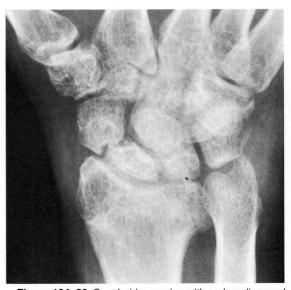

Figure 104–28. Scaphoid nonunion with early radiocarpal and midcarpal arthritic changes.

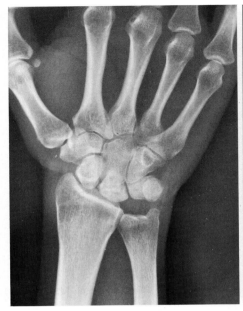 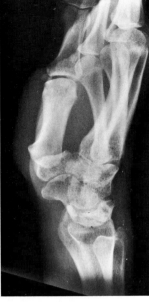

Figure 104–29. Stage III (Lichtman) Kienböck's disease in an ulnar minus variant wrist.

in a long arm cast for six weeks, followed by a short arm cast for six weeks. Union, if it occurs, should do so in approximately three months.

In 1910, Kienböck published his now classic description of lunatomalacia (Beckenbaugh and associates, 1980). His concept that this condition represented avascular necrosis has been accepted, and yet the true etiology of this condition remains a mystery. Most feel that the avascular necrosis results from a stress fracture of the lunate (Axelsson, 1971). Individuals who develop this disease (in other words, a stress fracture of the lunate) statistically are more likely to have "negative ulnar variance" (Fig. 104–29) (Hulten, 1928; Gelberman and associates, 1975; Palmer, Glisson, and Werner, 1982). They probably also have a tenuous blood supply to part of the lunate, and subject the wrist to repetitive loads in a position that leads to intermittent compromise of this tenuous blood supply (Lee, 1963).

Treatment. Treatment for Kienböck's disease is predicated upon the stage of the disease being dealt with. Stahl and Lichtman have both introduced classifications for this disease, based on the radiographic appearance of the wrist (Table 104–2) (Stahl, 1947; Lichtman and associates, 1977, 1982). Many surgical approaches to Kienböck's are now popular, including joint leveling procedures (ulnar lengthening, radial shortening); Silas-

tic replacement of the lunate; Silastic replacement of the lunate combined with limited intercarpal fusion; limited intercarpal fusion alone; vascularized bone grafts; and wrist denervation, to name only a few (Persson, 1950; Gillespie, 1961; Agerholm and Goodfellow, 1963; Tajima, 1966; Tillberg, 1968; Nahigian and associates, 1970; Moberg, 1974; Chuinard and Zeman, 1980; Almquist and Burns, 1982; Armistead and associates, 1982; Palmer, 1986; Watson, Ryu, and DiBella, 1985). All are reported to relieve pain in a large percentage of patients. However, in the words of Eric Moberg, "all procedures in use today are successful only in delaying the inevitable—progressive degenerative arthritis of the wrist" (Palmer, 1986).

For Stage I, the author prefers intermittent

Table 104–2. Radiographic Staging of Kienböck's Disease*

Stage	Stahl	Lichtman
I	Compression fracture	Linear or compression fracture
II	Sclerosis	Sclerosis
III	Sclerosis and mild collapse	Sclerosis and definite collapse
IV	Sclerosis, collapse, and fragmentation	Sclerosis, collapse, and associated degenerative changes
V	Sclerosis and DJD changes	

*As proposed by Stahl and Lichtman.

immobilization to deal with wrist discomfort and synovitis (Lichtman and associates, 1977, 1982). This stage may not progress to more advanced Kienböck's disease.

For Stages II and III, it is better to "unload" the lunate and allow for stress fracture healing and revascularization of the lunate. The author prefers an ulnar lengthening procedure in patients who are ulnar minus or ulnar neutral (Fig. 104–30). For the rare individual with ulnar positive variance and Kienböck's disease, a scaphotrapezial trapezoidal (STT) fusion is performed (see Chap. 106).

In Stage IV, the problem is no longer pure Kienböck's disease but an arthritic wrist (Fig. 104–31). For this problem, it is preferable to have a limited wrist fusion preserving the joints that are nonarthritic. If the arthritic process has advanced to the point where all joints of the wrist are involved, pan wrist fusion is performed.

The use of a Silastic lunate replacement has been reported to give satisfactory results in the treatment of all stages of Kienböck's disease (Swanson, 1970; Lichtman and associates, 1982). However, it has been revealed that a significant percentage of patients undergoing Silastic replacement of the lunate may eventually develop Silastic synovitis of the wrist (Fig. 104–32) (Smith, Atkinson, and Jupiter, 1985). To help avoid this, it is now recommended that if a Silastic lunate replacement is inserted, the carpus be addition-

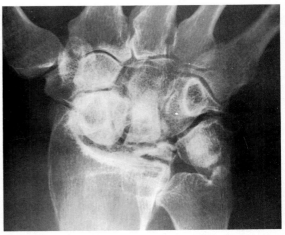

Figure 104–31. Stage IV Kienböck's disease with carpal collapse and advanced radiocarpal and midcarpal arthritis.

ally stabilized with a simultaneous intercarpal arthrodesis (Watson, Ryu, and DiBella, 1985).

Fractures of Hamate

Fractures of the hamate body are rare. They usually result from a direct blow to the carpus and are frequently associated with other carpal injuries (Bowen, 1973). Frac-

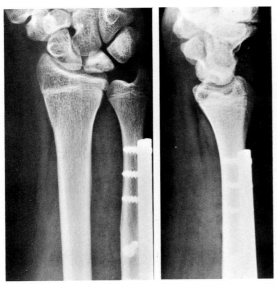

Figure 104–30. An ulnar lengthening procedure in this 15 year old male with Stage III Kienböck's disease gave complete relief of wrist pain.

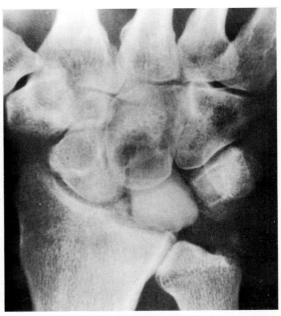

Figure 104–32. Six years after Silastic lunate replacement for Kienböck's disease, carpal cysts and associated increasing wrist pain are thought to be secondary to silicone synovitis.

tures of the hook of the hamate are uncommon, but not rare (Duke, 1963; Andress and Peckar, 1970; Bowen, 1973; Egawa and Asai, 1983; Foucher and associates, 1985). They result from a direct injury such as might be sustained while using a golf club, tennis racquet, or baseball bat. This injury should be suspected in a patient with deep, ill-defined pain on the ulnar side of the wrist (particularly a golfer). The diagnosis is best made with an external oblique radiograph of the wrist. The preferred method of treatment is excision of the hook of the hamate (Carter, Eaton, and Littler, 1977).

Other Carpal Fractures

Other carpal fractures are rare and frequently associated with other wrist injuries (Desault, 1805; Bonnin and Greening, 1944; Bartone and Grieco, 1956; Adler and Shaftan, 1962; Stein, 1971; Boe, 1979; Levy and associates, 1979; Bryan and Dobyns, 1980; Palmer, 1981; Rhoades and Reckling, 1983, Freeland and Finely, 1984). They are often missed because of the severity of the associated injuries. A good example is the fracture of the head of the capitate that is associated with a scaphoid fracture and a dislocation of the capitate head—the naviculocapitate syndrome (Fig. 104–33) (Fenton, 1956; March and Lampros, 1959; Vance, Gelberman, and Evans, 1980). In this instance, the scaphoid fracture and the capitate fracture may be obvious, but the dislocation or malrotation of

the proximal pole of the capitate may be missed unless suspected and specifically looked for. Here, distraction films may be helpful.

Treatment. Undisplaced fractures of the "other carpal bones" are best treated in a short arm cast or, in the case of trapezial and trapezoid fractures, a short arm thumb spica cast for six weeks. Displaced fractures are treated with open reduction and internal fixation with Kirschner wires to restore joint congruity. Immobilization is again in a short arm cast or short arm thumb spica for six weeks.

CARPAL DISLOCATIONS

As mentioned previously, all carpal dislocations must be thought of in terms of the associated ligamentous damage as well as the obvious loss of normal bony relationships (Thompson, Campbell, and Arnold, 1964; Fisk, 1980; Green and O'Brien, 1980; Johnson, 1980; Bilos and Hui, 1981). In treating carpal dislocations, one should strive for restoration of normal bony alignment, and immobilize to allow for ligamentous healing (Green and O'Brien, 1978). If proper ligamentous healing does not occur, late carpal instability will result and the inherently unstable proximal carpal row will be destabilized with load (Green and O'Brien, 1980).

With extremely rare exceptions, all carpal dislocations are perilunate or a variant thereof (Campbell, Lance, and Yeoh, 1964;

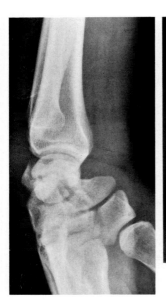 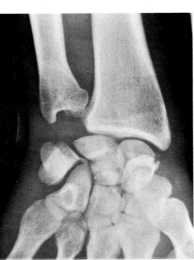

Figure 104–33. The naviculocapitate syndrome. Note that the proximal pole of the capitate is rotated 180 degrees.

Kauer, J. M. G.: Functional anatomy of the wrist. Clin. Orthop., *149*:9, 1980.

Kauer, J. M. G., and Landsmeer, J. M. F.: Functional anatomy of the wrist. *In* Tubiana, R. (Ed.): The Hand. Vol. 1. Philadelphia, W. B. Saunders Company, 1981, pp. 142–157.

Kienböck, R.: Uber traumatische Malazie des Mondbeins und ihre Folgezustande: Entartungsformen und Kompressionsfrakturen. Fortschr. Geg. Roentgenstr., *16*:78, 1910–1911.

Kleinman, W. B., Steichen, J. B., and Strickland, J. W.: Management of chronic rotary subluxation of the scapho-trapezio-trapezoid arthrodesis. J. Hand Surg., *7*:125, 1982.

Landsmeer, J. M. F.: Studies in the anatomy of articulation. I. The equilibrium of the "intercalated" bone. Acta Morphol. Neerl. Scand., *3*:287, 1961.

Lee, M. L. H.: The intraosseous arterial pattern of the carpal lunate bone and its relation to avascular necrosis. Acta Orthop. Scand., *33*:43, 1963.

Leslie, I, J., and Dickson, R. A.: The fractured carpal scaphoid: natural history and factors influencing outcome. J. Bone Joint Surg., *63B*:225, 1981.

Levinsohn, E. M., and Palmer, A. K.: Arthrography of the traumatized wrist. Radiology, *146*:647, 1983.

Levy, M., Fischel, R. E., Stern, G. M., and Goldberg, I.: Chip fractures of the os triquetrum: the mechanism of injury. J. Bone Joint Surg., *61B*:355, 1979.

Lewis, O. J.: The hominoid wrist joint. Am J. Phys. Anthropol., *30*:251, 1969.

Lewis, O. J., Hamshere, R. J., and Bucknill, T. M.: The anatomy of the wrist joint. J. Anat., *106*:539, 1970.

Lichtman, D. M., Alexander, A. H., Mack, G. R., and Ganther, S. F.: Kienböck's disease—update on silicone replacement arthroplasty. J. Hand Surg., *7*:343, 1982.

Lichtman, D. M., Mack, G. R., MacDonald, R. I., Gunther, S. F., and Wilson, J. N.: Kienböck's disease: the role of silicone replacement arthroplasty. J. Bone Joint Surg., *59A*:899, 1977.

Lichtman, D. M., Schneider, J. R., Swafford, A. R., and Mack, G. R.: Ulnar midcarpal instability: clinical and laboratory analysis. J. Hand Surg., *6*:515, 1981.

Linscheid, R. L., Dobyns, J. H., Beabout, J. W., and Bryan, R. S.: Traumatic instability of the wrist; diagnosis, classification and pathomechanics. J. Bone Joint Surg., *54A*:1612, 1972.

Marsh, A. P., and Lampros, P. J.: The naviculocapitate fracture syndrome. Am. J. Roentgenol., *82*:255, 1959.

Matti, H.: Uber die Behandlung der Naviculare-Fracture und der Refractura Patellae durch Plombierung mit Spongiosa. Zentralbl. Chir., *64*:2353, 1937.

Maudsley, R. H., and Chen, S. C.: Screw fixation in the management of the fractured carpal scaphoid. J. Bone Joint Surg., *54B*:432, 1972.

Mayfield, J. K.: Mechanism of carpal injuries. Clin. Orthop., *149*:45, 1980.

Mayfield, J. K., Johnson, R. P., and Kilcoyne, R. F: The ligaments of the human wrist and their functional significance. Anat. Rec., *186*:417, 1976.

Mayfield, J. K., Johnson, R. P. and Kilcoyne, R. F.: Carpal dislocations: pathomechanics and progressive perilinur instability. J. Hand Surg., *5*:226, 1980.

Mazet, R., Jr., and Hohl, M.: Conservative treatment of old fractures of the carpal scaphoid. J. Trauma, *1*:115, 1961.

McMurtry, R. Y., Youm, Y., Flatt, A. E., and Gillespie, T. E.: Kinematics of the wrist. II. Clinical applications. J. Bone Joint. Surg., *60A*:955, 1978.

Milch, H.: So-called dislocation of the lower end of the ulna. Ann. Surg., *116*:282, 1942.

Milch, H.: Colles' fracture. Bull. Hosp. Joint Dis., *11*:61, 1950.

Milch, H.: Treatment of disabilities following fracture of the lower end of the radius. Clin. Orthop., *29*:157, 1963.

Mino, D. E., Palmer, A. K., and Levinsohn, E. M.: The role of radiography and computerized tomography in the diagnosis of subluxation and dislocation of the distal radioulnar joint. J. Hand Surg., *8*:23, 1983.

Mino, D. E., Palmer, A. K., and Levinsohn, E. M.: Radiography and computerized tomography in the diagnosis of incongruity of the distal radioulnar joint. J. Bone Joint Surg., *67A*:247, 1985.

Moberg, E.: Treatment of Kienböck's disease by shortening of the radius. Presented at the joint meeting of Japanese and American Hand Surgeons, Hiroshima, 1974.

Murray, G.: Bone graft for non-union of the carpal scaphoid. Br. J. Surg., *22*:63, 1934.

Nahigian, S. H., Li, C. S., Richey, D. G., and Shaw, D. T.: The dorsal flap arthroplasty in the treatment of Kienböck's disease. J. Bone Joint Surg., *52A*:245, 1970.

Navarro, A., cited by Scaramuzza, R. F.: El moviomiento de rotacion en el carpo y su relacion con la fisiopatologia de sus lesiones traumaticas. Bol. Trabajos Soc. Argent. Ortoped Traumatol., *34*:337, 1976.

Palmer, A. K.: Trapezial ridge fractures. J. Hand Surg., *6*:561, 1981.

Palmer, A. K.: The distal radioulnar joint. Orthop. Clin. North Am., *15*:321, 1984.

Palmer, A. K.: Bunnell Traveling Fellowship Report 1984: J. Hand Surg., *11A*:94, 1986.

Palmer, A. K., Dobyns, J. H., and Linscheid, R. L.: Management of post-traumatic instability of the wrist secondary to ligament rupture. J. Hand Surg., *3*:507, 1978.

Palmer, A. K., Glisson, R. R., and Werner, F. W.: Ulnar variance determination. J. Hand. Surg., *7*:376, 1982.

Palmer, A. K., Levinsohn, E. M., and Kuzma, G. R.: Arthrography of the wrist. J. Hand Surg., *8*:15, 1983.

Palmer, A. K., Skahen, J. R., Werner, F. W., and Glisson, R. R.: The extensor retinaculum of the wrist: an anatomical and biomechanical study. J. Hand Surg., *10B*:11, 1985.

Palmer, A. K., and Werner, F. W.: The triangular fibrocartilage complex of the wrist: anatomy and function. J. Hand Surg., *6*:153, 1981.

Palmer, A. K., and Werner, F. W.: Biomechanics of the distal radioulnar joint. Clin. Orthop., *187*:26, 1984.

Persson, M.: Causal treatment of lunatomalacia. Further experiences of operative ulna lengthening. Acta Chir. Scand., *100*:531, 1950.

Reeves, B.: Excision of the ulnar styloid fragment after Colles' fracture. Int. Surg., *45*:46, 1966.

Rhoades, C. E., and Reckling, F. W.: Palmar dislocation of the trapezoid—case report. J. Hand Surg., *8*:85, 1983.

Rose-Innes, A. P.: Anterior dislocation of the ulna at the inferior radio-ulnar joint: case reports, with a discussion of the anatomy of rotation of the forearm. J. Bone Joint Surg., *42B*:515, 1960.

Ruby, L. K., Stinson, J., and Belsky, M. R.: The natural history of scaphoid nonunion. A review of 55 cases. J. Bone Joint Surg., *67A*:428, 1985.

Russe, O.: Fracture of the carpal navicular. J. Bone Joint. Surg., *42A*:759, 1960.

Sarrafian, S. K., Melamed, J. L., and Goshgarian, G. M.: Study of wrist motion in flexion and extension. Clin. Orthop., *126*:153, 1977.

Saunier, J., and Chamay, A.: Volar perilunar dislocation of the wrist. Clin. Orthop, *157*:139, 1981.

Sebald, J. R., Dobyns, J. H., and Linscheid, R. L.: The natural history of collapse deformities of the wrist. Clin. Orthop., *104*:140, 1974.

Smith, R. J., Atkinson, R. E., and Jupiter, J. B.: Silicone synovitis of the wrist. J. Hand Surg., *10A*:47, 1985.

Speed, J. S., and Knight, R. A.: Treatment of malunited Colles' fractures. J. Bone Joint Surg., *27*:361. 1945.

Sprague, H. H., Burandt, D., Dushuttle, R. P., and Koniuch, M. P.: The use of the Herbert screw in scaphoid injury. J. Hand Surg., *10A*:426, 1985.

Stahl, F.: On lunatomalacia (Kienböck's disease): clinical and roentgenological study, especially on its pathogenesis and late results of immobilization treatment. Acta Chir. Scand. Suppl., *126*:1, 1947.

Stein, A. H., Jr.: Dorsal dislocation of the lesser multangular bone. J. Bone Joint Surg., *53A*:337, 1971.

Stern, P. J: Transscaphoid-lunate dislocation: a report of two cases. J. Hand Surg., *9A*:370, 1984.

Swanson, A. B.: Silicone rubber implants for the replacement of the carpal scaphoid and lunate bones. Orthop. Clin. North Am., *1*:299, 1970.

Tajima, T.: An investigation of the treatment of Kienböck's disease (abstr.). J. Bone Joint Surg., *48A*:1649, 1966.

Taleisnik, J.: The ligaments of the wrist. J. Hand Surg., *1*:110. 1976.

Taleisnik, J.: Wrist: Anatomy, Function and Injury. AAOS Instructional Course Lectures, *27*:61, 1978.

Taleisnik, J.: Post-traumatic carpal instability. Clin. Orthop., *149*:73, 1980.

Taleisnik, J., Gelberman, R. H., Miller, B. W., and Szabo, R. M.: The extensor retinaculum of the wrist. J. Hand Surg., *9A*:494, 1984.

Taleisnik, J., and Kelly, P. J.: The extraosseous and intraosseous blood supply of the scaphoid bone. J. Bone Joint Surg., *48A*:1125, 1966.

Taleisnik, J., and Watson, H. K.: Midcarpal instability caused by malunited fractures of the distal radius. J. Hand Surg., *9A*:350, 1984.

Testut, J. L., and Laterjet, A.: Traite d'Anatomie Humaine. Vol. 1, 8th Ed. Paris, Doin, 1928.

Thompson, T. C., Campbell, R. D., Jr., and Arnold, W. D.: Primary and secondary dislocation of the scaphoid bone. J. Bone Joint Surg., *46B*:73, 1964.

Tillberg, B.: Kienböck's disease treated with osteotomy to lengthen ulna. Acta Orthop. Scand., *39*:359, 1968.

Vance, R. M., Gelberman, R. H., and Evans, E. F.: Scaphocapitate fractures: patterns of dislocation, mechanisms of injury, and preliminary results of treatment. J. Bone Joint Surg., *62A*:271, 1980.

Verdan, C., and Narakas, A.: Fractures and pseudarthrosis of the scaphoid. Surg. Clin. North Am., *48*:1083, 1968.

Watson, H. K.: Limited wrist arthrodesis. Clin. Orthop., *149*:126, 1980.

Watson, H. K., and Ballet, F. L.: The SLAC wrist: scapholunate advanced collapse pattern of degenerative arthritis. J. Hand Surg., *9A*:358, 1984.

Watson, H. K., and Hempton, R. F.: Limited wrist arthrodesis. I. The triscaphoid joint. J. Hand Surg., *5*:320, 1980.

Watson, H. K., Goodman, M. L., and Johnson, T. R.: Limited wrist arthrodesis. II. Intercarpal and radiocarpal combinations. J. Hand Surg., *6*:223, 1981.

Watson, H. K., Ryu, J., and DeBella, A.: An approach to Kienböck's disease: triscaphe arthrodesis. J. Hand Surg., *10A*:179, 1985.

Weber, E. R.: Biomechanical implications of scaphoid waist fractures. Clin. Orthop., *149*:83, 1980.

Weber, E. R., and Chao, E. Y.: An experimental approach to the mechanism of scaphoid waist fractures. J. Hand Surg., *3*:142, 1978.

Weigl, K., and Spira, E.: The triangular fibrocartilage of the wrist joint. Reconstr. Surg. Traumatol., *11*:139, 1969.

Werner, F. W., Palmer, A. K., and Glisson, R. R.: Forearm load transmission: the effect of ulnar lengthening and shortening. Transactions of the 28th Annual Meeting of the Orthopaedic Research Society. New Orleans, January, 1982, p. 273.

Weseley, M. S., and Barenfeld, P. A.: Trans-scaphoid, transcapitate, transtriquetral, perilunate fracture-dislocation of the wrist: a case report. J. Bone Joint Surg., *54A*:1073, 1972.

Wright, R. D.: A detailed study of movement of the wrist joint. J. Anat., *70*:137, 1936.

Youm, Y., and Flatt, A. E.: Kinematics of the wrist. Clin. Orthop., *149*:21, 1980.

Youm, Y., McMurtry, R. Y., Flatt, A. E., and Gillespie, T. E.: Kinematics of the wrist. I. An experimental study of radial-ulnar deviation and flexion-extension. *60A*:423, 1978.

Management of Stiff Metacarpophalangeal and Interphalangeal Joints

Stiffness is the restricted ability to range a joint freely through its normal excursion, either actively or passively. It may be due to internal obstruction of the joint itself or to extrinsic factors such as tendon adhesions, scar contracture, or simple edema. Colloquially, the term "stiffness" may be used by patients to describe true range limitation or the painful motion of arthritis. Stiffness due to burn scar, congenital anomalies, or the pain or architectural disruption of rheumatic disorders is discussed elsewhere in this book. Otherwise, surgeons deal primarily with the residua of trauma: mechanical, chemical, thermal, or biologic (sepsis).

ANATOMY AND PATHOPHYSIOLOGY

Metacarpophalangeal and interphalangeal joints are not pin or strap hinges, but are complex variations on ball and socket arrangements whose motion depends on the gliding surfaces of cartilage lubricated by synovial fluid. They are constrained by liga-ments and motored by musculotendinous units. Cartilage is nonvascularized mesothelial tissue and therefore depends on diffusion from synovial fluid for nutrition. The metabolism of articular cartilage is very sluggish, so that ranging an otherwise normal joint through a full excursion twice a day is sufficient to preserve cartilage health. Lubricating synovial fluid is produced from the single cell surface of the synovial lining of the joint capsule primarily as a dialysate of plasma with added hyaluronic acid. The lubricant forms a layer just a few molecules thick, and its lubricity involves a complex mechanism of intermolecular slippage. Eighty per cent of the energy involved in moving a joint is used to overcome the inertia and friction that resists the initiation of motion. As the fluid is non-newtonian it becomes less viscous (more slippery) with increasing temperature and when subjected to the shear forces of motion. In stationary or slowly moving joints the more viscous fluid can support higher loads. With higher rates of shear (and consequent increase in temperature), the viscosity decreases with the square of the speed, thus rapidly lessening the drag on the moving cartilage surfaces. Therefore, credence is given to the concept of "warming up" before activity or the sense of stiffness one feels in a cold environment. Finally, the nonconcentric shapes of the male and female joint surfaces produce a wedge-shaped fluid interface that is more conducive to slip or glide than a uniform film on parallel surfaces might be according to current theories of lubrication (Figs. 105–1, 105–2) (Barnett, Davis, and MacConaill, 1961).

The constraining ligaments are complex thickenings within and adjacent to the joint capsule wall consisting of linearly arranged

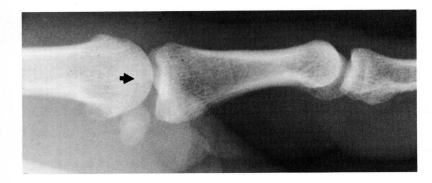

Figure 105–1. Radiograph of MP joint showing nonparallel joint surfaces *(arrow)*. (Wedge lubrication.)

collagen fibers. The anatomic configuration of the ligaments are unique to each joint and are structured to control its particular excursion. Ligaments are inelastic, but pleat and unfold as the position of their bony attachments alters with various anatomic postures. The rest of the joint capsule is structured of semirandomly oriented connective tissue that allows excursion partially by the internal stretch permitted by its irregularly oriented fibers, but mostly by accordion pleating or buckling of the full thickness of the capsule when compressed (Fig. 105–3).

Metacarpophalangeal and proximal interphalangeal joints have several anatomic similarities as well as some important architectural differences (Fig. 105–4). Both have eccentrically mounted collateral ligaments. The face of the proximal half of each joint flares or widens from dorsal to volar to provide a camlike action. The proximal interphalangeal joint ranges only in one plane, flexion and extension. It is stable laterally, being constrained both by its ligamentous arrangement and by its trochlear shape (Fig. 105–4*B*). The metacarpophalangeal joint is curved in two planes forming an abbreviated ball and socket to permit abduction, adduc-

tion, and some rotation as well as flexion and extension (Fig. 105–4*A*). Architectural differences between the volar plates of each have significant clinical implications (Bowers and associates, 1980). The metacarpophalangeal volar plate is composed of crisscrossing fibers that collapse like an accordion on flexion. The plate on the proximal interphalangeal joint is a thick rigid cartilage that permits little compression.

ETIOLOGY OF STIFFNESS

Immobility

As cartilage nutrition depends on the mechanical spread of synovial fluid, prolonged immobilization results in stiffness (Field and Heuston, 1970a, b). Even small degrees of motion can minimize stiffness and disuse osteoporosis, so that when in a cast a patient should be encouraged to range his joints within the constraints of the splint. The length of time that a joint can tolerate immobility diminishes with age. Salter (Salter and associates, 1980; Salter, 1983) has shown that in animals, continuous passive motion

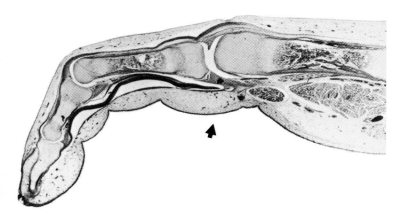

Figure 105–2. Cross section of digit, showing nonparallel joint surfaces *(arrow)*. (From Landsmeer, J. M. F.: Atlas of Anatomy of the Hand. Edinburgh, Churchill Livingstone, 1976, p. 246.)

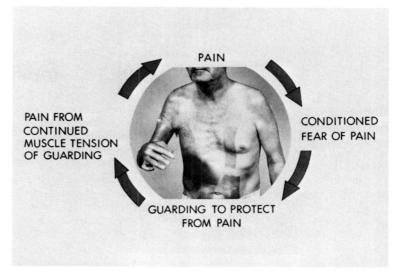

Figure 105–13. Healed burn patient in whom anxiety and conditioned fear of pain subconsciously support his otherwise mobile shoulder and elbow against gravity by active muscle guarding. Continuous active muscle action causes muscle fatigue and pain, producing a vicious cycle.

tients are very mechanistic and distrustful of any suggestion that their problems are psychologic, requiring all the tact and persuasive skills of a surgeon or therapist before they can even accept a referral.

TREATMENT

Anatomic Restoration

The first order of defense against stiffness is prevention. Early aggressive treatment of an injury should be directed toward minimization of further trauma and restoration of functional anatomy. Functional anatomy does not necessarily imply restoration of preinjury normalcy. Sometimes the treatment required for anatomic accuracy produces so much additional trauma and scar that the resultant function is less than if the injury was left untreated. Mild nonrotational displacements of metacarpal fractures and boxer's fracture of the fifth metacarpal head with less than 30 degrees of angulation are examples of bony injuries often best left displaced if surgery is required for reduction. Mild mallet deformities can also be made worse by aggressive operative intervention. Even the occasional displaced intra-articular fracture can function quite well without anatomic restoration (Fig. 105–14). A patient who presents several days after a displaced fracture into a digital joint and appears to have maintained a reasonable, pain-free range of motion can be immeasurably harmed

by a slavish need to restore everything to its preinjury anatomy. This is not to suggest that anatomic accuracy should not usually be restored following most injuries, but each situation must be individualized in light of the risks and benefits of the treatment recommended.

Mobilization versus Immobilization

Rest of the part, immobilization, is the first priority of treatment for acute inflammation. As the inflammation subsides, motion must be restored to prevent scar maturing into a dense restrictive mass. The posture of the digital chain plays a role in the ultimate outcome. As described above, edema and pain tend to posture the hand in the intrinsic minus position, and fixation in this posture is very difficult to correct. Occasionally, preventing disruption of fresh fractures, tendon, or nerve or other soft tissue repairs requires immobilization in specific postures that may be less than ideal for preservation of joint mobility. In order to best prevent joint stiffness, the metacarpophalangeal (MP) joint should be flexed and the proximal interphalangeal (PIP) fully extended (the intrinsic plus or positive position) (Fig. 105–15). The anatomic peculiarities of the volar plates and the forces available via muscle power determine that MP joints stiff in flexion are relatively easily mobilized, as are PIP joints that are stiff in extension. Conversely, MP exten-

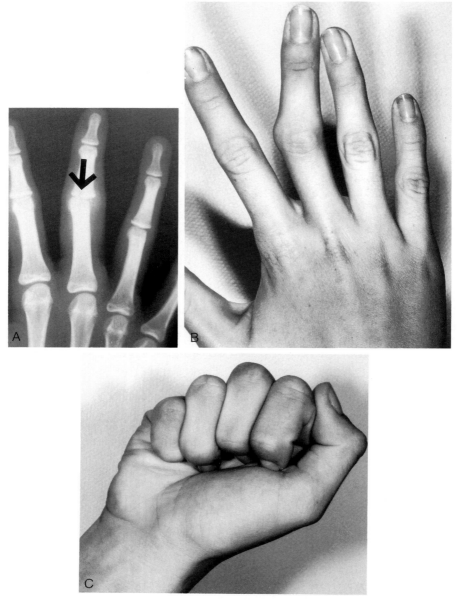

Figure 105–14. *A* to *C,* Radiograph and range of motion in PIP joint with neglected untreated condylar crush *(arrow).*

sion contractures and PIP flexion contractures are extremely difficult to overcome. Extension contractures of the little finger MP joint are exceptionally hard to correct because the flexibility of the intermetacarpal ligament inefficiently transfers some of the power of the long flexors to the metacarpal.

Perhaps nothing generates more controversy and depends more on individual intuition and experience than deciding when and how much to mobilize an injured part. Although general rules for each fracture, nerve, muscle, and tendon repair exist, there appears to be a substantial disparity among surgeons about the exact timing of progression from immobilization to full unrestricted activity. Often the particular injury and individual patient determine the specific procedures. In general, passive, apprehensive patients need to be pushed, while overaggressive, seemingly painfree patients require restraint. As demonstrated by Salter (Salter and associates, 1980; Salter, 1983) cartilage healing requires continuous motion, but how

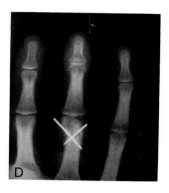

Figure 105–14 *Continued D to F,* Radiograph and range of motion after wedge osteotomy.

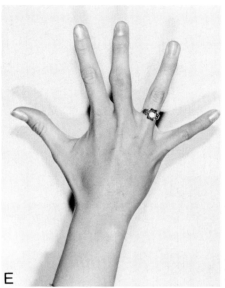

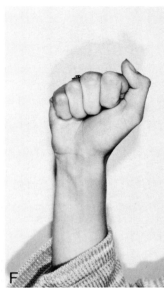

can this be done at the same time that a fracture, tendon, or nerve repair is being protected from disruption? How does one provide Kleinert-like flexor tendon motion in a complex injury that includes fragmented bone and an associated extensor tendon repair? Tendon gliding and joint flexibility are of no value without skeletal stability and a strong tendon anastomosis. Once the disrupted structures are solid, however, motion can often be recovered. Therefore, immobilization for stability and integrity must take priority over the initiation of motion. Fortunately, in normal repair, motion can often be recovered after healing is solid.

Hand Therapy (Fitzgerald, 1977; Hunter and associates, 1978)

Young, Wray, and Weeks (1978) pointed out the value of therapy in correcting stiffness. In their large series of 2,781 stiff joints in 749 patients, only 135 required surgery. Formal treatment by competent hand therapists has grown in popularity in the last decade. Sterling Bunnell was strongly opposed to what he called "fizzle" therapy, but in his time most therapy was of the bone-crushing, forceful, "shake loose the rusty hinge" school that often did more harm than good. Today, however, following the convincing developments of Paul Brand in Velore, India, whose work was introduced to the United States by Erle Peacock, the subspecialty of hand therapy has arisen among the ranks of occupational and physical therapists. Highly competent therapists with sophisticated understanding of hand function, wound healing, and splint construction, coupled with strong motivational skills, are available in most communities.

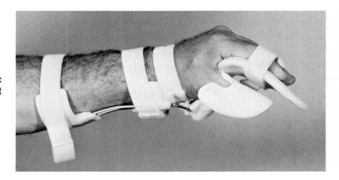

Figure 105–15. Appropriate splinting in intrinsic plus position to minimize risk of stiffness. Wrist dorsiflexed, MP's flexed, and IP's extended.

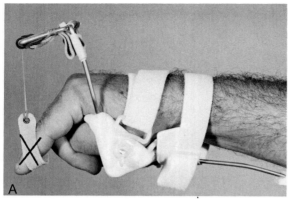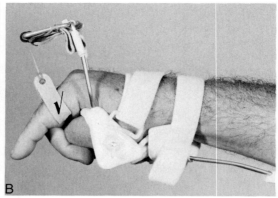

Figure 105–16. Dynamic splinting. *A,* Improper application of dynamic tension, creating too long a lever arm that magnifies the force excessively. *B,* Proper physiologic location to apply dynamic force.

Irene Hollis, who pioneered hand therapy in the U.S., divided patients as follows:

Smart Hands	Smart Head
Smart Hands	Dumb Head
Dumb Hands	Smart Head
Dumb Hands	Dumb Head

Intellectual and motivational skills are independent of physical or motor skills in varying degrees in any given person. Those with "smart heads and smart hands" probably do well no matter what the physician may do, while those with "dumb hands and dumb heads" seem hopeless. It would appear that those in the central two categories require and respond best to formal therapy. Even the smartest people require teachers and the most skilled athletes do better with coaches. Learning or relearning motor skills is time consuming, requiring several hours a day of instruction, supervision, and exercise. The thrice weekly "50 minute hour," half of which is spent in the whirlpool, is usually inadequate to help patients with significant problems. Some surgeons feel that the doctor should manage and control the patient doing his own rehabilitation, but this is wasteful of both time and skills, and in practice no surgeon has this much time to spare.

Attempts at mobilization of a stiff joint should begin with active and passive ranging as tolerated by the patient. If this fails, spring or elastic powered dynamic splinting by an appropriate custom-made or commercially available device should be tried (Fig. 105–16) (Colditz, 1983). Dynamic splinting has the advantage of permitting range augmented by the power of the spring. At rest the spring continues to apply force to the scar. Mechanically this represents a "creep" event (Fig. 105–17A). If this is not successful, serial plasters are the next order of treatment. Over a light coating of Vaseline or two thicknesses of Tube Gauze, several layers of 2 inch plaster strips are carefully applied while the joint is held at its extreme range. These are changed daily, and if this therapy is successful a little range will be gained at each application. The patient can often be taught to apply the strips himself (Fig. 105–18). In contrast to the "creep" of dynamic splinting, this represents a different mechanical event called "stress relaxation" (Fig. 105–17B). Serial plasters are more cumbersome, do not permit exercise, and in some resistant cases merely change the angle at which the joint is held and do not increase overall range. One compromise is to use dropout casts where practical.* Experience and laboratory data on the effects of "creep" and "stress relaxation" on scar document that serial casts have a greater stretching effect on cicatrix than do springs or rubber bands. In applying either splint or cast, the force point should be close to the joint, for the reasons explained later (see Fig. 105–16). As a general guide, one can be reasonably optimistic of success if the resisting scar feels rubbery when the joint is manipulated. If the resistance is firm and rigid, it will probably respond only to serial plasters or surgery.

---

*Another well-advertised and popular "stress relaxation" device is the Joint Jack. While this device permits the patient to remove it for hygienic reasons, it requires a much more compliant patient than does a serial plaster and is more cumbersome.

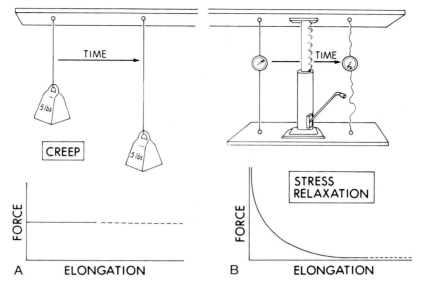

Figure 105–17. Diagrammatic representation showing typical curves of creep *(A)* and stress relaxation *(B)*.

CREEP

STRESS RELAXATION

FORCE

FORCE

A ELONGATION

B ELONGATION

Surgical Release (Curtis, 1970, 1978; Nicholson, 1979)

Surgery should be considered only as a last resort for those patients whose anatomic disruption or scar rigidity resists all nonsurgical effort. The degree of residual range restriction must be significant and the benefits anticipated worth the risk that the surgery may possibly increase the stiffness. Unless all circumstances are favorable, these procedures often fail to improve the range significantly. As a rule of thumb, if the joint has 60 degrees of range or more and other joints in the chain are normal, the hand is usually quite functional for most activities, and the risk of making the situation worse does not justify the possible gains. Several criteria must be present to justify surgical intervention: (1) a correctable anatomic defect; (2) viable, functional cartilage; (3) reasonably healthy soft tissues; (4) strong, functional motors; (5) adequate patient motivation; (6) reasonable sensation; and (7) stable skeleton.

Each of these factors can be variably weighted in importance depending on individual circumstances; if more than one is present, they are additive. Thus, for example, any attempt to mobilize an atrophic, insensate, heavily scarred digit is doomed to failure. However, on occasion, a highly motivated patient can surprisingly overcome significant anatomic hindrances. Rarely, one encounters a patient who works so hard in the therapeutic setting that he overcomes very resistant scar and recovers significant motion; when such a patient is seen several months after returning to a normal life style, these gains have disappeared. It would seem that such people are akin to "super athletes" who can accomplish prodigious physical feats in a controlled environment that are impossible to maintain in every day life. A clue to this situation is the need for the patient to work hard every morning to maintain the previous day's gains (Fig. 105–19).

The surgical plan must also consider and deal with associated adherent tendons, scar

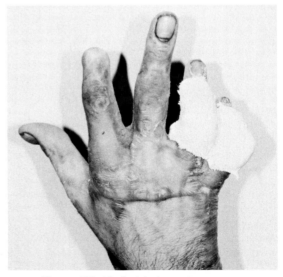

Figure 105–18. Serial plaster finger casts.

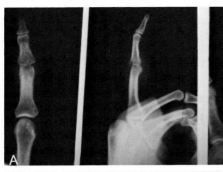
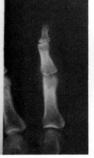
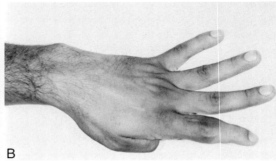
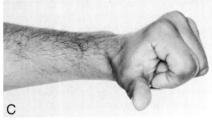

Figure 105–19. *A,* Destroyed index PIP joint from sepsis. *B,C,* Range of motion after capsular release and major therapeutic effort. Six months after discharge the range was minimal owing to the patient's inability to maintain the excessive effort required to preserve the range.

contractures, Dupuytren's contracture, or arthritis. Surgically one must release all restrictive scar including tight collateral ligaments, volar and dorsal capsules, tendon adhesions, and skin and fascial contractures.

Sometimes judicious manual manipulation can break up less resistant scar or the last few restrictive bands following surgical lysis. The force must be placed adjacent to the joint, as in Figure 105–20. Application of pressure at a distance from the joint tends to hinge open the joint space rather than gliding the distal cartilage face evenly over the proximal head in a physiologic manner. In addition, the longer lever arm magnifies the applied forces dramatically, which can be very damaging to soft tissues and may even fracture osteoporotic bone.

Both metacarpophalangeal and proximal interphalangeal joints are best approached through a longitudinal dorsal incision, especially when the entire joint capsule is involved and the scar releases required are almost circumferential around the joint. The volar capsule of the metacarpophalangeal joints can be reached by reflecting skin, soft tissue, and collateral ligaments. The volar capsule release should be done proximally, even into the proximal periosteum, in order to preserve a layer of tissue between the joint cartilage and the tendon when sliding forward with extension (Fig. 105–21).

If the flexor tendon also requires release, a midlateral or volar "Bruner" zigzag approach may be appropriate (Weeks, Young, and

Wray, 1980). A thorough understanding of the anatomy of the part and details of the injury permits individualization of the procedure. In general, the collateral ligaments, the volar or dorsal capsule, and any restricting scar should be sectioned. Tendon adhesions require lysis, and contractured skin scars may require Z-plasties, free grafts, or (very

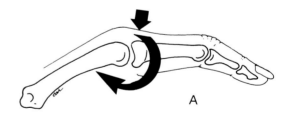
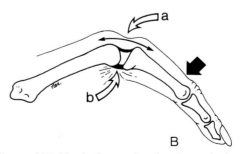

Figure 105–20. *A,* Proper location to apply force to manipulate a stiff joint. *B,* Improper application of force, causing hinging at volar adhesion *(b)* with distraction of dorsal joint. If the tissues are soft and supple, negative pressure in the joint produces a visible depression over the dorsum *(a).*

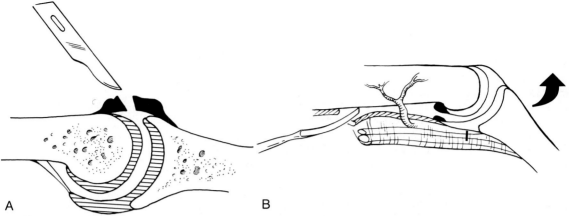

Figure 105–21. Diagrammatic representation of dorsal capsule release *(A)* and volar contracture release *(B)*.

rarely) pedicles. (Contrary to classical teaching, free skin grafts can be placed directly on tendons under certain circumstances without restricting motion.)

Any release must result in a free, easy joint ranging both actively and passively. If the joint still has a rubbery, resistant feel when manipulated, release is inadequate and it usually stiffens again very quickly.

Each joint has peculiarities specific to its unique anatomy and function.

Metacarpophalangeal Joints. The cam-like configuration of the MP joint permits lateral and some rotational motion in extension. In flexion the collateral ligaments tighten to stabilize any lateral or rotational motion. Individually each digit flexes to point directly at the navicular bone. When all the fingers flex together, they spread slightly to accommodate each other, and final locking is accomplished by the resultant tight fit. Because of this anatomic arrangement and the relative weakness of the volar plate, MP joints are seldom stiff in flexion. When they *are* stiff in extension, severance of the collateral ligaments from their proximal attachment is required, along with release of the dorsal capsule and any attendant restricting tendon or skin. *Caution:* Never section the collateral ligaments if the intrinsic muscles are paralyzed from an ulnar nerve palsy, or an unstable joint will result (Buch, 1974).

Proximal Interphalangeal Joints. In contrast to the MP joint, the PIP joints are more often stiff in flexion. Restricted extension is usually caused by the check rein effect of tight fibers originating on the proximal edge of the volar plate and diverging to attach to the "assembly line" ridge on the phalanx. In this circumstance the joint is first ap-

proached volarly through a zigzag incision in the skin, and then by reflecting a flap of flexor sheath to approach the offending tissues intrathecally (Figs. 105–21*B*, 105–22). The nutrient vessels to the vincular system pass beneath these check reins and must be preserved when the tight bands are sectioned (Fig. 105–22). If this does not provide sufficient release, the collateral ligaments should be severed. On occasion the lower fibers of the accessory collateral ligaments may require release.

Distal Interphalangeal Joints. Stiff DIP joints can rarely be improved surgically. Fortunately, very few tasks necessitate motion

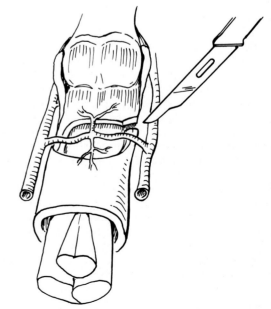

Figure 105–22. Check ligament release showing preservation of vincular circulation.

in this joint. Stability in a semiflexed position by arthrodesis, tenodesis, or simple pinning should constitute the only surgical intervention for this joint, in all but the most unusual circumstances.

It should be reiterated that stiffness restricted to the pericapsular structures is rare and can usually be managed by nonoperative means. Most circumstances that require surgical intervention are complex and demand release of many other adherent structures. Release should be extended until all restricting structures are freely mobile.

Postoperatively, the hand should be immobilized in the intrinsic plus posture and splinted (see Fig. 105–15). Very rarely, pins may be required if splinting is inadequate or the joint is unstable. Pins should be used very sparingly.

Finally, any surgical gains must be complemented by early active therapy until the scar is mature and the gains are secure. Therapy should begin as soon as the patient can tolerate the discomfort, even on the day of surgery. Treatment must be gradual, since excess pain leads to guarding and involuntary splinting, with recurrence of the rigid scar. The homily of "no pain, no gain" must be tempered by reason; too little force causes the scar again to restrict motion, while too much produces excess trauma and a similar result. How much force is correct? Experience suggests that the maximal amount of effort that a well-motivated patient who handles pain well can exert with his own musculature seems to produce the correct "window of force." This directs the healing tissues to produce optimally supple and flexible scar, which results in maximal excursion. This concept blends the effects of motivation with the final physical characteristics of the scar.

When all treatment fails, arthrodesis, or (in certain select patients) amputation, represents the final salvage. The choice of this final solution depends on determining which circumstance is best for the individual patient, both psychologically and functionally. As a general rule, a laborer or mechanic is much more functional with disarticulation through a stiff left ring proximal interphalangeal joint, while a young woman may be willing to accept much more disability to preserve this symbolic digit. Usually the patient's own wishes determine the final treatment. Currently available prosthetic joints almost never work for very long in posttraumatically stiff proximal interphalangeal joints, and are rarely indicated in metacarpophalangeal joints.

REFERENCES

Barnett, C. H., Davis, D. V., and MacConaill, M. A.: Synovial Joints—Their Structure and Mechanics. London, Longmans, Green & Company, 1961.

Bowers, W. H., Wolf, J. W., Nehil, J. L., and Bittinger, S.: The proximal interphalangeal joint volar plate. I. An anatomical and biomechanical study. J. Hand Surg., 5:79, 1980.

Brody, G. S., Peng, T. J., and Landel, R. F.: The etiology of hypertrophic scar contracture: another view. Plast. Reconstr. Surg., 67:673, 1981a.

Brody, G. S., Peng, T. J., and Landel, R. F.: The rheologic properties of human skin and scar tissue. In Marks, R. P. (Ed.): Bioengineering and The Skin. Boston, MTP Press, 1981b, pp. 141–158.

Buch, V. I.: Clinical and functional assessment of the hand after metacarpophalangeal capsulotomy. Plast. Reconstr. Surg., 53:452, 1974.

Colditz, J. C.: Low profile dynamic splinting of the injured hand. Am. J. Occup. Ther., 37:182, 1983.

Curtis, R. M.: Surgical restoration of motion in the stiff interphalangeal joints of the hand. Bull. Hosp. Joint Dis., 31:1, 1970.

Curtis, R. M.: Management of the stiff hand. In Hunter, J. M., Schneider, L. H., Mackin, E. J., and Bell, J. A. (Eds.): Rehabilitation of the Hand. St. Louis, C. V. Mosby Company, 1978, pp. 138–146.

Field, P. L., and Heuston, J. T.: Articular cartilage loss in long-standing immobilization of interphalangeal joints. Br. J. Plast. Surg., 23:186, 1970a.

Field, P. L., and Heuston, J. T.: Articular cartilage loss in long-standing flexion deformity of the proximal interphalangeal joints. Aust. N. Z. J. Surg., 40:70, 1970b.

Fitzgerald, J. A.: Management of the injured and postoperative hand. Physiotherapy, 63:282, 1977.

Hunter, J. M., Schneider, L. H., Mackin, E. J., and Bell, J. A.: Rehabilitation of The Hand. St. Louis, C. V. Mosby Company, 1978.

Kempin, L. S.: Psychological motivation in successful hand therapy. In Hunter, J. M., Schneider, L. H., Mackin, E. J., and Bell, J. A. (Eds.): Rehabilitation of The Hand. St. Louis, C. V. Mosby Company, 1978, pp. 662–664.

Nicholson, B. G.: Capsulectomy of the metacarpophalangeal and proximal interphalangeal joints. J. Hand Surg., 4:482, 1979.

Peacock, E. E.: Some biomechanical and biophysical aspects of joint stiffness. Ann. Surg., 164:1, 1966.

Peacock, E. E.: Wound Repair. 3rd Ed. Philadelphia, W. B. Saunders Company, 1984, pp. 263–266.

Salter, R. B.: Motion versus rest: why immobilize joints? Abbott Proceedings, 14:1, 1983.

Salter, R. B., Simmonds, D. F., Malcolm, B. W., Rumble, E. J., MacMichael, D., and Clements, N. D.: The biological effect of continuous passive motion on the healing of full thickness defects in articular cartilage. J. Bone Joint Surg., 62A:1232, 1980.

Young, V. L., Wray, R. C., and Weeks, P. M.: The surgical management of stiff joints in the hand. Plast. Reconstr. Surg., 62:835, 1978.

Weeks, P. M., Young, V. L., and Wray, R. C.: Operative mobilization of stiff metacarpophalangeal joints. Ann. Plast. Surg., 5:178, 1980.

Andrew J. Weiland

Small Joint Arthrodesis and Bony Defect Reconstruction

Arthrodesis is a well-established procedure, useful when joint function is decreased secondary to pain, deformity, instability, or loss of motor control. Many techniques to attain fusion of the wrist and small joints of the hand have been described, the goal of each being, to paraphrase Moberg, "to achieve a solid, painless arthrodesis in proper position in a reasonable time."

SMALL JOINT ARTHRODESIS

Indications

Metacarpophalangeal, Proximal Interphalangeal, and Distal Interphalangeal. Arthrodesis in the finger is generally reserved for the proximal and distal interphalangeal joints. It is particularly useful when the joint will be subjected to heavy stress or loading in a young individual. The metacarpophalangeal joint is not commonly fused, arthroplasty being the preferred method of treatment when destruction or degenerative changes are present.

Specific indications for arthrodesis of these joints are joint destruction secondary to rheumatoid disease or trauma, paralytic deformities, burn contractures, lesions of the flexor or extensor tendons (i.e., boutonnière, mallet deformities), osteoarthritis, and joint infections.

Metacarpophalangeal Joint of Thumb. Conditions mentioned above may similarly be indications for fusion of the metacarpophalangeal joint of the thumb. Arthrodesis is also useful in ulnar nerve paralysis when metacarpophalangeal joint hyperextension leads to decreased thumb function (Hill, 1969). Flexion deformities of the metacarpophalangeal joint with compensatory hyperextension of the interphalangeal joint are also successfully treated by fusion.

Carpometacarpal Joint of Thumb. The most common condition leading to arthrodesis of the trapeziometacarpal joint of the thumb is osteoarthritis. Post-traumatic conditions and rheumatoid arthritis may also produce painful motion that may be alleviated by fusion of this joint. Considerable controversy exists between advocates of fusion for these

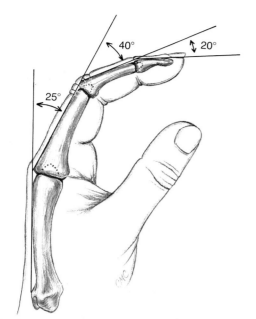

Figure 106–1. Recommended position for arthrodesis of the finger joints.

conditions and those proposing various arthroplasty techniques. Fusion is useful when preservation of thumb power is especially important (i.e., for heavy laborers) and when attenuated carpometacarpal capsular restraints are present. Possible contraindications to arthrodesis are a pre-operatively stiff or severely arthritic metacarpophalangeal joint and the presence of associated scaphotrapezial arthritis. These considerations are especially important since studies have shown (Leach and Bolton, 1968; Carroll and Hill, 1973) a compensatory increase in metacarpophalangeal and intercarpal motion with metacarpotrapezial arthrodesis. If these anatomic areas are compromised, less than optimal results may be obtained by the trapeziometacarpal fusion.

General Considerations

Many different techniques for achieving arthrodesis of the finger joints are described in the literature; the preference of the surgeon determines which procedure is used. A 90 to 100 per cent successful fusion rate is common with most techniques applicable to the various small joints of the hand. Several commonly employed and time-proven techniques are described in this chapter.

Regardless of which arthrodesis technique is used, the position of fusion should be as close as possible to the position of function. Particular requirements for individual patients may take precedence, but in general the angles recommended for various joints are those illustrated in Figures 106–1 and 106–2.

At the metacarpophalangeal joint, flexion increases slightly from the index to the small finger. The index metacarpophalangeal joint is fused in 25 degrees of flexion, with a 5 degree progressive increase per digit as one moves ulnarly. This is done because the radial digits are more important for pinch while the ulnar digits participate more in power grasp. A similar increase in flexion position is suggested for the proximal interphalangeal joint, with the index proximal interphalangeal placed at 40 degrees and advancing 5 degrees per digit from a radial to ulnar direction. The distal interphalangeal joints are usually positioned in 5 to 20 degrees of flexion. Fusion of this joint can be difficult, however, owing to the relatively small size of the opposing surfaces.

Since the thumb participates in all hand

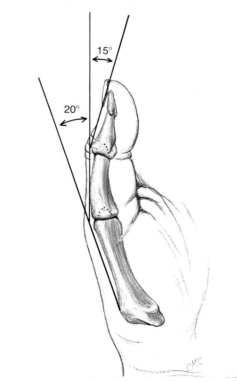

Figure 106–2. Recommended position for arthrodesis of the thumb interphalangeal and metacarpophalangeal joints.

lists are easily constructed from this type of material.

Patient problem lists are important at this phase of the rehabilitative process. Successful reconstruction demands that the patient and surgeon become equal partners in the patient's care. The surgeon can provide potential function. Only the patient can make the new hand perform properly. Postoperative therapy is often prolonged and uncomfortable. The patient's motivation must be high to complete the tasks. As a consequence, the patient should be encouraged to select reconstructions that will make a significant difference in his or her life.

ANALYSIS OF KINESIOLOGIC PROBLEMS

Although some functional abnormalities are simple to analyze, others are subtle and complex. An unstable or painful distal interphalangeal (DIP) joint is an obvious nuisance. However, if a woman with multiple fixed upper extremity deformities secondary to rheumatoid arthritis complains that she cannot comb her hair, the significant architectural problem could be at many levels. Can she hold the brush handle firmly? Can she pronate and supinate her wrist without discomfort? Are her shoulder joints adequate to allow the brush to touch the back of the head? If combing hair is the primary functional goal, accurate mechanical and physiologic assessment is essential.

The inability to perform manual tasks is the result of one or a combination of three factors: pain, power and position. Certain tasks require that the elements of the hand be properly *positioned* for function. For example, buttoning small buttons is impossible unless the fingernail or tip of the index or long finger can be brought accurately to the tip of the thumb. Holding a soft drink bottle requires that the volar surfaces of the fingers match the curve of the container and that the thumb be abducted adequately. If patients have *pain* during manipulations, they are asked to repeat the task until localization is accurate. Although pain and power problems are frequently related, careful questioning usually separates the two elements. If pain and weakness coexist, patients are asked to judge which element is more important. Finally, if *power* loss is a primary problem, the

precise reason for the weakness must be determined. Power losses result from ruptured tendons, weakness of motor units, joint stiffness, or joint instability. Unless the surgeon understands the reasons for power loss, function cannot be restored.

Each of the functional diary items must be analyzed. Frequently the patients must be observed doing specific tasks in order to define the abnormalities accurately. During this functional analysis, range of motion for each upper extremity joint is also measured and recorded. Power is measured objectively using pinch meters and power grip meters. Finally, if clumsiness and slowness are major complaints, timed functional testing may even be performed (Johnson, 1959; Perry, 1978a, 1978b).

At this point, excellent radiographs, an accurate physical examination, and the therapist's analysis of complaints usually reveal the anatomic and physiologic causes of the functional problems.

PATIENT EDUCATION

Once the functional problems have been defined and analyzed, patients must learn about the advantages and disadvantages of potential solutions. Starting with simple solutions first, patients are familiarized with assistive devices available to help with individual tasks. As an example, if a patient's primary problem involves opening jars, and a painful wrist is the disruptive factor, the patient is given a jar opener. If the assistive device corrects the functional abnormality, the goal is accomplished. On the other hand, if wrist pain is a major factor in other manipulative problems that cannot be assisted with external devices, or if the assistive device is inadequate, the patient is instructed about the various surgical procedures, from arthroplasty to arthrodesis, that would relieve the discomfort. If possible, the patient is allowed to try positional changes or stabilization procedures prior to surgery. For the wrist arthrodesis, for example, a well-fitting splint holding the radiocarpal joint in the desired position is provided and the patient does daily tasks. If the splint alone solves the problem, so much the better.

For excellent results, patients must be willing to become equal partners with the surgeon in their own care. The educational phase of the rehabilitative program allows patients to make decisions for reconstruction on the basis of information rather than hope. Frequently, introducing patients to others who have had the proposed reconstruction also helps. Discussing the proposed operation and its outcome with others who have had a personal experience provides needed psychologic support. Hand therapists are valuable to both patient and surgeon during the educational phase of the author's program.

CORRECTING ABNORMALITIES

Patients with systemic arthritis always have a multitude of abnormalities and complaints (Brewerton, 1957; Short, Bauer, and Reynolds, 1957). A plan for reconstructing the upper extremity must include lower extremity considerations as well. In general, hip and knee problems should be corrected prior to upper extremity reconstructions. During the process of hip and knee reconstructions, patients are required to support their body weight at least in part with their upper extremities. Complex upper extremity reconstructions deteriorate quickly if patients use reconstructed hands, wrists, or elbows to bear weight. Foot surgery done without postoperative crutch walking can be performed in conjunction with hand reconstruction.

If the hand surgeon is not prepared to reconstruct the lower extremity or even to evaluate lower extremity problems, a cooperative relationship with an orthopedist must be developed. Although managing patients by committee is an unsatisfactory endeavor, cooperation among specialists is important. The overall plan should include careful consideration of lower extremity difficulties.

Once the lower extremity problems are under good management, the upper extremity reconstructions must be carefully ordered. In general, hand reconstruction should begin proximally and proceed distally.

The shoulder joint provides a delivery mechanism for the hand. Although abduction and forward flexion of the shoulder are important, external rotation is equally valuable. Adding external rotation to a shoulder that can be abducted only to 90 degrees allows the patient to touch the back of the head (Codman, 1934).

The elbow is equally important in bringing the hand to useful position. In general, elbows must be stable and pain free to provide adequate function. The elbow must flex and extend sufficiently to bring the hand to the mouth and to the perineum. Although pronation must be adequate to place the palm on a flat surface, limited pronation can be aided by shoulder abduction. Unfortunately, a supinated position cannot be achieved with shoulder movement, and rotation at the elbow must be maintained.

Stability and lack of pain are more important to successful wrist function than full flexion and extension. As long as the wrist is pain free and axially aligned and has approximately 30 degrees of extension and 30 degrees of flexion, most tasks can be accomplished with ease (Palmer and associates, 1986). Even a fully immobilized wrist in the proper position provides an excellent platform for finger and thumb function (Nalebuff, 1983). Most activities are performed with the radiocarpal joint in a neutral position. Even power grip can be adequate and strong with the radiocarpal joint in neutral position. Perineal care, however, requires some wrist flexion in most individuals.

Finally, finger and thumb correction should be designed specifically to provide the functional requests of the patient. Reconstruction can never provide an extremity adaptable to all manipulative tasks. Joint reconstructions should be designed to provide the specific functions the patient requires (Ansell, 1969).

MAINTAINING RECONSTRUCTIONS

In cases of traumatic injury, the event that produced the pathology is a one-time occurrence. Maintaining a post-traumatic reconstruction means being concerned with potential complications of artificial parts or with wear and tear on joints given abnormal loading. In contrast, in patients with ongoing systemic arthritis, reconstruction maintenance after surgery requires concern not only about the individual surgical procedures and potential complications, but also about the progression of the disease process. Because each joint in the upper extremity is linked functionally, abnormalities at one level influence other levels. For example, an excellent metacarpophalangeal (MP) joint reconstruction in a patient with severe ulnar deviation will provide stable long-term function if the wrist maintains axial alignment. If the wrist begins to translocate toward the ulnar side or rotate to produce radial deviation of the metacarpals, recurrent extensor tendon misalignment will inevitably occur. In general, once the postoperative therapy for any reconstruction is complete, the patient should be examined at yearly intervals indefinitely.

DEGENERATIVE ARTHRITIS

Osteoarthritis is a localized degenerative process occurring in one or several joints. Although the etiology is unknown, osteoarthritis seems to represent a wear process (Barnet, 1956; Radin, 1975–76; Howell and associates, 1978–79). Essentially all men and women over the age of 60 years show some physical or radiologic evidence of osteoarthritis. Only a small percentage of these individuals, however, are symptomatic. Occupational factors may have a great deal to do with the involvement of specific joints (Mintz and Fraga, 1973; Burke, Fear, and Wright, 1977). The spontaneous degenerative changes in the hand affect the distal interphalangeal (DIP) joints, the metacarpocarpal joint of the thumb, and, less frequently, the proximal interphalangeal (PIP) joints. For the purpose of this discussion, degenerative arthritis includes traumatic arthritis. Although sometimes considered a separate entity, traumatic arthritis differs from osteoarthritis only in the fact that the individual joint surface changes occur at an earlier stage in life. Finally, erosive osteoarthritis will also be included in this section. Erosive osteoarthritis is an inflammatory polyarthritis affecting women more frequently than men. The process attacks the distal interphalangeal, proximal interphalangeal, and trapezio–first metacarpal joints, but rarely attacks the metacarpophalangeal joints. This condition produces locally destructive erosive synovitis, but no systemic symptoms (Bauer and Bennett, 1936).

Degenerative arthritic changes attack the distal interphalangeal joints in most individuals. By the eighth decade, 90 per cent of women have radiographic evidence of distal interphalangeal joint osteoarthritis. The trapezio–first metacarpal joint is the next most commonly involved joint (Carstam, Eken, and Andren, 1968), followed by the proximal interphalangeal, carpocarpal, and radiocarpal joints.

Distal Interphalangeal Joints

Although the arc of motion of the distal interphalangeal joint represents less than 5 per cent of the total arc of motion of the finger, position of the tip is critical to finger function (Littler, 1960). The flexor digitorum profundus tendon, the flexor of the distal interphalangeal joint, also provides over half the power for flexion of the proximal interphalangeal joint. Degenerative arthritis of the distal interphalangeal joint can produce pain, misalignment, instability, or an unattractive appearance.

Early in the course of distal interphalangeal joint involvement, pain can be managed by nonsteroidal anti-inflammatory drugs. Pain in these joints is usually intermittent. Once the bony surfaces erode to a point at which the joint is unstable, pain is usually not a primary functional complaint.

When instability or cosmetic deformity of the distal interphalangeal joint becomes significant or pain cannot be managed adequately with drugs, arthrodesis is an ideal solution. Fusion eliminates discomfort. In the process of arthrodesis, the tips can be made narrow and attractive. The large exostoses (Heberden's nodes) are trimmed, and the finger tips reshaped. Finally, arthrodesis preserves the flexor profundus function but redirects the flexion power to the proximal interphalangeal joint.

The position of the arthrodesis depends entirely on the specific manipulative requirements of the patient. In general, for aesthetic reasons, distal interphalangeal joints should be fused in extension, because patients prefer the extended position much more than a flexed one. In contrast, patients who need to grip handled objects may require a few degrees of flexion in the distal interphalangeal joints of the small, ring, and long fingers. Fusing the distal interphalangeal joint of the index finger in full extension allows excellent pulp to pulp pinch, but eliminates tip to tip pinch. Buttoning buttons and picking up small objects from flat surfaces are difficult with the distal interphalangeal joint of the index finger held in extension. If the interphalangeal joint of the thumb is normal, however, the patient can compensate.

The interphalangeal joint of the thumb is frequently involved with osteoarthritic changes (Clayton, 1962). In this instance, flexion and extension are valuable. Fingernail to fingernail pinch cannot be achieved without some interphalangeal joint flexion. If the collateral ligament structures are intact, the interphalangeal joint of the thumb can be reconstructed using resection implant arthroplasty techniques. If the collateral structures are destroyed, however, pain and instability can be eliminated by arthrodesis.

Mucous cyst formation may be a complication of osteoarthritis in the distal and proximal interphalangeal joints. The cysts are the result of small sharp osteophytes producing persistent small openings in the joint capsule (Kleinert and associates, 1973). If a cyst extends distally, pressure on the nail bed can produce an unsightly nail deformity. Attempts to remove the cyst by evacuation, excision, or even skin grafting almost always fail. In order to prevent recurrence, the osteophyte at the joint line must be debrided (Eaton, Dobranski, and Littler, 1973).

Proximal Interphalangeal Joints

The proximal interphalangeal joint contributes approximately 20 per cent to the arc of motion of the finger (Littler, 1960). Movements of this joint determine the relative position of the tip of the finger to the distal palm and thumb. The ability to change position of the proximal interphalangeal joint is important in almost all fine manipulative tasks. Changes in proximal interphalangeal joint position alter the longitudinal arch of the finger, adapting the digit to objects of various size during power gripping. In order to be useful, the joint must be axially aligned, pain free, and stable. Degenerative arthritis may destroy all three requisites. An unstable, painful proximal interphalangeal joint with 90 degrees of flexion and extension cannot be used effectively.

Early in the course of degenerative changes at the level of the proximal interphalangeal joint, nonsteroidal, anti-inflammatory drugs can manage discomfort adequately (Moskowitz, 1981). In addition, simply changing the way in which objects are manipulated can solve functional abnormalities. Most patients with significant degenerative arthritis of the proximal interphalangeal joint have limited range of motion. As a rule, however, provided that the arc is reasonable (− 20 degrees of extension to 60 degrees of flexion), a limited range of motion produces little functional impairment. Pain, instability, and axial misalignment are the primary dysfunctional elements in prehension. If the pain cannot be controlled with anti-inflammatory drugs, reconstruction using either resection implant arthroplasty techniques or arthrodesis can restore useful finger function (Swanson, 1973a).

Arthrodesis of a single proximal interphalangeal joint is always less than satisfactory. With the joint fused in position to allow the tip of the finger to be brought to the thumb and provide a reasonable longitudinal arch, a significantly flexed position is required. With the joint fused in flexion, patients invariably adjust the tensions on their extensor tendons to bring the tips of the fingers into alignment. This brings the distal segments of the affected finger out of the palmar space, but produces hyperextension at the metacarpophalangeal joint. The proximal interphalangeal joint is always prominent on the dorsum of the hand with the fingers in extension and is constantly irritated by the environment. Reaching out to put the hand in a small place or even placing the hand in a tight pocket irritates the dorsum of the joint. In contrast, arthrodesis of all four proximal interphalangeal joints in proper position provides excellent finger function if metacarpophalangeal joint function is satisfactory.

To be seriously considered for reconstruction of the proximal interphalangeal joint, the finger must have an excellent flexor mechanism with normal gliding and reconstructible collateral ligaments. Resection implant arthroplasty relieves pain effectively (Swanson, 1968; McDowell, 1971). Although postoperative motion is never normal, most surgeons report postoperative ranges of approximately 60 degrees.

Each proximal interphalangeal joint is subjected to different stresses. The index finger joint and, to a lesser extent, the long finger joint are stressed strongly toward the ulnar side in key pinch. To prevent ulnar deviation, many surgeons recommend fusing the proximal interphalangeal joint of the index finger and reconstructing the proximal interphalangeal joints of the ulnar three digits (Steinbrocker, 1969; Millender and Nalebuff, 1975c, 1975d; Moberg, 1975; Zancolli, 1975).

Resection implant arthroplasty using polysiloxan rubber implants is currently the reconstruction of choice, if motion is to be preserved at the proximal interphalangeal joint level. The technical aspects of this procedure have been described in detail elsewhere (Urbianak, McCollum, and Goldner,

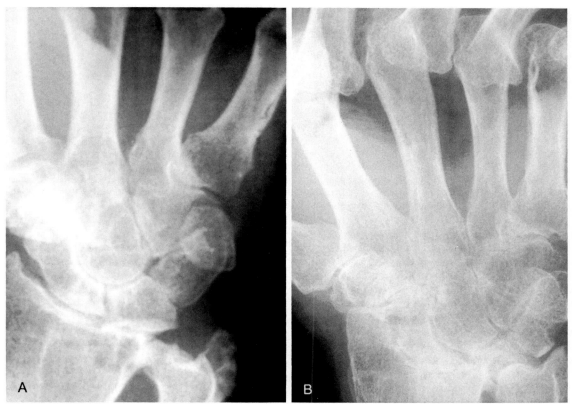

Figure 107–10. Radiograph of hand of patient with rheumatoid arthritis. *A,* Note the synovial cyst of the radius at the radioscapholunate ligament insertion (cyst of Testut). *B,* Five years later. Note that the radial cyst has collapsed, dislocating the lunate.

the long run. Essentially all hand activities can be performed with total radiocarpal motion of 40 to 60 degrees (Palmer and associates, 1985). In active synovitic states, limiting radiocarpal motion postoperatively with casting and splinting for up to six weeks reduces the development of future deformities. If a radial subchondral cyst is present (cyst of Testut), the cyst should be scraped with a curette and grafted with cancellous bone obtained from the radius. Postoperatively, patients in whom grafts were used are treated as if they had synovectomies alone.

Once ulnar translocation of the carpus begins, with its accompanying radial deviation of the metacarpals, synovectomy alone reduces discomfort but does not stop the progression of the deformity. If the carpus can be relocated passively, and the radial deviation corrected passively or actively, synovectomy with limited carpal arthrodeses has proved effective in eliminating pain, instability, and progression of the deformities (Myerdierks, Mosher, and Werner, 1987). Fusing

the lunate to the ulnar aspect of the radius realigns the carpus, eliminates radial deviation of the metacarpals, and prevents subsequent ulnar translocation. If the distal radioulnar joint is unstable, the radiolunate arthrodesis can be combined with a Lauenstein procedure, creating a firm bony base for finger and thumb function (see Fig. 107–9). Arthrodeses are held in place with Kirschner wires, and the addition of cancellous bone grafts usually yields a firm union within eight to 12 weeks. The hand and wrist are held in a cast until the arthrodesis is complete and then splinted protectively while motion is regained (Clayton, 1965; Dupont and Vainio, 1968). Flexion and extension, as well as radial and ulnar deviation of the carpus, are usually excellent following radiolunate arthrodesis (Fig. 107–11). Flexion and extension occur through the midcarpal joint. As a rule, the carpocarpal architecture is quite abnormal on plain radiograph at this point, but in spite of appearance, pain is usually minimal, and motion excellent.

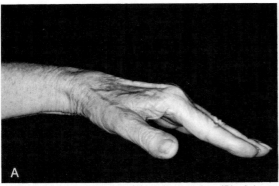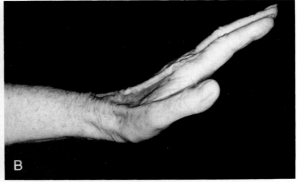

Figure 107–11. Flexion *(A)* and extension *(B)* of the radiocarpal joint following lunoradial arthrodesis and Lauenstein procedure. Radiograph of this patient shown in Figure 107–9.

As the magnitude of carpal collapse and subluxation increases, reconstructive choices become more limited. If ulnar translocation and radial deviation of the metacarpals are not passively correctable, or if the radiocarpal joint is subluxated, synovectomy and limited arthrodesis are inadequate. The wrist must be stable and pain free for the fingers and thumb to function. Although a mobile radiocarpal joint is extremely useful, most hand functions can be performed adequately with the radiocarpal joint fixed in a neutral position. In an unstable or abnormally positioned wrist, fusing the carpus in a neutral position restores power, eliminates pain, and maximizes finger and thumb function.

The arthrodesis of the wrist should be performed using remnants of local bone and cancellous bone grafts from the radius, if possible. Although the ilium is a superb source of cancellous bone grafts, patients with hip and knee abnormalities find it difficult to manage with sore hips and one arm. A wide variety of techniques have been described to fuse the carpal bones; however, stabilization using a single, longitudinal, large diameter stainless steel pin has been shown to be the most effective technique (Millender, Nalebuff, and Feldon, 1982). In all arthrodeses in which small pieces of bone are used for fusion, longitudinal collapse is inevitable. The single pin prevents longitudinal collapse while external casting provides immobilization. Unless block bone grafts are employed to increase length in complex reconstructions, arthrodesis is usually complete within 12 weeks. Postoperatively, patients must establish finger and thumb motion quickly, while the bony elements are kept immobile.

Although arthrodesis in a neutral position optimizes finger and thumb function, lack of radiocarpal motion does make some activities difficult or impossible. Most activities of daily living and even productive work functions can be performed with the wrist in a neutral position. Perineal care, however, requires a flexed wrist position. Independent living requires reaching both ends of the gastrointestinal tract. If one radiocarpal joint is fused in the neutral position, the other wrist must be mobile or fused in a position compatible with perineal management. If both wrists are unstable and painful, at least one wrist should move following reconstruction (Meuli, 1972).

Although a number of total wrist arthroplastic devices are available, all require fixation of the proximal and distal portions of the device using bone cement (Voltz, 1977). If the initial reconstruction using an arthroplastic device is adequate and progression of the disease or wear is minimal, results can be quite satisfactory. Unfortunately, reconstructions in patients with rheumatoid disease are rarely stable. The disease progresses in joints proximal and distal to the reconstruction, and many joint reconstructions in rheumatoid patients require revision. Revision or salvage following cemented arthroplasty procedures is extremely difficult. Removing the cement, changing the angles of the articulating pieces, and even rebalancing tendons over mobile devices may be impossible. Currently, the use of total wrist arthroplastic devices should be limited to investigative studies or centers specializing in this type of reconstruction.

Resection implant arthroplasty, which has been used for many years as an alternative to arthrodesis, can be an extremely useful procedure (Swanson, 1973e). Although the procedure uses an implantable Silastic part, the operation should be considered a resection arthroplasty. The concept is to bring the component parts of the wrist and forearm into proper alignment, fusing small components as necessary and allowing a stable carpal mass to articulate axially to a stable radial platform. The implant device simply separates the bone ends of the carpus and radius to create a plane of motion, not a wrist joint. The reconstruction should be designed to create a stable, pain free wrist with a markedly limited range of motion. Functionally, the patient should be able to bring the radiocarpal joint into a few degrees of extension and have enough flexion to reach the perineum.

Late failures in resection implant arthroplasty are always due to imbalance or instability created by large ranges of motion. Soft tissues, particularly the dorsal and volar capsular ligament remnants, should be reconstructed to prevent more than 60 degrees of active motion. An attempt should be made to conserve as much of the bony substance as possible. As in all resection arthroplasties, there is an inverse relationship between the amount of bone removed or lost and the stability of the reconstruction. Soft tissue balancing is the key to stable reconstructions. Without at least two excellent wrist extensors, successful results using this technique are unusual. At the time of surgery, the extensors of the wrist must be balanced for neutral flexion and extension. If the extensor carpi ulnaris is attenuated or ruptured, the extensor carpi radialis longus should be transferred to the insertion of the extensor carpi ulnaris.

The ultimate range of motion in each reconstruction is determined by the postoperative care as well as the surgical technique. If the capsular remnants are minimally adequate or if a great deal of bone has been lost as a result of the disease process or has been resected to restore axial alignment, the wrist should be immobilized following reconstructions long enough to limit motion. The longer the wrist is immobilized, the more limited the range of motion on completion. Soft tissue reconstruction and postoperative management should be combined to create a rigid reconstruction with minimal motion and excellent balance. Finally, the balance of this reconstruction must be followed for at least 24 months. If the disease process alters the balance of the radiocarpal reconstruction, the joint should be rebalanced by adjusting ten-

don positions. If the range of motion in a resection implant arthroplasty is restricted adequately and balance remains neutral, reconstructions can be satisfactory for long intervals (Fig. 107–12).

One of the most valuable attributes of the resection implant arthroplasty technique is the ability to revise or salvage failures relatively easily. In contrast to the techniques using fixed implant stems and cement, implant arthroplasties are almost always salvageable. If resection implant arthroplasty of the radiocarpal joint fails owing to progressive disease, tendon imbalance, or rupture, excellent function can be obtained by converting the implant arthroplasty to an arthrodesis. The remnants of the implant material should be removed completely, and the sclerotic bone and synovial material debrided. Length can be restored by a block bone graft from the iliac crest tailored to fit the implant cavity. Careful fixation using a single longitudinal Steinmann pin along with external immobilization results in a solid arthrodesis. Because block bone grafts are slow to acquire

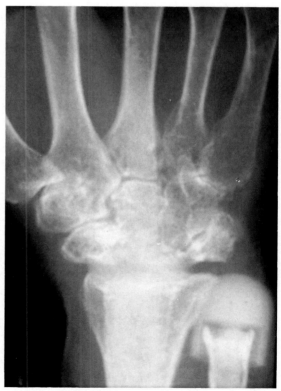

Figure 107–12. Radiograph of patient with rheumatoid arthritis 11 years after resection implant arthroplasty of the radiocarpal and distal radioulnar joints.

new blood supply, arthrodesis can be accelerated significantly by using large quantities of cancellous bone grafts on both sides of the block bone graft. The living cells in the cancellous bone graft usually bridge the defect long before the block bone graft is incorporated (Madden, 1970).

FINGER JOINTS

Rheumatoid disease can produce imbalance abnormalities or bony destruction and instability in all three finger joints. As a rule, however, the proximal interphalangeal and metacarpophalangeal joints are most severely affected. The distal interphalangeal joint abnormalities rarely produce primary functional problems, and as discussed in the section devoted to osteoarthritis, fusing this joint in the proper position is an ideal correction for most problems.

With some exceptions, proximal interphalangeal and metacarpophalangeal destructive problems rarely exist equally in the same digit. Psoriatic arthritis is an obvious exception. In psoriatic disease, spontaneous arthrodeses are extremely common. Proximal interphalangeal joints in particular progress to spontaneous arthrodesis. If these joints can be maintained in a functional position as they fuse, the hands remain relatively functional (McMaster, 1972).

Reconstructing both the proximal interphalangeal and metacarpophalangeal joints in a single digit is rarely possible. If both joints are reconstructed, the metacarpophalangeal joint usually moves adequately but the proximal interphalangeal joint becomes fixed around a small arc of motion. In most patients with rheumatoid arthritis, small joint reconstruction of the fingers should be limited to the metacarpophalangeal joint (Smith and Kaplan, 1967). Soft tissue rebalancing procedures, synovectomy for discomfort, and arthrodesis for instability should be used to place proximal interphalangeal joints in functional positions. Reconstructing the proximal interphalangeal joint itself, however, is rarely indicated. The metacarpophalangeal joint provides the greatest arc of motion in the finger. Proximal interphalangeal joints must be stable, pain free, and fixed in a functional position, but they need not be fully mobile for excellent hand function.

The development of satisfactory reconstructive techniques for the metacarpophalangeal joint represents an important advance in rheumatoid reconstructive surgery. Although function can be improved by fusing misaligned metacarpophalangeal joints in patients with excellent proximal interphalangeal joint motion, fixing the metacarpophalangeal joint severely limits gross gripping and fine manipulative function. Many techniques of resection arthroplasty at the metacarpophalangeal joint level have been developed. Results of resection arthroplasty alone are inconsistent, and the excellent results reported by some surgeons are difficult to reproduce. If the reconstruction is designed to restore a wide range of motion, the metacarpophalangeal joints become unstable, and deformities recur rapidly. On the other hand, if the reconstruction is designed to produce stability, gross gripping functions are compromised.

Initial attempts by Flatt (1960) to reconstruct metacarpophalangeal joints used metal implant devices. These experimental reconstructions produced some remarkably functional hands, but the reconstructions deteriorated rapidly and became fixed in single positions (Flatt, 1961). The experimental results did encourage other investigators, however.

Many attempts have been made to design "total joint" implantable devices at the metacarpophalangeal joint level equivalent to the total joint replacements of the lower extremity. In commercially available devices, the stems of the implants must be cemented into the metacarpals and proximal phalanges. Because the stems are fixed, the axis of rotation of the implant device must be perfectly positioned in order to balance the forces moving around the mobile structure and to prevent breakdown of the reconstruction. In an ongoing disease state, even if perfect balance can be achieved initially, changes in the kinesiology of the extremity with time unbalance most reconstructions. Should imbalance occur, the implant device must be replaced or revised. Revision or replacement has proved difficult or impossible in most instances. As a consequence, the use of cemented or fixed stemmed implant devices should be restricted to experimental studies and to centers specializing in this type of reconstruction.

The development of resection implant arthroplasty at the metacarpophalangeal joint level has proved to be an excellent and efficacious technique of reconstruction. Adding a flexible internal splint and spacer to the resection arthroplasty allows controlled movement immediately after operation. Early active and passive movement controls the architecture of scar tissue formed between the associated bones. The implant device plus the remodeled capsule produces a functional pseudojoint (Backhouse, 1969; Allende, 1971; Bolton, 1971).

Resection implant arthroplasty should be thought of as a soft tissue procedure. Enough bone is resected to bring the osseous elements back into normal alignment, but the deforming forces unbalancing the metacarpophalangeal joint must be analyzed, and each deforming force reconstructed appropriately. All forces working around the metacarpophalangeal joint reconstruction need to be rebalanced—extension forces, flexion forces, and intrinsic muscle forces. Attempts should be made to reconstruct the static elements around the joint as well, although the active forces are more important. Ultimately, the movement of resection implant arthroplastic reconstructions depends not only on the mechanical reconstruction at the time of surgery, but also on postoperative management.

In all resection arthroplasties, there is an inverse relationship between the amount of bone resected and the stability of the ultimate reconstruction. The more bone resected, the greater the instability; the less bone removed, the greater the stability. Thus, altering the surgical technique and the postoperative management can create a joint for each patient appropriate for individual life style and needs. For example, in patients whose metacarpophalangeal joints are subluxated, ulnarly deviated, and translocated toward the ulnar side but whose proximal interphalangeal joints are excellent, the metacarpophalangeal joints need to be stabilized, axially aligned, and given modest ranges of active motion. In contrast, patients with fixed proximal interphalangeal joints require large ranges of motion at the metacarpophalangeal joint level for adequate function. Varying the amount of bone resected and the postoperative immobilization program determines the ultimate range of motion at each joint.

As a rule, patients presenting for metacarpophalangeal joint reconstruction demonstrate ulnar deviation and translocation as well as subluxation of the joint. The radial sagittal band fibers of the extensor mechanism are severely attenuated, displacing the extensor tendons toward the ulnar side. The radial metacarpal phalangeal collateral ligaments are ruptured or attenuated, eliminating static radial support. The intrinsic muscles have rested in a shortened position long enough to alter length relationships. Ulnar intrinsic muscles are often too short to allow passive repositioning of the fingers in axial alignment. An adequate metacarpophalangeal joint resection implant arthroplasty must correct all of these dynamic imbalance abnormalities, or the deformities will recur (Swanson, 1973e).

Metacarpophalangeal reconstructions are performed under conduction block anesthesia. A transverse incision at the level of the new joint line gives excellent exposure and good aesthetic result as well. Only enough bone is resected from the metacarpal head and the base of the proximal phalanx to allow each finger to be brought up into axial alignment. Static forces are reestablished by reinsertion of the attenuated radial collateral ligaments. If the radial collateral ligament is completely destroyed, the static element can be reconstructed using a portion of the volar plate. Once enough bone is resected to reestablish normal position, the intrinsic musculature must be rebalanced, and in some cases, the ulnar intrinsic tendons must be lengthened to achieve an intrinsic-minus position with the finger axially aligned. Supination of the index finger toward the thumb in pulp to pulp pinching is a useful and necessary function. The first volar interosseous muscle is a principal supinator of the index finger and is usually left attached. If the muscle is too short, removing additional bony material from the metacarpal or proximal phalanx reestablishes balance. The extensor tendons are then centralized over the metacarpophalangeal joint reconstruction by reefing the radial sagittal band fibers (Smith and associates, 1966).

The postoperative management of resection implant arthroplasties at the metacarpophalangeal joint level is as important to the ultimate result as the surgical procedure (Swanson, 1973e; Madden, Arem, and De-Vore, 1976; DeVore, Muhleman, and Sasarita, 1986). As the scar forms around the implant devices, the fingers must remain axially aligned for at least 12 weeks for adequate healing. Patients are required to keep their fingers in functional splints all day for at least six weeks, and in night splints for six to 12 weeks longer. Although the operative and postoperative care of these reconstructions is tedious and time consuming, the results are usually gratifying (Fig. 107–13).

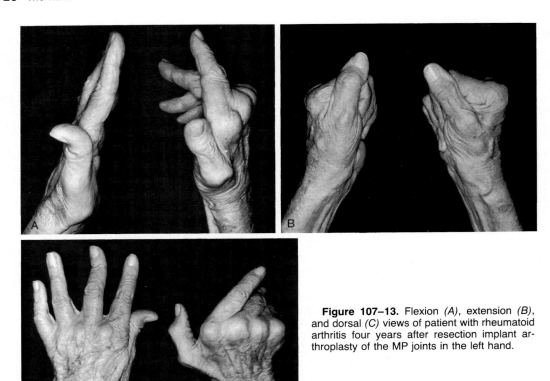

Figure 107–13. Flexion *(A)*, extension *(B)*, and dorsal *(C)* views of patient with rheumatoid arthritis four years after resection implant arthroplasty of the MP joints in the left hand.

Finally, because rheumatoid disease is a progressive, destructive process, joint reconstructions must be maintained indefinitely following their completion. Patients must be seen every six to 12 months to make sure that the forces acting across the reconstructed joints remain balanced. For example, if the disease at the wrist progresses, radial deviation of the metacarpals develops. The ulnar deviation vectors at the metacarpophalangeal joint are increased geometrically. Unless the radial deviation of the metacarpals is controlled, the metacarpophalangeal joint reconstructions will fail, and the ulnar deviation position will be reestablished. If the volar synovitis of the flexor mechanism progresses to the point that flexor tendons can no longer glide adequately within the digital theca, all flexion forces will be concentrated at the metacarpophalangeal joint level, and subluxation deformities will recur. One of the advantages of the resection implant arthroplasty technique is the fact that revision of the reconstructions can be performed at any time. For example, if the dorsal scar capsule around the implant device prevents adequate flexion, the scar tissue can be excised at six to 12 months, improving flexion significantly.

SUMMARY

Reconstructing the upper extremities of patients with arthritic deformities represents the highest level of the reconstructive surgeon's art. Although no surgical technique is unique to arthritic reconstruction, the magnitude of the reconstructive problem requires comprehensive functional evaluation and careful planning. Because all tissues in the upper extremity can be affected by systemic synovitic conditions, the surgeon must be prepared to solve functional problems in any system. Patient education plays a critical role in the reconstructive process. Specific goals at all levels must be shared by the patient, the patient's family, the hand therapist, and the surgeon. In spite of the inherent difficulties, however, rehabilitative programs including upper extremity reconstructive surgery can improve and maintain manipulative function throughout the patient's lifetime.

REFERENCES

Allende, B. T.: Artritis rheumatoidea en la articulacion metacarpofalangiea. Rev. Orthop. Traum. Lat.-Am. 16:111, 1971.

American Society of Hand Therapists, Incorporated, 1977, Philadelphia, PA.

Ansell, B. M.: Hand assessment in rheumatoid arthritis. Ann. Rheum. Dis. (Suppl.) 28:77, 1969.

Backdahl, M.: The caput ulnae syndrome in rheumatoid arthritis. Acta Rheum. Scand. (Suppl.) 51:1, 1963.

Backhouse, K. M.: Mechanical factors influencing normal and rheumatoid metacarpalphalangeal joints. Ann. Rheum. Dis. (Suppl.) 28:15, 1969.

Backhouse, K. M., and Catton, T. R.: An experimental study of the function of the lumbrical muscles in the human hand. J. Anat. 88:133, 1954.

Barnet, C. H.: Wear and tear in joints: An experimental study. J. Bone Joint Surg. 38B:567, 1956.

Bauer, W., and Bennett, G. A.: Experimental and pathological studies in degenerative type of arthritis. J. Bone Joint Surg. 18A:1, 1936.

Bayles, T. B.: The history of the treatment of rheumatoid arthritis (1939–1975). Orthop. Clin. North Am. 6:603, 1975.

Beevor, C.: Croonian Lectures on Muscular Movement. Delivered in 1903. Edited and reprinted for the guarantors of "Brain." New York, Macmillan Company, 1951.

Belin, D. C., Abeles, M., and Weinstein, A.: Rheumatoid markers in the absence of arthritis. J. Rheumatol. 6:293, 1979.

Bolton, H.: Arthroplasty of the metacarpophalangeal joints. Hand 3:131, 1971.

Bowers, W. H.: Distal radioulnar joint. In Green, D. (Ed.): Operative Hand Surgery. New York, Churchill Livingstone, 1982.

Boyes, J. H.: The role of the intrinsic muscles in rheumatoid arthritis. In Tubiana, R. (Ed.): The Rheumatoid Hand. Group d'étude de la main, No. 3. Paris, L'Expansion Scientifique Francaise, 1969.

Boyes, J. H., and Stark, H. H.: Flexor tendon grafts in the fingers and thumb. A study of factors influencing results in 1,000 cases. J. Bone Joint Surg. 53A:1332, 1971.

Braley, S.: The chemistry and properties of the medical-grade silicones. J. Macromol. Sci.-Chem. A-4:529, 1970.

Brattstrom, M.: Evaluation of the arthritic patient. Analysis of functional handicap. In Principles of Joint Protection in Chronic Rheumatic Disease. Chicago, Year Book Medical Publishers, 1973.

Brewerton, D. A.: Hand deformities in rheumatoid arthritis. Ann. Rheum. Dis. 16:183, 1957.

Brewerton, D. A., and Daniel, J. W.: Return to work: Experience of a hospital rehabilitation officer. Br. Med. J. 2:240, 1969.

Burke, M. J., Fear, M. C., and Wright, V.: Bone and joint changes in pneumatic drillers. Ann. Rheum. Dis. 36:276, 1977.

Carroll, R. E., and Hill, N. A.: Small joint arthrodesis in hand reconstruction. J. Bone Joint Surg. 51A:1219, 1969.

Carroll, R. E., and Hill, N. A.: Arthrodesis of the carpometacarpal joint of the thumb—a clinical and cineroentgenographic study. J. Bone Joint Surg. 55B:292, 1973.

Carstam, N., Eiken, O., and Andren, L.: Osteoarthritis in the trapezio-scaphoid joint. Acta Orthop. Scand. 39:354, 1968.

Chao, E. Y., Opgrande, J. D., and Axmear, F. E.: Three dimensional force analysis of finger joints in selected isometric hand functions. J. Biomech. 9:387, 1976.

Christie, A. J., Weinberger, K. A., and Dietrich, M.: Silicone lymphadenopathy and synovitis: Complications of silicone elastomer finger joint prosthesis. J.A.M.A. 237:1463, 1977.

Clayton, M. L.: Surgery of the thumb in rheumatoid arthritis. J. Bone Joint Surg. 44A:1376, 1962.

Clayton, M. L.: Surgical treatment of the wrist in rheumatoid arthritis: A review of thirty seven patients. J. Bone Joint Surg. 47A:741, 1965.

Codman, E. A.: The Shoulder. Boston, 1934.

Conaty, J. P., and Nickel, V. L.: Functional incapacitation in rheumatoid arthritis: A rehabilitative challenge. J. Bone Joint Surg. 53A:624, 1971.

Crosby, E. B., and Linscheid, R. L.: Rupture of the flexor profundus of the ring finger secondary to ancient fracture of the hook of the hamate. J. Bone Joint Surg. 56A:1076, 1974.

Cystekar, R. G., Davie, J. M., and Cattell, H. S.: Foreign body reaction to silicone rubber. Complication of a finger joint implant. Clin. Orthop. 98:231, 1974.

Darrach, W., and Dwight, K.: Derangements of the inferior radioulnar articulation. Med. Rec. 87:708, 1915.

DeCeulaer, K. -P.: Drug allergy to prednisolone in rheumatoid arthritis. Scott. Med. J. 24:218, 1979.

DeVore, G. L., Muhleman, C. A., and Sasarita, S. G.: Management of pronation deformity in metacarpal phalangeal joint implant arthroplasty. J. Hand Surg. 11A:859, 1986.

Disease Control Programs: Arthritis. U.S. Dept. of Health, Education and Welfare, 1966.

Dolphin, J. A.: The extensor tenotomy for chronic boutonniére deformity of the finger. J. Bone Joint Surg. 47A:161, 1965.

Duchenne, G. B.: Physiology of motion. Demonstrated by means of electrical stimulation and clinical observation as applied to the study of paralysis and deformities (translated by E. B. Kaplan). Philadelphia, J. B. Lippincott Company, 1949.

Dupont, M., and Vainio, K.: Arthrodesis of the wrist in rheumatoid arthritis. Ann. Chir. Gynaecol. Fenn. 57:513, 1968.

Eaton, R. G., Dobranski, A. I., and Littler, J. W.: Marginal osteophyte excision in treatment of mucous cysts. J. Bone Joint Surg. 55A:570, 1973.

Edmonds, M. E., Jones, T. C., Saunders, W. A., and Sturrock, R. D.: Autonomic neuropathy in rheumatoid arthritis. Br. Med. J. 2:173, 1979.

Eiken, O., and Carstam, N.: Functional assessment of basal joint fusion of the thumb. Scand. J. Plast. Reconstr. Surg. 4:122, 1979.

Elliot, R. A.: Injuries to extensor mechanism of the hand. Orthop. Clin. North Am. 1:335, 1970.

Ellison, M. R., Kelly, K. J., and Flatt, A. E.: The results of surgical synovectomy of the digital joints in rheumatoid disease. J. Bone Joint Surg. 52A:1041, 1976.

Eyler, D. L., and Markee, J. E.: The anatomy and function of the intrinsic musculature of the fingers. J. Bone Joint Surg. 36A:1, 1954.

Ferlic, D. C., Clayton, M. L., and Holloway, M.: Complications of silicone implant surgery in the MP joint. J. Bone Joint Surg. 57A:991, 1975.

Fernandez-Palazzi, F., and Vainio, K.: Synovectomy of the carpal joints in rheumatoid arthritis. A report of

47 cases. AIR Arch. Interam. Rheum. (Rio de Janeiro) 8:249, 1965.

Flatt, A. E.: The prosthetic replacement of rheumatoid finger joints. Rheumatism 16:90, 1960.

Flatt, A. E.: Restoration of rheumatoid finger-joint functions; interim report on trial of prosthetic replacement. J. Bone Joint Surg. 43A:753, 1961.

Flatt, A. E.: The Care of the Rheumatoid Hand. St. Louis, C. V. Mosby Company, 1963.

Flatt, A. E.: Some pathomechanics of ulnar drift. Plast. Reconstr. Surg. 37:295, 1966.

Flatt, A. E.: Prosthetic replacement of joints in the rheumatoid joint. In Tubiana, R. (Ed.): The Rheumatoid Hand. Paris, GEM Publication, 1969.

Flatt, A. E., and Fischer, G. W.: Biomechanical factors in the replacement of rheumatoid finger joints. Ann. Rheum. Dis. (Supp.) 28:36, 1969.

Fleischer, A., and McGrath, M. H.: Rheumatoid nodules of the hand. J. Hand Surg. 9A:404, 1984.

Freeman, M. A., Swanson, S. A., and Heath, J. C.: Study of the wear particles produced from cobalt-chromium-molybdenum-manganese total joint replacement prosthesis. Ann. Rheum Dis. (Suppl.) 28:29, 1969.

Froimson, A. L.: Tendon arthroplasty of the trapezial metacarpal joint. Clin. Orthop. 70:191, 1970.

Gervis, W.: Excision of the trapezium for osteoarthritis of the trapezial metacarpal joint. J. Bone Joint Surg. 31B:537, 1949.

Goldman, R.: Finding jobs for arthritic patients. J. Rehabilitation 25:21, 1959.

Goncalves, D.: Correction of disorders of the distal radioulnar joint by artificial pseudoarthrosis of the ulna. J. Bone Joint Surg. 56B:462, 1974.

Gordon, M., and Bullough, P. G.: Synovial and osseous inflammation in failed silicone rubber prosthesis. J. Bone Joint Surg. 64A:574, 1982.

Gordon, T.: Osteoarthritis in U. S. adults. In Population Studies of the Rheumatic Diseases. Proceedings of the Third International Symposium. New York, Excerpta Medica Foundation, 1966.

Granowitz, S., and Vainio, K.: Proximal interphalangeal joint arthrodesis in rheumatoid arthritis: A follow up study of 122 operations. Acta Orthop. Scand. 37:301, 1966.

Harrison, K. M.: Rheumatoid deformities of the proximal interphalangeal joints of the hand. Ann. Rheum. Dis. (Suppl.) 28:20, 1969.

Heather, A. J.: A two year follow up study of the patients admitted to the Rehabilitation Center of the Hospital of the University of Pennsylvania. Am. J. Phys. Med. 37:237, 1958.

Hijmans, W. D. P., and Hershel, H.: Early Synovectomy in Rheumatoid Arthritis. Amsterdam, Excerpta Medica Foundation, 1969.

Homsy, C. A.: Proplast: Chemical and biological considerations. In Biomaterials in Reconstructive Surgery, 1983.

Howell, D. S., Woessner, J. F., Jiminez, S., Seda, H., and Schumacher, H. R.: A view on the pathogenesis of osteoarthritis. Bull. Rheum. Dis. 29:996, 1978–79 series.

Hunter, J. M., and Salisbury, R. E.: Use of gliding artificial implants to produce tendon sheaths—technique and results in children. Plast. Reconstr. Surg. 45:564, 1970.

Hunter, J. M., and Salisbury, R. E.: Flexor tendon reconstruction in severely damaged hands. J. Bone Joint Surg. 53A:829, 1971.

Jayasanker, M., Schoene, H. R., and Joseph, C. H.: Trapezialmetacarpal arthritis—results of tendon interpositional arthroplasty. J. Hand Surg. 6:442, 1981.

Johnson, L. C.: Kinetics of osteoarthritis. J. Lab. Invest. 8:1223, 1959.

Kaplan, E. B.: Anatomy, injuries and treatment of the extensor apparatus of the hand and the digits. Clin. Orthop. 13:24, 1959.

Kellgren, J. H., and Ball, J.: Tendon lesions in rheumatoid arthritis: A clinicopathologic study. Ann. Rheum. Dis. 9:48, 1950.

Kelsey, J. L., Pastides, H., Kreiger, N., Harris, C., and Chernow, R. A.: Upper Extremity Disorders—A Survey of Their Frequency and Costs in the United States. St. Louis, C. V. Mosby Company, 1980.

Kessler, I., and Hecht, O.: Present application of the Darrach procedure. Clin. Orthop. 72:254, 1970.

King, G. J., McMurtry, R. Y., Rubenstein, J. D., and Gertzbein, S. D.: Kinematics of the distal radioulnar joint. J. Hand Surg. 11A:798, 1986.

Kleinert, H. E., Kutz, J. E., Atasoy, E., and Stormo, A.: Primary repair of flexor tendons. Orthop. Clin. North Am. 4:865, 1973.

Kleinert, H. E., Kutz, J. E., and Cohen, M. J.: Primary repair of Zone II flexor tendon lacerations. In AAOS Symposium on Tendon Surgery in the Hand. St. Louis, C. V. Mosby Company, 1975.

Kleinert, H. E., Kutz, J. E., Fishman, H., and McGraw, L. H.: Etiology and treatment of the so-called mucous cyst of the finger. J. Bone Joint Surg. 54A:1455, 1972.

Kleinert, H. E., and Frykman, G.: The wrist and thumb in rheumatoid arthritis. Orthop. Clin. North Am. 4:1085, 1973.

Laine, V. A. I., and Vainio, K.: Spontaneous rupture of tendons in rheumatoid arthritis. Acta Orthop. Scand. 24:250, 1955.

Landsmeer, J. M. F.: Anatomy of the dorsal aponeurosis of the human finger and its functional significance. Anat. Rec. 104:31, 1949.

Leddy, J. P., and Packer, J. W.: Avulsion of the profundus tendon insertion in athletes. J. Hand Surg. 2:66, 1977.

Linscheid, R. L.: Surgery for rheumatoid arthritis—timing and technique: The upper extremity. J. Bone Joint Surg. 50A:605, 1968.

Linscheid, R. L., and Chao, E. Y. S.: Biomechanical assessment of finger function in prosthetic joint design. Orthop. Clin. North Am. 4:317, 1973.

Lipscomb, P. R.: Surgery for the rheumatoid hand—timing and technique. Summary. J. Bone Joint Surg. 50A:614, 1968.

Littler, J. W.: The physiology and dynamic function of the hand. Surg. Clin. North Am. 40:259, 1960.

Littler, J. W.: The finger extensor mechanism. Surg. Clin. North Am. 47:415, 1967.

Littler, J. W., and Eaton, R. G.: Redistribution of forces in the correction of boutonnière deformity. J. Bone Joint Surg. 49A:1267, 1967.

Long, C.: Viscoelastic characteristics of the hand in spasticity. A quantitative study. 45th Annual Session, American Congress Rehabilitation Medicine, Miami Beach, FL, Aug. 27–Sept. 1, 1967.

Long, C.: Intrinsic-extrinsic muscle control of the fingers. Electromyographic studies. Annual Meeting of the American Society of Surgery of the Hand, Chicago, Jan. 19, 1968.

Long, C., and Brown, M. E.: Electromyographic kinesiology of the hand. Muscles moving the long finger. J. Bone Joint Surg. 46A:1683, 1964.

Long, C., Thomas, D. H., and Crochetiere, W. J.: Objective measurements of muscle tone in the hand. Clin. Pharmacol. *5*:909, 1964.

Mackin, E. J.: Hand therapy comes of age. J. Hand Ther. *1*:1, 1987.

Madden, J. W.: Current concepts of wound healing as applied to hand surgery. Orthop. Clin. North Am. *1*:325, 1970.

Madden, J. W., Arem, A., and DeVore, G. L.: A rational postoperative management program for metacarpophalangeal implant arthroplasty. J. Hand Surg. *2*:358, 1976.

Madsen, E.: Delayed primary suture of flexor tendons cut in the digital sheath. J. Bone Joint Surg. *52B*:264, 1970.

Mannerfelt, L., and Malmsten, M.: Arthrodesis of the wrist in rheumatoid arthritis. A technique without external fixation. Scand. J. Plast. Reconstr. Surg. *5*:124, 1971.

Mannerfelt, L., and Norman, O.: Attrition ruptures of flexor tendons in rheumatoid arthritis caused by bony spurs in carpal tunnel. J. Bone Joint Surg. *51B*:270, 1969.

Marks, J. S.: Motor polyneuropathy associated with chloroquine phosphate. Postgrad. Med. J. *55*:569, 1979.

Martel, W., Hayes, J. T., and Duff, I. F.: The pattern of bone erosion in the hand and wrist in rheumatoid arthritis. Radiology *84*:204, 1965.

McDowell, C. L.: Experimental Silastic implants in small joints. Clin. Orthop. *80*:21, 1971.

McEwen, C., and O'Brian, W. B.: A multi-center evaluation of early synovectomy in the treatment of rheumatoid arthritis. J. Rheumatol. (Suppl.) *1*:107, 1974.

McFarland, G., and Hoffer, M. M.: Rheumatoid nodules in synovial membranes and tendons. Clin. Orthop. *58*:165, 1968.

McMaster, M.: The natural history of the rheumatoid metacarpal phalangeal joint. J. Bone Joint Surg. *54B*:687, 1972.

McMaster, P. E.: Late rupture of extensor and flexor pollicis longus following Colles' fracture. J. Bone Joint Surg. *14*:93, 1932.

Meuli, H. C.: Reconstructive surgery of the wrist joint. Hand *4*:88, 1972.

Millender, L. H., and Nalebuff, E. A.: Evaluation and treatment of early rheumatoid hand involvement. Orthop. Clin. North Am. *6*:697, 1975a.

Millender, L. H., and Nalebuff, E. A.: Preventive surgery—tenosynovectomy and synovectomy. Orthop. Clin. North Am. *6*:765, 1975b.

Millender, L. H., and Nalebuff, E. A.: Surgical treatment of the boutonnière deformity in rheumatoid arthritis. Orthop. Clin. North Am. *6*:753, 1975c.

Millender, L. H., and Nalebuff, E. A.: Surgical treatment of the swan neck deformity. Orthop. Clin. North Am. *6*:733, 1975d.

Millender, L. H., Nalebuff, E. A., and Feldon, P. G.: Boutonnière deformity. *In* Green, D. P. (Ed.): Operative Hand Surgery. Vol. II. New York, Churchill Livingstone, 1982.

Millender, L. H., Nalebuff, E. A., and Feldon, P. G.: Combined wrist arthrodesis and metacarpal phalangeal joint arthroplasty operative technique. *In* Green, D. P. (Ed.): Operative Hand Surgery. Vol. II. New York, Churchill Livingstone, 1982.

Millroy, P.: Surgery of the rheumatoid hand. *In* Proceedings of the Australian Orthop. Assoc. J. Bone Joint Surg. *48B*:593, 1966.

Mintz, G., Fraga, A.: Severe osteoarthritis of the elbow in foundry workers. Arch. Environ. Health *27*:78, 1973.

Moberg, E.: Surgical treatment for the absence of single hand grip and elbow extension in quadriplegia. J. Bone Joint Surg. *57A*:196, 1975.

Moskowitz, R. W.: Management of osteoarthritis. Bull. Rheum. Dis. *31*:31, 1981.

Myerdierks, E. M., Mosher, J. F., and Werner, F. W.: Limited wrist arthrodesis. J. Hand. Surg. *12A*:526, 1987.

Nalebuff, E. A.: Diagnosis, classification and management of rheumatoid thumb deformities. Bull. Hosp. Joint Dis. *29*:119, 1968.

Nalebuff, E. A.: Restoration of balance in the rheumatoid thumb. *In* Tubiana, R. (Ed.): The Rheumatoid Hand. Paris, GEM Publication, 1969a.

Nalebuff, E. A.: Surgical treatment of finger deformities in the rheumatoid hand. Surg. Clin. North Am. *49*:833, 1969b.

Nalebuff, E. A.: Surgical treatment of rheumatoid tenosynovitis in the hand. Surg. Clin. North Am. *49*:799, 1969c.

Nalebuff, E. A.: Rheumatoid hand surgery. J. Hand Surg. *8*:678, 1983.

Nalebuff, E. A., and Millender, L. H.: Surgical treatment of the swan neck deformity in rheumatoid arthritis. Orthop. Clin. North Am. *6*:733, 1975.

Nalebuff, E. A., and Potter, T. A.: Rheumatoid involvement of tendons and tendon sheaths in the hand. Clin. Orthop. *59*:147, 1968.

Nalebuff, E. A., Potter, T. A., and Tomaselli, R.: Surgery of the swan neck deformity in the rheumatoid hand. A new approach. Arthritis Rheum. *6*:289, 1963.

Napier, J. R.: The prehensile movements of the human hand. J. Bone Joint Surg. *38B*:902, 1956.

National Center for Health Statistics: Rheumatoid arthritis in adults, United States, 1960–1962. Series II, No. 17, 1966.

National Center for Health Statistics: Prevalence of chronic skin and musculo-skeletal conditions, United States, 1976. Series 10, No. 124, 1978.

Niebauer, J. J., and Landry, R. M.: Dacron-silicone prosthesis for the metacarpophalangeal and interphalangeal joints. Hand *3*:55, 1971.

Palmer, A. K., Dobyns, J. H., and Linscheid, R. L.: Management of post-traumatic instability of the wrist secondary to ligament rupture. J. Hand Surg. *3*:507, 1978.

Palmer, A. K., Werner, F. W., Murphy, D., and Glisson, R.: Functional wrist motion. A biomechanical study. J. Hand Surg. *10A*:39, 1985.

Peimer, C. A., Medige, J., Eckert, B. S., Wright, J. R., and Howard, C. S.: Reactive synovitis after silicone arthroplasty. J. Hand Surg. *11A*:624, 1986.

Perry, J.: Normal upper extremity kinesiology. J. Physical Ther. *58*:265, 1978a.

Perry, J.: Pathomechanical relationship between lesion specificity and residual function. Motor insufficiency I: Pathomechanics. J. Physical Ther. *58*:279, 1978b.

Pinner, J. I.: Placement of arthritic applicants. Arch. Environ. Health *4*:492, 1962.

Radin, E. L.: Mechanical aspects of osteoarthrosis. Bull. Rheum. Dis. *26*:862, 1975–76 series.

Robinson, H. S.: The cost of rehabilitation in rheumatoid disease. J. Chronic Dis. *8*:713, 1958.

Savill, D. L., and Duthie, J. J. R.: Synovectomy of the wrist. *In* Early Synovectomy in Rheumatoid Arthritis Symposium. Amsterdam, Excerpta Medica Foundation, 1967.

Schneider, L. H., Hunter, J. M., Norris, T. R., and Nadeau, P. O.: Delayed flexor tendon repair in no man's land. J. Hand Surg. *2*:452, 1977.

Second Hand Club (Britain): Inaugural Meeting, Royal Infirmary, Derby, Great Britain, May 11, 1956.

Shapiro, J. S., Heijna, W. M., Nasatir, S., and Ray, R. S.: The relationship of wrist motion to ulnar phalangeal drift in the rheumatoid patient. Hand *3*:68, 1971.

Short, C. L., Bauer, W., and Reynolds, W. E.: Rheumatoid Arthritis. A Definition of the Disease and a Clinical Description Based on a Numerical Study of 293 Patients and Controls. Cambridge, MA, Harvard University Press, 1957.

Smith, R. J., and Kaplan, E. B.: Rheumatoid deformities of the metacarpal phalangeal joints of the finger. A correlative study of anatomy and pathology. J. Bone Joint Surg. *49A*:31, 1967.

Smith, R. J., Atkinson, R. E., and Jupiter, J. B.: Silicone synovitis of the wrist. J. Hand Surg. *10A*:47, 1985.

Smith, E. M., Juvinall, R. C., Bender, L. F., and Pearson, J. R.: Flexor forces and rheumatoid metacarpophalangeal deformity. J.A.M.A. *198*:150, 1966.

Social Security Administration: Social Security Disability Applicant Statistics, 1973.

Spinner, M., and Kaplan, E. B.: Extensor carpi ulnaris—its relationship to stability of the distal radioulnar joint. Clin. Orthop. *68*:124, 1970.

Stack, H. G.: Muscle function in the fingers. J. Bone Joint Surg. *44B*:899, 1962.

Stark, H. H., Boyes, J. H., and Wilson, J. N.: Mallet finger. J. Bone Joint Surg. *44A*:1061, 1962.

Stark, H. H., Moore, J. F., Ashworth, C. R., and Boyes, J. H.: Fusion of the first metacarpo-trapezial joint for degenerative arthritis. J. Bone Joint Surg. *59A*:22, 1977.

Steinbrocker, O.: Prognosis for employability in the major arthritides: Rheumatoid arthritis, osteoarthritis and gout. Penn. Med. *72*:82, 1969.

Stern, W. K.: Cutaneous rheumatoid vasculitis. Int. J. Dermatol. *18*:394, 1979.

Straub, L. R., and Wilson, E. H., Jr.: Spontaneous rupture of extensor tendons in the hand associated with rheumatoid arthritis. J. Bone Joint Surg. *38A*:1208, 1956.

Swanson, A. B.: Surgery of the hand in cerebral palsy and the swan neck deformity. J. Bone Joint Surg. *42A*:951, 1960.

Swanson, A. B.: Pathomechanics of the swan-neck deformity. J. Bone Joint Surg. *47A*:636, 1965.

Swanson, A. B.: Silicone rubber implants for replacement of arthritic or destroyed joints of the hand. Surg Clin. North Am. *48*:1113, 1968.

Swanson, A. B.: Silicone rubber implants in trapezio-metacarpal joint arthritis. J. Bone Joint Surg. *51A*:799, 1969.

Swanson, A. B.: The results of silicone rubber implant arthroplasty in the digits. J. Bone Joint Surg. *53A*:807, 1971.

Swanson, A. B.: Treatment of the stiff hand and flexible implant arthroplasty in the fingers. The AAOS Instructional Course Lectures, Vol. 21. St. Louis, C. V. Mosby Company, 1972.

Swanson, A. B.: The ulnar head syndrome and its treatment by implant resection arthroplasty. J. Bone Joint Surg. *54A*:906, 1972.

Swanson, A. B.: Flexible Implant Resection Arthroplasty in the Hand and Extremities. St. Louis, C. V. Mosby Company, 1973a.

Swanson, A. B.: Flexible implant resection arthroplasty of radiocarpal joint. In Swanson, A. B. (Ed.): Flexible Implant Resection Arthroplasty in the Hand and Extremities. St. Louis, C. V. Mosby Company, 1973b.

Swanson, A. B.: Implant arthroplasty for disabilities of the distal radioulnar joint. Orthop. Clin. North Am. *4*:373, 1973c.

Swanson, A. B.: Implant resection arthroplasty of the proximal interphalangeal joint. Orthop. Clin. North Am. *4*:1007, 1973d.

Swanson, A. B.: Proximal interphalangeal and metacarpophalangeal joint flexible implant arthroplasty results. In Swanson, A. B. (Ed.): Flexible Implant Resection Arthroplasty in the Hand and Extremities. St. Louis, C. V. Mosby Company, 1973e.

Testut, L., and Latarjet, R. A.: In Tratado de Anatomia Jumana. Ed. 9. Vol. I. 1951. Salvat Editores SA, Buenos Aires.

Tubiana, R., and Valentin, P.: Anatomy of the extensor apparatus and the physiology of the finger extensor. Surg. Clin. North Am. *44*:897, 1964.

Urbaniak, J. R., McCollum, D. E., and Goldner, J. L.: Metacarpal phalangeal and interphalangeal joint reconstruction. Use of silicone rubber–Dacron prosthesis for replacement of irreparable joints of the hand. South. Med. J. *63*:1281, 1970.

Vaughn-Jackson, O. J.: Rupture of extensor tendons by attrition of the inferior radioulnar joint. Report of two cases. J. Bone Joint Surg. *30B*:528, 1948.

Vaughn-Jackson, O. J.: Attrition ruptures of tendons as a factor in the production of deformities of the rheumatoid hand. Proc. Roy. Soc. Med. *52*:132, 1959.

Vemireddi, N. K., Reford, J. B., and Pombejar, C. N.: Serial nerve conduction studies in carpal tunnel syndrome secondary to rheumatoid arthritis. Arch. Phys. Med. Rehabil. *60*:393, 1979.

Voltz, R. G.: Total wrist arthroplasty. A new approach to wrist disability. Clin. Orthop. *128*:180, 1977.

Wolff, B. B.: How do rheumatic diseases relate to economic potential as influenced by: Personal attitude and motivation. Penn. Med. *72*:68, 1969.

Worsing, R. A., Engber, W. D., and Lange, T. A.: Reactive synovitis from particulate Silastic. J. Bone Joint Surg. *64A*:581, 1982.

Younger, C. P., and DeFiore, J. C.: Rupture of flexor tendons to the fingers after a Colles' fracture. J. Bone Joint Surg. *59A*:828, 1977.

Zancolli, E.: Surgery for the quadriplegic hand with active strong wrist extension preserved. Clin. Orthop. *112*:101, 1975.

tents, and therefore the stenosing tenosynovitis (Meachim and Roberts, 1969).

De Quervain's tenosynovitis clinically presents with the gradual onset of pain, and sometimes swelling, in the area of the radial styloid and first extensor compartment. The pain is exaggerated by the simultaneous flexion of the thumb and ulnar deviation of the wrist. This maneuver is the basis for the so-called Finkelstein test (Fig. 108–8). A palpable thickening of the tenosynovium can frequently be appreciated at the entrance to the first compartment. In severe cases, occasional crepitus or a snapping sensation similar to that seen in flexor tenosynovitis can be felt, as the swollen nodule of tenosynovium pops to and fro under the dorsal retinaculum.

In the chronic situation, adjacent structures such as the branches of the radial sensory or lateral antebrachial cutaneous nerves may be involved by secondary adhesion formation and fibrosis (Rask, 1978). These patients may have numbness and paresthesias in the sensory distributions, in addition to the other clinical features of de Quervain's disease.

Bunnell (1944) believed that the high incidence of de Quervain's disease in women was explained by their increased ability to deviate the wrist ulnarly. Conklin and White (1960) considered that the angulation of tendon pull with wrist motion was exaggerated in women. The frequent coincidence of postmenopausal degenerative arthritis and stenosing tenosynovitis also undoubtedly has some influence (Weilby, 1970).

Wartenberg's syndrome is an entrapment disorder of the radial sensory nerve at the junction of the brachioradialis and extensor carpi radialis longus. Saplys, Mackinnon, and Dellon (1987) stressed that this entity is commonly confused with de Quervain's disease. Both disorders can produce pain in the dorsoradial wrist that is aggravated by ulnar wrist deviation, and both often produce a positive Finkelstein test; the two can be distinguished by the area of maximal tenderness. In Wartenberg's syndrome, tenderness is localized more proximally at the brachioradialis–extensor carpi radialis longus junction, and commonly also shows a positive Tinel's sign at this point. Conversely, de Quervain's disease is characterized by tenderness primarily over the first dorsal wrist compartment. In addition, pain associated with Wartenberg's disease is more commonly of a burning, searing variety and associated with denser changes in sensibility testing of the radial nerve (Saplys, Mackinnon, and Dellon, 1987).

X-ray examination should usually be performed in suspected cases of de Quervain's disease. Most radiographic results are normal, but several authors have suggested that osteoporosis, periosteal reaction, and arthritic changes about the radial styloid may be more common than previously thought (Leao, 1958; Nyska, Floman, and Fast, 1984). More importantly, x-ray examination helps to rule out other common causes of radial wrist pain, such as arthritis of the basal joint of the thumb, occult scaphoid fractures or nonunions, and other intercarpal abnormalities. Basal joint arthritis of the thumb can also be differentiated from de Quervain's disease by the more distal location of pain and tender-

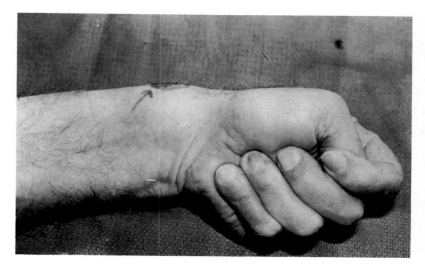

Figure 108–8. Finkelstein's test for de Quervain's disease is performed with the thumb held in a flexed position by the other digits, and the wrist simultaneously deviated in an ulnar direction. This maneuver usually reproduces the pain in the first dorsal compartment.

ness about the metacarpal base. Basilar arthritis is also characterized by a positive "grind" test in which where pain and crepitus is reproduced by longitudinal compression and rotation of the thumb carpometacarpal joint. Scaphoid non-unions can occasionally be confused with de Quervain's disease. However, a more discrete history of wrist trauma, tenderness in the anatomic snuffbox, and appropriate radiographic studies should eliminate any misunderstanding.

Anatomically, the tendons of the extensor pollicis brevis and abductor pollicis longus occupy the first dorsal compartment of the wrist. This tunnel is formed by a groove in the radial styloid below and the thick dorsal retinacular ligament above (Fig. 108–9).

The arrangement of the tendons within the first dorsal compartment has been extensively studied (Finkelstein, 1930; Lacey, Goldstein, and Tobin, 1951; Loomis, 1951; Leao, 1958). Anomalies of the tendinous slips, their insertions, and the compartment itself are the rule rather than the exception. Aber-

rant tendinous slips can exist in up to 75 per cent of cases (Lacey, Goldstein, and Tobin, 1951). The abductor pollicis longus tendon usually has two separate slips, but may have as many as six (Strandell, 1957). The classic teaching of a single abductor pollicis longus tendon is seen in only 10 to 20 per cent of individuals.

Parsons and Robinson (1899) studied 127 forearms and found that only 10 per cent of their dissections had an abductor pollicis longus insertion exclusively at the base of the thumb metacarpal (Loomis, 1951). The other 90 per cent had dual insertions, the second insertion being found, in decreasing order of frequency, to the abductor pollicis brevis, trapezium, opponens pollicis, proximal phalanx of the thumb, and carpometacarpal joint. This study is consistent with Wagenseil's (1936) findings of a dual insertion in 69 per cent of his cases.

The extensor pollicis brevis has been described by Strandell (1957) as a phylogenetically young muscle. It exists as a separate

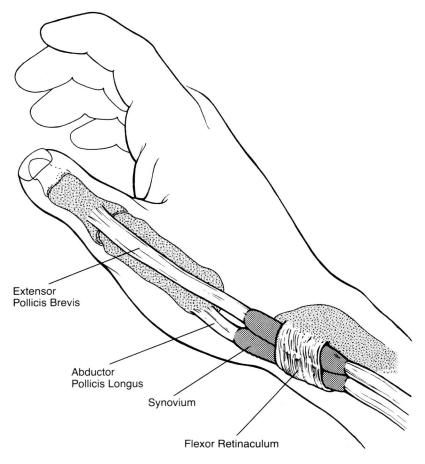

Extensor
Pollicis Brevis

Abductor
Pollicis Longus

Synovium

Flexor Retinaculum

Figure 108–9. The first dorsal compartment of the wrist. The abductor pollicis longus and extensor pollicis brevis tendons pass through the first extensor canal lined by a nourishing tenosynovium. The roof of the compartment is the dorsal retinaculum, the wall is its vertical septa, and the floor is formed by a groove in the radial styloid. Frequent anatomic variations may be the rule rather than the exception.

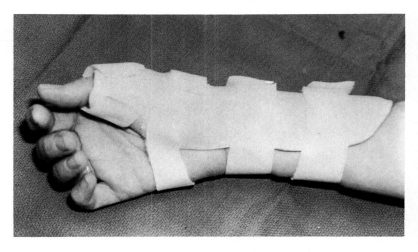

Figure 108–10. Wrist splint for de Quervain's disease. A custom-made Orthoplast splint from the distal forearm to just short of the interphalangeal joint has allowed this 43 year old physician, distrustful of both surgery and steroids, to manage for seven years with intermittent symptoms of dorsal stenosing tenosynovitis.

muscle only in man and gorillas. It is commonly a slender tendon, considerably thinner than the abductor pollicis longus. In contrast to the abductor pollicis longus, the extensor pollicis brevis is a single tendon in 90 per cent (Leao, 1958), a double tendon in only 5 per cent, and absent in 5 per cent (Wood, 1868; Parsons and Robinson, 1899). However, its insertion can also be quite variable. Parsons and Robinson found 72 per cent inserted into the proximal phalanx, 21 per cent into both phalanges, and 7 per cent into the distal phalanx alone.

In addition to the variability of the tendons of the first dorsal compartment, there are common abnormalities of the compartment itself. The most common variation is a longitudinally oriented ridge that separates the first compartment into two separate tunnels (Muckart, 1964; Viegas, 1986). An aberrant third tunnel can occasionally be found anywhere in the fibrous walls of the main compartment (Loomis, 1951; Burman, 1952; Lapidus and Fenton, 1952; Strandell, 1957).

Other anatomic anomalies such as aberrant muscle bellies of the long abductor or short extensor within the compartment can produce the same clinical picture as de Quervain's stenosing tenosynovitis (Patel and Desai, 1988).

Persistent symptoms following attempted surgical release of the first dorsal compartment are commonly seen with this degree of anatomic variability, especially if a systematic search and release of all involved tendinous slips is not carried out. Louis (1987) described a clinical test to distinguish an unreleased extensor pollicis brevis tendon

postoperatively. With the thumb metacarpal held passively in maximal abduction, neutralizing the effect of the abductor pollicis longus tendon, passive flexion of the proximal phalanx reproduces the characteristic wrist pain.

Treatment

The same treatment principles apply to flexor and extensor stenosing tenosynovitis. Splinting and nonsteroidal, anti-inflammatory drugs seem more helpful for de Quervain's disease than for trigger fingers. A well-crafted splint, immobilizing only the radial wrist and thumb base, often gives symptomatic relief yet allows enough mobility for a modified work schedule (Fig. 108–10).

The other primary, nonoperative therapy for de Quervain's disease is a local steroid injection into the first dorsal compartment. The most common injection technique involves entering the compartment proximal to the dorsal retinacular ligament near the point of maximal tenderness. Before needle puncture, active thumb extension helps to localize the position of the tendon accurately. Great care is taken to inject the tendon sheath and to avoid intratendinous infusion. When localization of the synovial sheath is difficult, puncture down to the distal radius periosteum, followed by slow withdrawal of the needle with concomitant gentle plunger pressure, will reveal free flow when the proper space is entered. After a certain volume has been injected, the observer often sees a bulging of the tenosynovium distal to

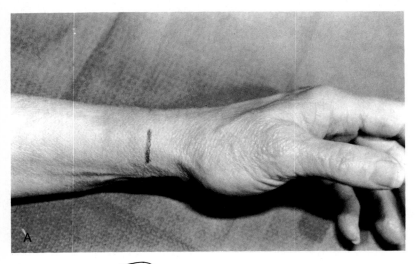

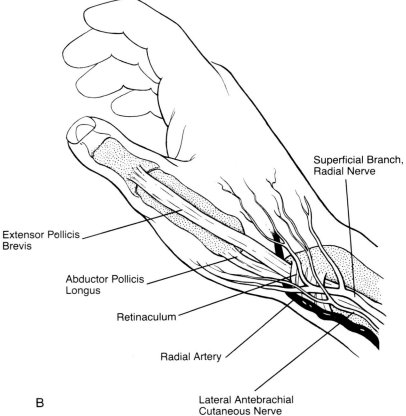

Superficial Branch,
Radial Nerve

Extensor Pollicis
Brevis

Abductor Pollicis
Longus

Retinaculum

Radial Artery

Lateral Antebrachial
Cutaneous Nerve

B

Figure 108–11. Potential incisions for release of de Quervain's disease. *A,* Transverse incisions provide the best possible scar but exposure may be limited. *B,* Any incision must be kept superficial in order to avoid injury to branches of the radial sensory or lateral antebrachial cutaneous nerves.

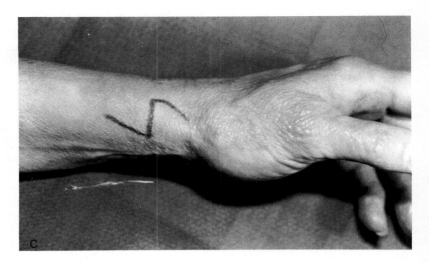

Figure 108–11 *Continued C,* Modified Z-plasty incisions offer improved exposure but intermediate-quality scars. Longitudinal incisions should be avoided because of their tendency to hypertrophy.

the first compartment if the technique has been precise. McKenzie (1972) reported a 93 per cent incidence of complete symptom relief in 30 patients treated in this manner and followed for 18 months. Other authors have not been so successful, but still demonstrate impressive improvement with local steroids, varying from 50 to 70 per cent in retrospective studies (Christie, 1955; Phalen, 1982). Unfortunately, in spite of the popularity of this treatment, there are few controlled studies documenting its efficacy (McGrath, 1984).

Patients should be instructed that after steroid injection, especially if the longer-acting corticosteroids are used, there may be a one or two week time lag between the injection and relief of symptoms. They also need to be advised of possible local side effects such as skin atrophy and pigmentation change (Gray, Kiem, and Gottlieb, 1978).

Although these agents are designed to maximize local improvement and avoid systemic side effects, some leakage and systemic absorption have been noted with their use. To minimize the rare, potential suppression of the hypothalamic-pituitary axis, usually only one synovial sheath (or joint) should be injected at a time. A hiatus of several weeks, depending on the duration of action of the agent used, should be observed between repeat injections. With these precautions, systemic complications should be minimal. Only one case of iatrogenic Cushing's syndrome was reported by Gray, Tenenbaum, and Gottlieb (1981). Strict adherence to sterile technique also minimizes potential septic complications. The Mayo Clinic reported no cases of sepsis after 3000 intra-articular and periar-

ticular steroid injections (Fitzgerald, 1976). The risk of tendon rupture after steroid injection is small, but the precise incidence is difficult to quantify (Halpern, Horowitz, and Nagel, 1977). Since many patients receiving local steroids also have rheumatoid arthritis or a sports-related trauma, a cause and effect relationship between tendon rupture and the steroid injection is often difficult to establish. Gray, Kiem, and Gottlieb (1978) reported no instances of flexor tendon rupture in 300 tendon sheath injections in patients with various forms of digital tendinitis. They also cautioned against frequent injections and stressed accurate injection technique.

Before the popularity of local corticosteroids, many initial reports urged early surgical intervention in the treatment of de Quervain's disease (Piver and Raney, 1952; Woods, 1964). Finkelstein in his review (1930) found no previous descriptions of operative failure or recurrent symptoms, but did observe two such cases himself. Other authors stressed the simplicity of the procedure and minimal complications (Patterson, 1936; Lipscomb, 1951).

More recent investigators have warned of a myriad of potential complications and treatment failures, and a high incidence of associated disease processes (Arons, 1987). Saplys, Mackinnon, and Dellon (1987) reported 17 patients with radial sensory nerve entrapment previously misdiagnosed as de Quervain's disease. Five of these 17 patients had neuromas after the inappropriate release of the first dorsal compartment.

In addition to misdiagnosis and nerve injury, several other complications have been recorded, including hypertrophic scar formation (Lipscomb, 1951), tendon adhesions, and restricted motion (Conklin and White, 1960). One of the most common problems is recurrent symptoms due to incomplete retinacular release or tendon subluxation (Alegado and Meals, 1979; White and Weiland, 1984). Arons (1987) emphasized the need for a careful search for other associated conditions that may complicate the management of patients with de Quervain's disease. His series included patients with trigger fingers, the carpal tunnel syndrome, arthritis, bursitis, tendinitis, fibromyositis, and generalized nonarticular rheumatism.

With these possible pitfalls, combined with the frequently anomalous anatomy, surgery for de Quervain's disease is clearly not as simple as previously thought. Surgical release of the first dorsal compartment is therefore best performed in a bloodless field. Local anesthesia may be adequate for straightforward cases, but intravenous regional or axillary block anesthesia affords the luxury of increased tourniquet time.

Transverse incisions over the compartment are recommended by many because they leave the most forgiving scar (Fig. 108–11A, B). If this approach is chosen, after incising the dermis, the remaining dissection should be a longitudinally oriented, spreading technique to isolate and protect the multiple branches of the radial sensory and lateral antebrachial cutaneous nerves. Belsole (1981) pointed out other potential shortcomings in terms of safe exposure. Longitudinal incisions

should be avoided because of their propensity for forming hypertrophic, painful scars. Curvilinear and modified Z-plasty exposures provide maximal exposure and intermediate quality scars (Fig. 108–11C) (Bruner, 1966; Arons, 1987).

The handling of the dorsal carpal ligament is controversial. De Quervain recommended simply incising the dorsal sheath. Similar advice was given by Conklin and White (1960) and Woods (1954). Others suggested excision of the roof of the canal for more complete decompression (Lipscomb, 1951; Leao, 1958). This latter approach increases the risk of palmar subluxation of the abductor pollicis longus and extensor pollicis brevis tendons (White and Weiland, 1984).

The author's preferred technique is that described by Burton and Littler (1975). Incision of the dorsal ligament is performed over the extensor pollicis brevis tendon, and all intracompartmental septa are released or excised (Rosenthal, 1987). A careful search is made to ensure that all tendinous slips are adequately freed. This technique leaves a radially based flap of retinaculum attached to the radius, which inhibits volar subluxation of the tendons with wrist flexion (Fig. 108–12) (Burton and Littler, 1975; Alegado and Meals, 1979).

In cases with extreme peritendinous fibrosis and dorsal ligament hypertrophy, portions of the retinaculum may need to be excised. After release of the first compartment, a dorsal fibrous ridge occasionally remains that needs to be removed to prevent subluxation

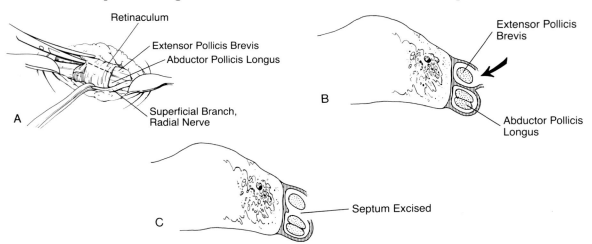

Figure 108–12. Surgical release of the first dorsal compartment for de Quervain's disease. *A,* The dorsal retinaculum is incised over the extensor pollicis brevis tendon, after careful identification and retraction of any overlying sensory nerve branches. *B,* A search must be made for any anomalous tendinous slips, and any accessory intracompartmental septa released. *C,* A radially based cuff of retinaculum is preserved, after compartment decompression, to prevent volar subluxation of the tendons. In severe cases, tenosynovectomy and partial excision of the retinacular roof may be required.

of the tendons and a radial neuritis (Alegado and Meals, 1979). The selective use of local tenosynovectomy and tenolysis are other helpful adjuncts.

Postoperatively, the wrist is splinted for comfort for two to three weeks, but free motion of the thumb and fingers is encouraged immediately.

INTERSECTION SYNDROME

The intersection syndrome was described as early as 1841 by Velpeau. Its current name was coined by Dobyns in 1978. The entity is characterized by pain and swelling where the muscle bellies of the abductor pollicis longus and extensor pollicis brevis cross the two radial wrist extensor tendons. Crepitus in the same area of the distal forearm can often be appreciated with alternating wrist flexion and extension. In the past, most authors considered that the basic pathologic process involves friction at this intersection of tendons and muscle bellies precipitating a local tendinitis (Thompson, Plewes, and Shaw, 1951; Wood and Linscheid, 1973; Dobyns, 1978). More recently, Grundberg and Reagan (1985) reviewed their experience in 13 patients. Each revealed a stenosing tenosynovitis of the extensor carpi radialis longus and brevis within the second dorsal compartment of the wrist. All patients were relieved of their symptoms by release of the second compartment, with no surgery directed at the more proximal muscle bellies. It is noteworthy that no pain or swelling was seen over the second compartment preoperatively; it only became obvious after incising the retinacular sheath intraoperatively. Like other forms of stenosing tenosynovitis, the majority do not require surgery. Most respond to splinting and long-acting, local corticosteroid injection provided that the proper diagnosis is made.

ASSOCIATED DISORDERS

Other Forms of Dorsal Tenosynovitis

Stenosing tenosynovitis has been described in essentially all other dorsal compartments in addition to the first two (Finkelstein, 1930; Dickson and Luckey, 1948; Burman, 1952; Drury, 1960; Spinner and Olshansky, 1973; Ambrose and Goldstone, 1975; Hooper and McMaster, 1979; Mogensen and Mattsson, 1980; Hajj and Wood, 1986).

Tenosynovitis of the extensor digiti minimi has been interestingly described as a mirror image of de Quervain's disease. In both instances the tendon may be duplicated in a majority of cases (Schenk, 1964), and the primary risk of surgical release is a debilitating neuroma. In the case of extensor digiti minimi compression, however, the dorsal ulnar sensory nerve branches are in potential jeopardy, rather than the radial sensory and lateral antebrachial cutaneous nerves, as in de Quervain's (Hooper and McMaster, 1979).

Because of the increased difficulty of establishing the diagnosis of stenosing tenosynovitis of the second through the sixth compartments, surgical exploration may be required more frequently as both a diagnostic and a therapeutic tool. If, on the other hand, the diagnosis is accurately made, most cases should respond to routine, conservative measures effective in other forms of stenosing tenosynovitis.

Early decompression has been suggested by Froimson (1988) for tenosynovitis of the extensor pollicis longus. This entity presents with pain and swelling just distal to Lister's tubercle where the tendon changes direction. The tendon is thought to be particularly prone to spontaneous rupture at this point, especially if related to rheumatoid arthritis or an old Colles' fracture. Incision of the dorsal hood, transposition of the tendon out of its tunnel, and subsequent suturing of the dorsal ligament to prevent subluxation back into the compartment is the recommended treatment.

Rheumatoid arthritis is one of the most frequent causes of tendon and nerve entrapment of the hand and wrist (Phalen, 1972). Its proclivity toward synovial proliferation often leads to de Quervain's disease, trigger fingers, and the carpal tunnel syndrome. In rheumatoid arthritis and other diffuse forms of tenosynovitis, an extensive tenosynovectomy may be indicated to prevent tendon rupture and improve motion. These synovectomies are commonly combined with the release of overlying restraining ligaments to decompress nerves, as in the carpal tunnel syndrome, or tendons, as in dorsal stenosing extensor tenosynovitis. The basic surgical approach suggested for dorsal wrist tenosynovectomy is outlined below; see also Chapter 107.

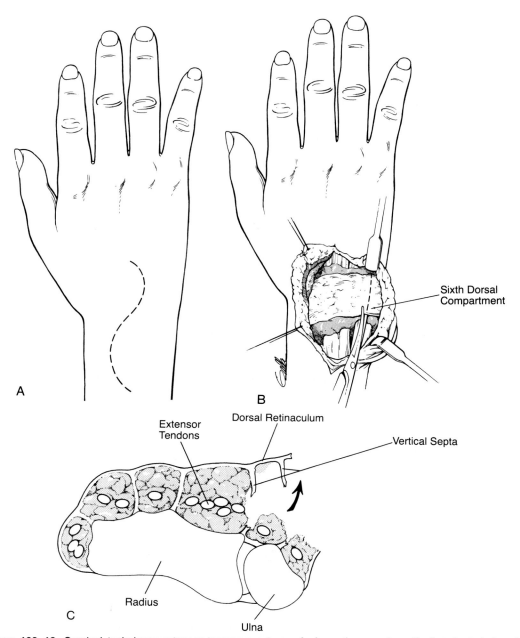

Figure 108–13. Surgical technique: extensor tenosynovectomy. *A,* A gently curved, vertically oriented dorsal wrist incision is used. Large dorsal veins and sensory nerve branches are preserved in the skin flaps. *B,* The dorsal retinaculum is incised through either the sixth or fourth compartment, and the retinacular flaps are developed. *C,* The vertical septa between compartments are released.

appears to be a modified joint fluid (gélee de pomme), which is more mucinous and viscous than normal (McEvedy, 1962). Whether the fluid is produced from the wrist joint or from multifunctional mesenchymal cells within the ganglion is uncertain (Psaila and Mansel, 1978).

Adult women are most frequently affected, as in stenosing tenosynovial disorders. However, ganglia are also seen commonly in men and occasionally in children (MacCollum, 1977). Most cases appear to arise spontaneously, a specific history of trauma being detected in less than 10 per cent of patients (Nelson, Sawmiller, and Phalen, 1972). McEvedy's 1962 study of 150 ganglia revealed no increased risk in occupations that involve work of a repetitive nature.

The most frequent presentation is a rounded, firm, painless mass (Barnes, Larsen, and Posch, 1964). However, in some cases pain may be severe. Small or occult dorsal wrist ganglia commonly have more pain symptoms than large bulbous cysts, for unclear reasons (Gunther, 1985; Angelides 1988). The close relationship of the posterior interosseous nerve to dorsal ganglia has been suggested by Dellon and Seif (1978) as a possible explanation for ganglion-related pain. Gunther believes the pain to be a pressure phenomenon within the scapholunate ligament.

Ganglia, by simple mass effect, have been common causes of significant compression of all three major nerves of the upper extremity, especially the median nerve in the carpal tunnel and the ulnar nerve in Guyon's canal (Mass and associates, 1982; Lucas, 1984; Kerrigan, Bertoni, and Jaeger, 1988; Kuschner, Gelberman, and Jennings, 1988). They also occasionally coexist with tendon entrapment syndromes (Constantian, Zuelzer, and Theogaraj, 1979).

The pathogenesis of ganglia has been obscure and controversial. Most early hypotheses included some form of synovial abnormality, such as synovial herniation, synovial neoplasia, mucinous degeneration of connective tissue, adventitial bursae from the joint capsule, synovial desmoids, and retention cyst formation (McEvedy, 1962).

Andrén and Eiken (1971) demonstrated that injection of ganglia with contrast material reveals no filling of the underlying joint. Conversely, arthrographic injection of the wrist usually communicates with the cyst.

This unidirectional flow has led to the postulation of a one-way valve mechanism. Angelides and Wallace (1976), in their extensive study of 500 ganglia, showed that the larger, clinically evident cyst communicates with a complex, tortuous system of smaller, intracapsular cysts and ducts. This network of serpentine cysts and ducts has been suggested as the possible valvular connection from the main cyst to the scapholunate joint. These authors demonstrated that all their dorsal wrist ganglia were attached to the scapholunate ligament. Most volar ganglia arise from the scaphotrapezial or radiocarpal ligaments. The concentration of ganglia on either side of the wrist, near the scaphoid, is speculated to be no mere coincidence. Chronic stress and scaphoid shear forces may play some role in their frequent formation in these locations (Angelides and Wallace, 1976; Gunther, 1985; Angelides, 1988). This irritation may lead to hyaluronic acid production. Mucin development may then dissect through the ligament and capsule to form small capsular ducts and cysts, which eventually merge to create the principal ganglion.

The most common treatment for ganglia is no treatment. Most patients are asymptomatic, and many never seek medical attention. Another large subgroup present because they are concerned that the new lump may represent a malignancy, and these simply need reassurance. Furthermore, some series have reported spontaneous regression in 40 to 58 per cent of patients (Carp and Stout, 1928; McEvedy, 1962; Zachariae and Vibe-Hansen, 1973). MacCollum (1977) found a 64 per cent resolution in 14 untreated children.

For patients with pain, cosmetic concerns, or symptoms consistent with concomitant entrapment syndromes, a variety of treatment options have been suggested.

The most popular non-operative modalities have included cyst rupture by external compression and needle aspiration, with or without the injection of corticosteroids or sclerosing agents.

Carp and Stout (1928) reported a 78 per cent success rate in nine patients treated by manual rupture. In the literature review of Barnes, Larsen, and Posch (1964), a recurrence rate of approximately 50 per cent was cited in most series treated in a similar manner. It was also suggested that only the more superficial ganglia could be easily broken. McEvedy (1962) estimated that one-half of all ganglia can be ruptured, and that one-half of these will recur.

Nelson, Sawmiller, and Phalen (1972) noted a 66 per cent cure rate in 44 patients treated with digital pressure and rupture. This study also showed a 65 per cent success rate in 46 patients treated with aspiration and triamcinolone injection, compared with a 57 per cent cure in those treated with hyaluronidase injection. McEvedy (1962) noted only an 18 per cent recurrence rate in his series of patients treated with sclerosing agents. The use of steroids and sclerosing medications has declined for several reasons (Mackie, Howard, and Wilkins, 1984). Many of these agents are painful on injection. The current concept of communication between the cyst and the wrist joint raises the possibility of joint sepsis or articular damage, in addition to concerns about skin and tendon atrophy. Finally, the success rates seem only slightly better than the natural history of the cystic process. Corticosteroid injection still is sometimes helpful for short-term pain relief.

The only available prospective study treating ganglia by cyst puncture and aspiration was performed by Richman and associates (1987). Thirty-six per cent of all ganglia treated in this way were cured. If three weeks of immobilization was added, the successful outcome improved to just under 50 per cent. Palmar digital ganglia and those of recent onset do even better (Bruner, 1963). This is the author's currently preferred treatment before recommending surgical excision. Patients must be warned of the possibility of recurrence and that repeat aspiration or surgery may be required. The aspiration is performed with strict aseptic technique. The skin overlying the ganglion is given local anesthesia with a 30 gauge needle. A larger needle (18 or 20 gauge) is then used to puncture the cyst and aspirate its contents (Fig. 108–16). Gentle pressure on the adjacent subcutaneous tissue with the opposite hand helps promote the gelatinous flow. For ganglia of the Al pulley, at the base of the digit, it is sometimes helpful to outline their extent with a marking pencil (Fig. 108–17). This aids in accurately locating the cyst before any soft tissue distortion results from the local anesthetic, and helps prevent puncturing too far laterally toward a digital nerve.

Until recently, the surgical excision of ganglia was plagued by relatively high recurrence rates. Zachariae and Vibe-Hansen (1973) reported a 34 per cent recurrence rate in a series of 347 cases. McEvedy's literature review (1962) summarized a 24 per cent relapse in 163 patients. Several authors speculated that smaller, unrecognized cysts may account for these difficulties (Andrén and Eiken, 1971; Zachariae and Vibe-Hansen, 1973). Clarification of the anatomic connection between the main cyst and multiple smaller intracapsular cysts and ducts has led to a new surgical approach with a recurrence rate of less than 1 per cent (Angelides and Wallace, 1976).

Dorsal wrist ganglia are usually excised through a small transverse incision. Care must be taken to identify and preserve branches of the radial sensory nerve (Fig. 108–18). A bloodless field and magnification are clearly helpful in this regard. The adjacent extensor tendons are retracted, and the main cyst is gently dissected down to the dorsal wrist capsule. The radial side of the

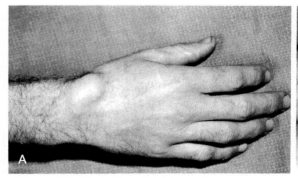 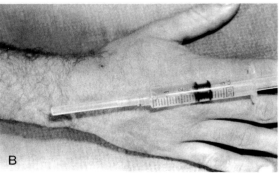

Figure 108–16. *A,* Dorsal wrist ganglia are aspirated under strict sterile technique. *B,* After the skin has been anesthetized with 1 per cent lidocaine and a 30 gauge needle, the cyst is punctured and aspirated with a larger-bore needle. Multiple punctures and counterpressure with the opposite hand are useful adjuncts.

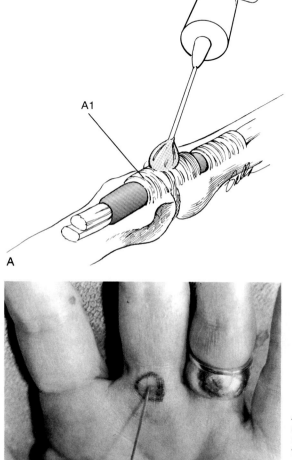

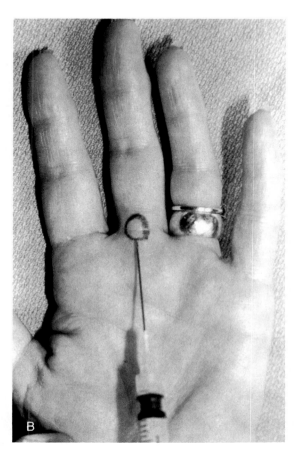

Figure 108–17. Flexor tendon sheath ganglion aspiration. *A,* The treatment of choice for most digital ganglia is simple needle aspiration. *B,* Most digital ganglia present as a tender, rounded mass in the distal palm, in this case the long finger flexor sheath. Outlining the ganglion with a marker aids in subsequent needle localization, after any distorting effect of the local anesthetic. *C,* The needle enters the skin directly over the flexor tendon sheath to avoid digital nerve injury. Usually a single puncture and aspiration is required.

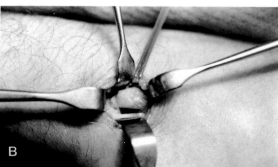

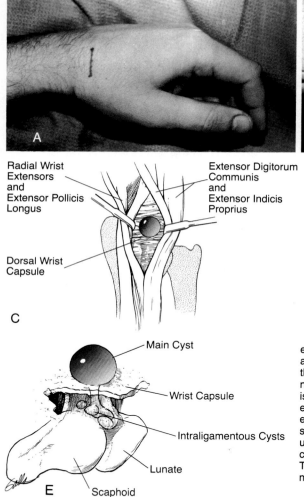

Radial Wrist
Extensors
and
Extensor Pollicis
Longus

Extensor Digitorum
Communis
and
Extensor Indicis
Proprius

Dorsal Wrist
Capsule

C

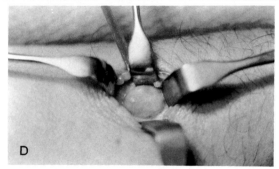

Main Cyst

Wrist Capsule

Intraligamentous Cysts

Lunate

Scaphoid

E

Figure 108–18. Surgical technique: dorsal wrist ganglion excision. *A,* Transverse incisions offer excellent scars and adequate exposure for most dorsal ganglia originating from the scapholunate joint. *B,* Branches of the radial sensory nerve must be identified and preserved. *C,* The main cyst is exposed by retracting the radial wrist extensors and extensor pollicis longus radially, and the fourth compartment extensors ulnarly. *D,* The main cyst may be rounded and smooth or multiloculated, as in this case. *E,* The main cyst usually communicates with a series of smaller intra-articular cysts and ducts attached to the scapholunate ligament. These smaller cysts and a circular window of joint capsule must be excised to minimize the possibility of recurrence.

capsule is incised, and small cysts and duct connections to the scapholunate ligament are searched for and excised en bloc with the main cyst. This usually requires the removal of a small circular window of capsule and a thin shave of the ligament, exposing the wrist joint. Overgenerous ligament excision should be avoided to prevent postoperative wrist instability. The joint is left open, and the skin simply closed after obtaining hemostasis.

Volar-radial ganglia, like their dorsal counterparts, must be traced down to the scaphotrapezial or radioscaphoid ligaments, and all secondary cysts and ducts removed. Preoperatively, an Allen's test is crucial, and the integrity of the ulnar artery must be ensured. These ganglia are frequently adherent to the radial artery. With caution, they can almost always be dissected safely from the artery with routine microsurgery technique. An alternative, suggested by Lister and Smith (1978), is to leave a thin portion of the cyst wall attached to the vessel. If the radial artery is injured, the author prefers to repair it microsurgically. On the other hand, the artery can be safely ligated, if necessary, provided the hand is adequately profused through the ulnar side. Volar radial ganglia can sometimes be confused with pseudoaneurysms of the radial artery (Fig. 108–19). Pseudoaneurysms usually have a history of specific trauma. Expansile pulsations from the aneurysm can usually be palpated in all directions. The radial artery pulse, stretched over a ganglion, is usually more localized. Pseudoaneurysms also frequently have a bluish tint and positive Allen's test. If differentiation is still unclear, ultrasonography, MRI scanning, or angiography, on rare occasions, may be required.

Transverse incisions are inadequate for safe exposure of volar wrist ganglia and preservation of the radial artery and radial sensory and palmar cutaneous nerves. Curvilin-

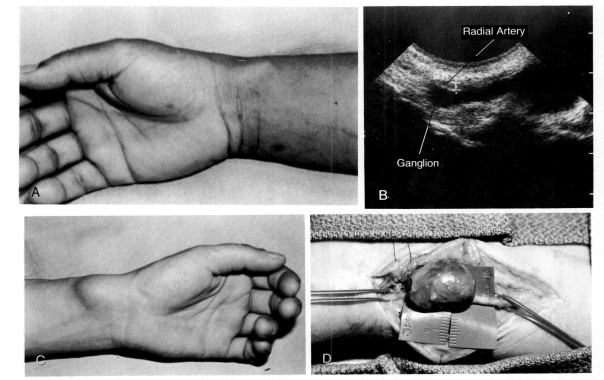

Figure 108–19. A careful history and physical examination can usually distinguish between a volar wrist ganglion and a pseudoaneurysm of the radial artery. In ambiguous cases, certain radiologic techniques may be helpful. *A,* Volar wrist mass in an active electrician with a history of frequent minor wire puncture wounds. *B,* Preoperative ultrasonography demonstrates a volar wrist ganglion independent of the radial artery. *C,* Large volar-radial mass in a former drug addict. *D,* Digital subtraction angiography allowed full preoperative identification and counseling prior to resection and vein grafting of this radial artery pseudoaneurysm.

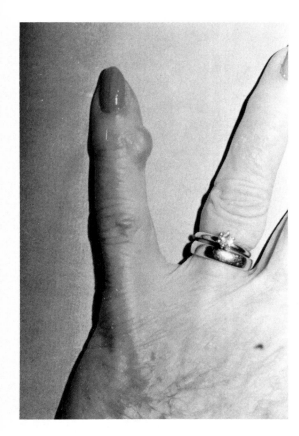

Figure 108–20. Mucous cysts are ganglia originating from the distal interphalangeal joint. They present as a rounded mass to the side of the extensor insertion.

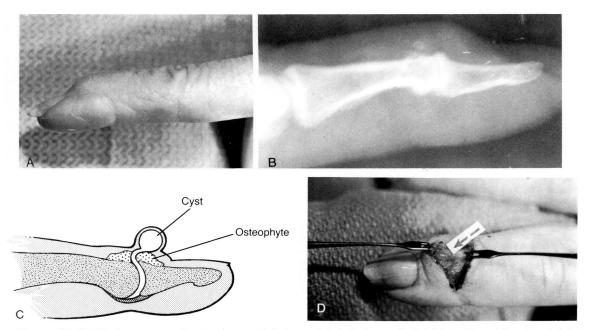

Figure 108–21. Most mucous cysts arise from an irritative, osteophytic focus. *A,* Painful swelling of the dorsal distal interphalangeal joint with a mild extension lag in a 67 year old woman. *B,* Lateral radiograph demonstrates a large osteophyte dorsal to the joint. *C,* The overlying mucous cyst communicates with the joint and is adjacent to the bone spur. *D,* Proper excision requires removal of both the cyst and the spur.

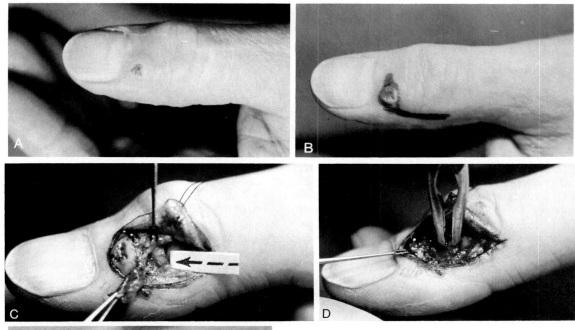

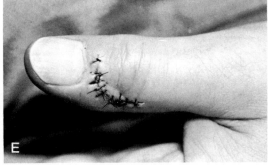

Figure 108–22. Surgical technique: mucous cyst excision. The patient decompressed the mucous cyst with a needle, after two failed excisions by his local doctor. *B,* A gently curved incision, including an elliptic excision of adherent, attenuated skin, is designed. This can be extended proximally as needed. *C,* All soft tissue between the extensor tendon and collateral ligament should be excised down into the distal interphalangeal joint. *D,* Bone irregularities are excised with a small rongeur. *E,* Simple closure is preferred. Complicated flaps or grafts are rarely needed.

ear or zigzag-type incisions across the wrist crease provide better visibility and allow for extension into the carpal tunnel or under the thenar musculature if necessary.

Most volar digital ganglia disappear with simple aspiration. Those that require excision are simply handled by removing a small, rectangular portion of the A1 pulley in continuity with the cyst. Dissection should not stray laterally toward the neurovascular bundles, and the continuity of the A2 pulley must be preserved distally.

Mucous Cysts (See also Chap. 133)

Mucous cysts are histologically identical to ganglia in other locations. They arise on the dorsum of the finger, at or distal to the distal interphalangeal joint (Fig. 108–20). The earliest sign may be longitudinal grooving of the nail, due to pressure on the nail matrix. More characteristically, they present as a small, firm, rounded mass to the side of the extensor tendon insertion. The skin overlying the cyst is frequently adherent and attenuated. These masses tend to occur in an older age group than wrist ganglia, and are frequently associated with osteoarthritic changes. Careful cyst dissections almost invariably reveal some communication with the underlying distal interphalangeal joint (Kleinert and associates, 1972; Newmeyer, Kilgore, and Graham, 1974). Most modern authors believe that osteophytic irritation is the primary nidus for cyst formation (Eaton, Dobranski, and Littler, 1973; Angelides, 1988). Appropriate radiographic examination is therefore indicated in all cases before surgery (Fig. 108–21).

Before the 1970's, many forms of treatment were tried with frustrating results, including aspiration, incision and drainage, irradiation, sclerosing injection, and cauterization. Careful excision of the cyst alone commonly resulted in recurrence rates between 25 and 50 per cent (Eaton, Dobranski, and Littler, 1973). At the time, the most commonly recommended treatment was excision and skin grafting; this led to a significant number of complications, including joint stiffness, nail deformity, and tender grafts (Constant and associates, 1969).

The appreciation by Newmeyer, Kilgore, and Graham (1974) of the connection between the cyst and the joint, and by Eaton, Dobranski, and Littler (1973) and Kleinert and associates (1972) of the association with degenerative joint disease, changed current treatment concepts. Careful cyst excision, including any stalklike connection to the joint, combined with removal of the osteoarthritic bone spicules dramatically reduced recurrence rates to under 3 per cent (Kleinert and associates, 1972; Eaton, Dobranski, and Littler, 1973).

Mucous cysts are removed to control pain, to improve the cosmetic appearance, and to reduce the risk of septic arthritis. Patients frequently pick at these cysts and occasionally try to "pop" them with a needle. Difficult joint infections have been reported as a sequela (Rangarathnam and Linscheid, 1984). Transverse incisions for small cysts, or gently curved incisions that can be converted into a modest rotation flap, are best (Fig. 108–22). More elaborate flaps or skin grafts usually are not required and may lead to unnecessary joint stiffness and increased scarring (Constant and associates, 1969; MacCollum, 1975). If the overlying skin is severely thinned and adherent, a small skin ellipse is usually excised at the same time. Occasionally, intentional preoperative needle puncture can be helpful, allowing the skin to contract for several days before the formal excision is made. If this method is used, meticulous sterile technique and wound care is important, and the patient should be started on oral antibiotics.

The cyst and all soft tissue between the collateral ligament and extensor insertion should be cleared down into the distal joint. The nail matrix must be preserved; nail deformities usually resolve after proper cyst removal. The extensor tendon is gently mobilized, and bone spurs are leveled with a fine power bur or bone rongeur. Inspection of the entire joint is mandatory to rule out occasional accessory cysts connected by an isthmus, under the extensor tendon, to the main cyst (Newmeyer, Kilgore, and Graham, 1974).

Adequate excision of osteophytes not uncommonly results in minor tears of the extensor tendon. These should be repaired with nonabsorbable sutures, and the distal interphalangeal joint should be splinted in extension. In the usual case with no extensor tendon damage, early motion is encouraged after solid wound healing.

this topic. In the course of these studies, Sunderland examined the major peripheral nerves of the upper and lower extremity, and described the topographic relationship of their fascicles. This was done by positively identifying known branches and then tracing them into the substance of the main trunk of the nerve. The nerves under investigation were then serially sectioned so that the positively identified branches could be followed within the nerve as far as possible. This was the point where they merged with other fascicles within the substance of the nerve. Unfortunately (at least for surgeons), Sunderland chose to illustrate his work with a three-dimensional reconstruction of the musculocutaneous nerve. In this he showed the intermingling and crossover of fibers as they traveled from one bundle to the other, stressing the consequent change in the cross sectional appearance of the nerve (Fig. 109–2).

Sunderland's observations are of course true, but readers extrapolated from this work and it was widely interpreted by surgeons to mean that accurate alignment of fascicles is

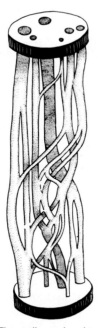

Figure 109–2. Three-dimensional reconstruction of the musculocutaneous nerve (Sunderland). The changing cross sectional relationship and interconnections between fascicles are evident. Despite this variable structure, groups of bundles tend to occupy more or less the same quadrant, making repair and functional recovery still possible. (Reproduced with kind permission from Sidney Sunderland and Churchill Livingstone.)

not possible. This may be so from a pure anatomic standpoint, but *it does not necessarily pertain from the standpoint of nerve repair,* where a successful outcome is measured by functional recovery (Jabaley, Wallace, and Heckler, 1980).

It is necessary to consider briefly the nature of the musculocutaneous nerve to understand the amount of crossing over that is seen there and to appreciate why this phenomenon may be less significant in other peripheral nerves more distal in the extremity, where injury frequently occurs.

The musculocutaneous nerve is a mixed motor and sensory nerve that originates mostly from C5 and C6 of the brachial plexus and, to a variable extent, from C7. It then runs a relatively short course to its target muscles in the upper arm: the coracobrachialis, biceps, and brachialis. Thereafter, it continues as a sensory nerve, the lateral antebrachial cutaneous nerve of the forearm. Because of its multiple level origin and its short course, considerable sorting of motor and sensory fibers into appropriate branches must occur before the musculocutaneous nerve reaches its target areas. This most likely accounts in part for the shifting of fibers observed between fascicles of this nerve, but the phenomenon is probably less dramatic elsewhere.

Relative to the musculocutaneous nerve, the other major nerves of the upper extremity travel a longer (and more leisurely) course, and migration of fibers between fascicles seems to occur much more gradually in the median, ulnar, and radial nerves. Even though various bundles may change their appearance and position relative to each other, it is even more significant that fibers within the bundles seem to run in more or less the same quadrant for considerably longer distances. From a practical standpoint, this means that the cross sectional appearance of a nerve may be constantly changing, but that *it is still possible to make a reasonable estimate for functional alignment purposes and at least connect appropriate quadrants with the expectation that some degree of recovery may occur.* Needless to say, the longer the segment of nerve that is missing, the less precise such match-ups become. On the other hand, this internal convolution may be partly offset by the fact that the major nerves in the upper arm are made up in such a way that, as one proceeds proximally, dispersal of fibers is greater and all bundles seem to contain some fibers destined for every location. Although accurate alignment becomes impossible, a few fibers may still be correctly connected and some recovery is possible. (The reader should recall the work of Sherren, who is said to have had 25 per cent of his own ulnar nerve in the upper arm purposely cut with no apparent loss of function, presumably because the remaining 75 per cent contained fibers destined for all target areas).

INTERNAL ANATOMY

As is often the case in an evolving and dynamic system, new discoveries produce new structures to be named, and earlier titles may not be completely appropriate. Not unlike an archaeologic dig, one can trace back through the nomenclature of nerve anatomy and nerve repair and appreciate each generation of surgeons and its problems. Nevertheless, if we are to make significant headway in the treatment of nerve injuries, we must have a common language. The terminology in the following section is based on the report of the Committee on Nomenclature of the International Society of Reconstructive Microsurgery and is modified slightly (Millesi and Terzis, 1983, 1984).

A peripheral nerve consists of both nervous and non-nervous tissue (Kuczynski, 1974). The nervous tissue is ectodermal in origin, conducts impulses, and is the transmitting part of the nerve. The non-nervous portion is mesodermal in origin, serves a supportive and nutritional role, and is not directly involved in impulse conduction. When a nerve is transected and repaired, it is the non-nervous portion that "heals," permitting the conducting fibers to grow back across this bridge of scar.

The functional part of a nerve is the *fiber* (synonym: axon). Fibers are long extensions of cell bodies that lie in the dorsal root ganglia or the anterior horn cells of the spinal cord. They are the longest cells in the body, literally reaching all the way to the tips of the fingers or toes. Groups of fibers that travel together and are enclosed are known as *fascicles* (or funiculi), and two or more fascicles form a *bundle*. One or more bundles constitute a peripheral nerve (Fig. 109–3).

The non-neural tissue is of three types:

epineurium, perineurium, and endoneurium. *Epineurium* is thin and filmy, loosely attached, and easy to dissect. Within it are the blood vessels, the lymphatics, and a considerable amount of collagen and fibroblasts. When nerves are sutured, epineurial fibroblasts are the primary source of collagen for healing. It is important to appreciate that epineurium can be divided into external (epifascicular) epineurium and internal (interfascicular) epineurium. External epineurium is that layer which encompasses the whole nerve, while internal epineurium lies between individual fascicles or bundles of fascicles.

Perineurium is a more definite structure, has greater strength, and is made up of six to nine lamellae arranged in different directions, not unlike the plies of a tire. It separates the internal and external environment of the nerve and is clearly a functional barrier. Within the perineurium is the *endoneurium* and the functioning axons, their Schwann cells, and myelin. The *milieu* within the perineurium differs in chemical composition and pressure from that without. It is important that perineurium be preserved if further damage to the already injured nerve is to be avoided. As noted earlier, from a surgical as well as a functional standpoint, the internal epineurium is the plane of dissection within a nerve. It now appears that one can incise epineurium, remove it as necessary, and use it in any way that seems appropriate without danger and without damage to the functioning portion of nerve, so long as perineurium is not violated. Although authors may disagree about the technique of suture placement, epineurium is the tissue of repair.

PHYSIOLOGY

In the normal nerve, conduction occurs at various speeds, ranging from 2.0 to 150 m per sec. Conduction velocity is directly related to the amount of myelin about the fibers and fiber diameter. In general, the thicker the myelin, the faster the nerve conducts. Conduction in myelinated nerves is fastest (3 to 150 m/sec) and occurs from node of Ranvier to node of Ranvier by the process of saltatory conduction. In unmyelinated fibers, the process is slower (2 to 2.5 m/sec).

When a nerve is physically transected, all

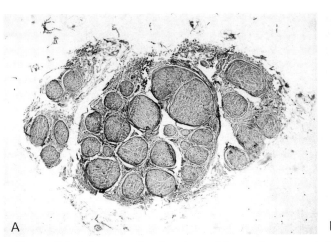 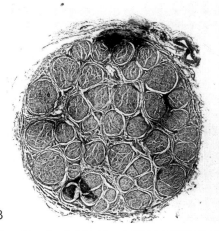

Figure 109–3. Cross sectional anatomy of the median nerve at different levels. *A,* Wrist level. The variation in size of fascicles and fascicular groups is evident. At this level, there is considerable internal epineurium between portions of the nerve because it is dividing into its terminal branches. Individual branches and bundles are easily identifiable and associated with specific function. Separate repair is indicated. *B,* A section from the same nerve at the midforearm level where there are no branches. Fascicles are tightly packed and a minimum of epineurium is evident. A blood vessel is visible in the external epineurium at the 1 o'clock position. Group fascicular repair at this level would produce satisfactory alignment.

its axons are divided. (For practical purposes, peripheral nerves consist only of axons and their surrounding tissue. The cell body of first order neurons as well as the remainder of the central nervous system are not within the purview of the peripheral nerve surgeon.) The axons distal to the level of transection degenerate and die; their myelin degenerates and is absorbed. The structural tissue surrounding these axons remains in place and undergoes a slower process of degeneration. This sequence was first described by Waller and is still called *wallerian degeneration.* When a nerve is completely transected, the process is easily understood, but it is important to understand that wallerian degeneration may also occur in a nerve that is clinically intact. In a crush or stretch injury, the epineurium or both epineurium and perineurium may survive but axons may still degenerate distal to the injury.

Both Sunderland and Seddon offered classifications of nerve injury that take into account that varying degrees of nerve damage may occur. Although their classifications are different, the import is the same. Other than in transection, the degree of nerve damage may not be apparent at the time of initial inspection. Practically speaking, one should understand that the degeneration does not occur immediately upon injury and may not

be apparent in nerves that have been crushed, stretched, torn, or twisted. For this reason, a surgeon may unwittingly repair nerve that is destined to degenerate and may have little or no potential for recovery. (This point is explored in greater detail in the section on Nerve Repair.) For the present, it is sufficient to appreciate that one cannot always accurately evaluate the degree of damage to a nerve at the time of injury.

A number of laboratory models for studying nerve recovery have been based on nerves that are crushed and allowed to degenerate, and then regenerate. Such studies have the advantage of eliminating malalignment as a factor and permitting study of the rate of regeneration in a relatively simpler model. Once transection is introduced, the matter becomes instantly more complicated and difficult to study. Whenever wallerian degeneration occurs, whether as the result of crush or of transection, recovery follows in a more or less predictable fashion. The cell body becomes metabolically hyperactive and axons begin to sprout and divide at the injury site. These axons are then drawn along solid substrates into the distal nerve. They appear to be selectively attracted by Schwann cells, but will follow other available structures, such as vessels or even collagen fibers. Although there is no evidence at present to suggest

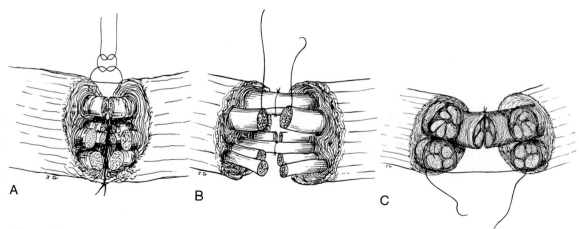

Figure 109–4. Three accepted techniques of nerve suture. *A,* External epineurial suture. Landmarks, such as blood vessels, are identified on the external surface of the nerve and stitches are placed in the external epineurium only. The disadvantages of such a technique are either that fascicles may retract away from each other and produce a gap, or sutures may be placed very far from the edges, allowing fascicles to overlap each other, owing to the telescoping. Since no stitches are placed in individual fascicles or bundles, alignment is not reliable. *B,* Interfascicular repair. Individual fascicles are identified and joined by stitches placed in their perineurium. This technique offers the advantage of accurate alignment, but at the expense of surgical trauma and foreign body. Sutures placed in perineurium may result in localized loss of function at that site. *C,* Group fascicular repair. Groups or bundles of fascicles, such as those seen in Figure 109–3, are identified by their anatomic separation or by function and joined as groups. The technique has the advantage of less surgical trauma and fewer stitches while still permitting accurate alignment of subcomponents.

tactic forces that select motor sensory fibers, their presence cannot be ruled out. For the present, however, the surgeon must rely on accurate alignment if there is to be functional recovery.

TECHNIQUE OF NERVE REPAIR

Simply put, the goal of nerve repair is to construct a juncture across which regenerating axons can advance. This is currently achieved with stitches, but it is becoming increasingly apparent that "nerve suture" may not always be the best possible technique. Despite some research to the contrary, suture remains the procedure of choice for joining nerve ends. For this reason, it is useful to define the ideal nerve repair, realizing that it may not be possible to attain but that it can serve as a model to guide the technique.

The ideal nerve repair should be performed as a primary procedure between viable nerve ends. There should be minimal tension, so that the ends lie in actual contact and remain there during the healing phase. Alignment between appropriate fascicles and bundles should be perfect, to permit fiber regeneration. There should be no foreign body, no hematoma, and no bacterial inoculum at the juncture. The repair should lie in a well-vascularized bed that contains as little scar as possible, and it should be mobilized early so that it glides freely through surrounding tissue.

In an effort to avoid the obligatory foreign body reaction associated with suture material, some surgeons have recently used fibrin glue to join nerve ends. Although this technique is not presently available in the United States (the theoretical risk of viral infection and AIDS makes acceptance unlikely), a modification of it will likely become so in the future. Fibrin is presently being used in Europe and other parts of the world and appears to have promise.

Other investigative efforts along these lines use the laser as a form of "spot-welding" to bond the nerve ends. Its advantages are that the "burn" created can be precisely located and produced in such a way that it is confined to the epineurium and does not affect the perineurium or the fibers contained therein. Laser technique is highly experimental and is not recommended for nerve repair in humans at this time.

Practically speaking, three techniques for nerve repair have been described (Fig. 109–4). From a technical standpoint, they differ in suture placement, but all have in common an attempt to align fascicles accurately. Al-of the median and ulnar nerves. Results in young children are better but still do not achieve normalcy.

When root avulsions are present, the results at best may be only partly acceptable. This is so when damage involves more than 6 cm of the upper, 4 cm of the medial, 3 cm of the lower trunks, the origins of the median and ulnar nerves, and to a lesser extent the origin of the radial nerve. In massive root avulsions at best only one or two of the numerous functions of the upper limb will be partially restored. Normal function of the hand cannot be expected when fascicles originating from the three lower roots have been injured.

Knowing these facts, the surgeon has to decide whether amputation in severe cases or musculotendinous transfers and other reconstructive measures in milder cases will yield a better result than complex nerve reconstruction. An association of all reconstructive methods and nerve repair has to be considered every time. In addition, experience shows that for manual workers and for most intellectually active people, results have to be excellent or at least very good in order to qualify surgery as successful. All other results, however satisfying to the surgeon, will be considered by the patient as poor or of very little use. There will be no parallelism between the functional result achieved and professional rehabilitation. The patient will act mostly as a one-handed individual. This means that in very severe lesions, sophisticated surgery, restoring a little function, or no treatment at all have the same impact in relation to economic activity. It must be stressed, however, that pain syndromes that can ruin the life of a patient with a BPI are half as frequent in individuals who have undergone surgery as in those with severe pain syndromes caused by root avulsion who have not had surgery. In this regard, the advantages of nerve repair are even more marked in patients with extraforaminal lesions; over 90 per cent of these will be cured of their pain.

Root Avulsion C5–T1. In complete avulsion of all five roots of the brachial plexus alternatives are (1) to do nothing specific and to help the patient to accept the situation and resort to some rehabilitation procedures, (2) to fit the patient with an active or passive splint, (3) to amputate the extremity as low as sensitive skin permits it, or (4) to proceed to various nerve transfers (neurotization).

Conservative Measures. These have matured over many years and have proved their usefulness. Whatever the type of treatment chosen, the various steps undertaken should relate to the prognosis. When the dominant arm is affected, contralateral side activity should be fostered as soon as possible and professional rehabilitation should be oriented to the activity of a single extremity if the prognosis is poor. It is of paramount importance to build up the patient's hopes of obtaining future economical and personal independence. This approach is similar to that adopted for paraplegic individuals.

Splinting. Acceptance of splints varies according to their bulk and usefulness. Patients may keep them only for certain activities. When scapular control improves with time, a secondary shoulder fusion will reduce the size of the splint and improve its use.

Amputation. Amputation can be considered only in exceptional conditions in which the patient insists on it. The patient should be encouraged to talk to an amputee and to inspect a prosthesis. Amputation is almost always refused by women and should not be proposed to the parents of a young patient. Current fashions in dressing and the frequency of outdoor activities are factors that may attract more attention to a missing limb than to a paralyzed extremity. Deafferentation pain syndromes and a painful phantom, which are frequent in massive root avulsions, are contraindications to amputation, which might make the pain worse. Patients may have false ideas about the performances of prostheses in high amputations, and will discard them unless they are essential for their activities, or use them only for cosmetic reasons.

Recovery of some scapular control and some protective sensation in the arm may allow a lower amputation with a longer humeral stump combined with a shoulder arthrodesis. This will enhance the usefulness of prosthetic fitting. When considering amputation, it may therefore be worthwhile to delay and wait for maximal recovery, even if this disturbs full rehabilitation. Selective amputation at the level of the arm has been performed in only five of the author's patients (4 per cent) out of 130 with very severe BPI. One patient committed suicide later on; he was a drug addict and had a persisting deafferentation pain syndrome that increased after removal of his arm. The author has not performed any

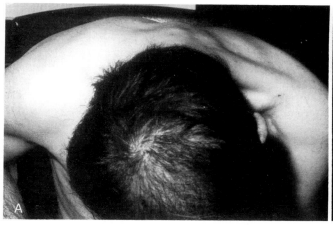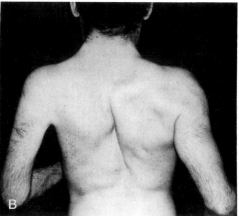

Figure 110–1. In this patient with avulsion of all roots on the left side, the XIth nerve has been used for neurotization of the musculocutaneous with a 12 cm intermediate graft. Elbow function is at M3$^+$. Intercostals could not be used because of numerous rib fractures and a phrenic nerve palsy. It is interesting to note that the upper trapezius is partially affected, lower and middle portion being atrophic (*A*). Active posterior projection of the shoulder shows flexion of the elbow and the partial atrophy of the trapezius (*B*).

amputations in the last ten years, even though the possibility has been discussed very openly with patients.

Neurotization. Motor donor nerves for transfer are the spinal accessory (XIth), to a lesser extent the dorsalis scapulae (if it depends totally or mainly on a healthy C4), and the intercostal nerves. The C2–C4 posterior rami to the deep muscles of the neck, as well as the great occipital nerve, have proved impractical because of difficulty of access. There are no motor nerves in the area other than those mentioned or those combining to form the XIth nerve. The use of the so-called deep cervical plexus is limited to the above. Sensory donor nerves are rami of the cervical plexus and intercostal nerves.

The usual recipients in C5–T1 avulsions are the suprascapular nerve, sometimes the long thoracic nerve, the musculocutaneous nerve or lateral cord, and the lateral origin of the median nerve.

Several alternatives are available for the use of each neurotizer.

The *spinal accesory nerve* is transferred as distally as possible via an intermediate graft to the musculocutaneous nerve, in order to allow elbow flexion. A shoulder arthrodesis is not always necessary, as the reinnervated biceps stabilizes this joint to some degree, and through its long head produces a few degrees of active internal rotation of the humerus. An M3$^+$ or even M4 elbow flexion is obtained in this manner, but the brachio-thoracic "pinch" or "grasp" remains paralyzed and relies on the weight of the arm alone. Arthrodesis of the shoulder may improve its stability and provide an active brachiothoracic grasp so long as the rhomboids and the middle trapezius remain innervated. The spinal accessory is not taken entirely but in its anterior and distal portion, thus only partially denervating the upper and middle trapezius (Fig. 110–1). This denervation has as a consequence an improved cosmetic appearance of the shoulder as it will not be permanently elevated, a compulsory deformity when shoulder depressors remain paralyzed. The XIth nerve does not provide any sensory fibers to the neurotized area. The author favors the transfer of the spinal accessory nerve not on the musculocutaneous but onto the suprascapular nerve, either by suturing or gluing it directly to the recipient, or by using a very short (2 to 4 cm) fascicular graft. Arthrodesis of the shoulder will not be considered in cases treated in this way, and thoracobrachial pinch is reconstructed by transferring one intercostal nerve onto the anterior thoracic nerves innervating the pectoralis major. Patients obtain about 40 degrees of real abduction in the shoulder, bring their forearm about 15 to 25 degrees away from the thorax, and can actively hold large flat objects between their extremity and the chest (Fig. 110–2).

Elbow flexion is reconstructed in these cases by the use of two to four intercostal

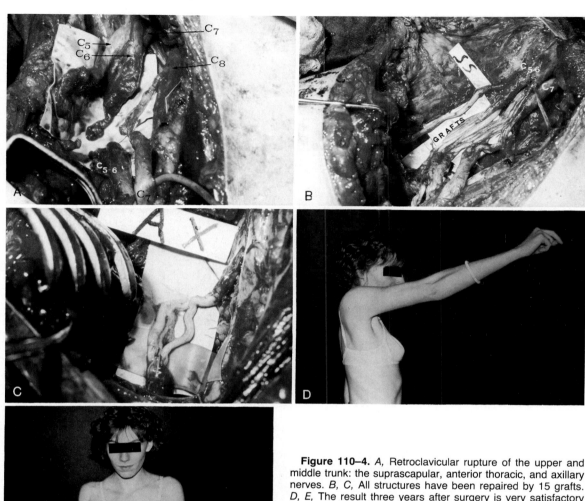

Figure 110–4. *A,* Retroclavicular rupture of the upper and middle trunk: the suprascapular, anterior thoracic, and axillary nerves. *B, C,* All structures have been repaired by 15 grafts. *D, E,* The result three years after surgery is very satisfactory even if shoulder abduction is limited. There is always a possibility that this function may be supplemented with musculotendinous transfers, but the patient prefers to delay this further operation.

form the sides of a triangle, C6 being on the short leg, thus having a shorter capacity for elongation and a more direct course toward the spinal cord, while C5 is protected by stronger foraminal ligaments and makes a more acute angle on the fulcrum represented by the bony gutter. At present, the best was to repair C5 rupture and C6 avulsion is to make a combined nerve transfer. The XIth nerve is connected to the suprascapular nerve, and the remaining distal upper trunk is grafted onto the proximal stump of C5 alone. The patients demonstrate a partial

"trumpet sign" frequent in obstetric Erb's palsies; i.e., abduction in the shoulder (mostly reaching the horizontal level) produces compulsory elbow flexion and wrist extension. If the elbow is kept extended by action of the triceps, global abduction and/or elevation in the shoulder does not exceed 60 degrees. However, the elbow can be flexed fully with the arm held against the thorax, which in most instances of obstetric palsy with a marked trumpet sign is not possible. Actually, in this type of repair, C5 simultaneously does its own job and that of C6. Dissociation of func-

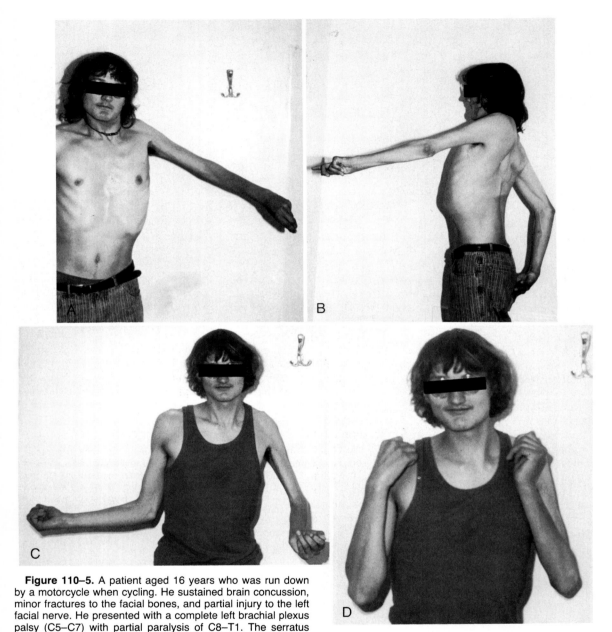

Figure 110–5. A patient aged 16 years who was run down by a motorcycle when cycling. He sustained brain concussion, minor fractures to the facial bones, and partial injury to the left facial nerve. He presented with a complete left brachial plexus palsy (C5–C7) with partial paralysis of C8–T1. The serratus anterior was at M2 and there was a palsy of the levator scapulae. The function of the XIth nerve was almost normal. At surgery six months post-trauma a root avulsion C5–C6–C7 was found with C8–T1 in continuity. The spinal accessory was used to neurotize the suprascapular and partially neurotize the axillary nerves; four intercostals (T3 and T6) were used to neurotize the musculocutaneous nerve. The photographs show the result obtained five years and eight months after the operation. Global abduction in the shoulder is 65 degrees (*A*), forward flexion is 60 degrees (*B*), and external rotation is 50 degrees (*C*) away from the thorax. There is no posterior projection. The global function of that joint is evaluated at 3, 3, 2, and 0 points, a total of 8 points. Elbow flexion is complete (*D*). The patient can lift at 90 degrees more than 3 kg (4 points). Extension is complete with 1 kg (2 points). Pronosupination scores 2 points, wrist function 6, and hand function 14. The total score is 36 points. Residual function before operation was 15 points; thus, the gain was 21 points. In fact, only the gain in shoulder function and elbow flexion (12 points) can be attributed to surgery; the rest of the gain is due to spontaneous recovery of C8 and T1, which were unusually large. Evaluation of this case demonstrates how difficult it is to assess corresponding contributions of regeneration obtained by surgical means and by spontaneous repair.

OSTEOTOMY OF THE CLAVICLE

In some cases the lesions or the stumps lie behind the clavicle or cannot be properly detached from the subclavian vessels because the view is restricted. An osteotomy of the clavicle is then helpful. A suitable plate is snugly adapted. Holes are drilled eccentrically away from the osteotomy site in order to obtain an interfragmentary compression when osteosynthesis is performed. The holes are measured and taped. The central hole is drilled only in the superficial cortical and its direction is oblique, as it will receive an interfragmentary lag screw. The clavicle is cut by an oscillating saw. The superior scapular vessels running parallel to it and the subclavian muscle may be spared, although the fascia of it has to be incised. It is then possible to move the clavicular ends upward and downward to inspect the plexus. If the exposure is insufficient, vessels and muscle are cut or the latter detached from the clavicle for later reinsertion. In children, two periosteal flaps extending beyond the osteotomy site are made before the clavicle is cut, and osteosynthesis is made with simple suture, a pin, or a plate according to age of the child. The plate is easy to put in place at the end of the operation.

PREPARATION OF NERVE STUMPS

The destroyed stumps are trimmed until healthy tissue is obtained. In injuries less than two days old the distal stumps are not degenerated and can be stimulated to obtain a muscular response. Orthodromic and antidromic sensory conduction can also be tested with appropriate equipment. This is a definite advantage, particularly in fresh gunshot wounds, in order to know how much of the traumatized nerve has to be resected. In fresh injuries the macroscopic appearance of the damaged nerve area corresponds to the extent of nerve tissue that will not respond to appropriate electrical stimulation. The proximal stump can be stimulated and sensory potentials recorded at the spinal or cortical level. Even motor potentials can be recorded in the deep muscles of the neck for lesions close to the foramina. However, this method is not always reliable as false-negative results may be obtained. When recordings produce a clear averaged curve, an inapparent intraforaminal avulsion inside the vertebral canal can be excluded, but it is difficult to correlate the tracings with the extent of proximal damage. Histologic examination of the last slice taken when trimming the proximal stump is not very reliable when rapid frozen sections are made. The usual staining techniques of the last slice taken in supraclavicular traction injuries show that 20 to 80 per cent of fibers were trimmed in a still damaged area. This demonstrates that in these injuries, nervous tissue is often injured very proximally and well above the site of apparent rupture.

SUTURING

Suturing can be performed in sharp lacerations only when the stumps have not retracted more than 2 cm because they were tethered to the vicinity, and in crush lesions when the plexus is caught between the clavicle and first rib. It is possible to mobilize the plexus and lessen the gap by bringing the arm in forward elevation (flexion) to 70 to 90 degrees and by shortening the clavicle by 2 cm. In stretch injuries direct suture is always impossible, because gaps usually exceed 4 cm after resection of damaged tissue. However, an avulsed root can be sutured directly to one portion of the trimmed proximal stump of a neighboring spinal nerve ruptured outside the foramen. Usually it is an avulsed C6 that is sutured to a ruptured C7 or vice versa, and sometimes C8 to a ruptured C7. This is called an intraplexal nerve transfer or neurotization. This method can be used in less than 5 per cent of the author's operated cases. One or two 6-0 or 7-0 epineural stay sutures are used approximately 1.0 to 1.5 cm above and below the apposition site, and 9-0 or 10-0 epifascicular nylon microsutures to maintain the fascicles or fascicular groups together. Since 1980 the number of microsutures has been limited to two or three, the repair being complemented with a sleeve of fibrin glue.

GRAFTING

Autologous nerve grafting is performed in the usual manner with a few variations. Since 1982, instead of using interfascicular nerve grafting as introduced by Millesi (1977a), the author has returned to cable grafting at the level of the plexus. However, the cable is made in a different way from the one described by Seddon (1947). The grafts are obtained from sural nerves, the medial cutaneous nerve of the arm, or rarely the superficial sensory ramus of the radial nerve in the forearm. They are covered by thick adventitial and epineural tissue. This tissue takes up a lot of space on the section of the cable, and possibly impedes sprout progression. Therefore, this tissue is cut away at the end of the grafts on a length of 5 to 7 mm to obtain "naked" fasciculi. They are glued together laterally to form cables that match the much larger fascicles or fascicular groups of the plexus. The end of this cable is then trimmed sharply with a special cutting device developed by Meyer and Smahel (1980), and sutured in place with two loose 9-0 nylon sutures. After the fascicular alignment is perfected, glue is applied circumferentially as a thin layer of fibrin. The grafts in the cable are of unequal length in order to be spread on the bed that will revascularize them. This method requires grafts with an excess length of 20 per cent. A few millimeters are lost for the trimming of the cable (Fig. 110–4*C*).

Free vascularized ulnar nerve grafts have been used in lower root avulsion to repair the upper and middle trunk, but the author prefers to use a pedicled ulnar nerve when conditions demand it, preparing the upper lateral vascular pedicle of the nerve in a way that it may be used if the pedicle at the origin of the ulnar nerve proves to be insufficient. The danger of using such a trunk as a graft, pedicled or revascularized by a microanastomosis, lies in the possible failure of blood supply. This is usually caused by a venous thrombosis. The graft is then lost and becomes fibrotic, impeding nerve regeneration. The author has also successfully used nerve trunks as grafts (ulnar, radial nerves), taking down the epineurium and using "naked" fascicles so that they may be easily revascularized.

TOPOGRAPHIC ORIENTATION OF GRAFTS

Erroneous reinnervation producing undesired synkinesias is the rule in lesions of the BP implying ruptures of the perineurium (degrees of severity of injury 3 to 5 according to Sunderland) under conservative or after operative treatment. Unsatisfactory functional results seem to depend on three major factors. The first is age: the younger the patient, the less rigid is the body image, the higher is the plasticity of the central nervous system, and the more likely is adaptation to the distortion of reinnervation. The second is the dispersion of erroneous input and output. It will be more easily compensated when it is concentrated on agonists-antagonists, such as biceps and triceps, than when several sometimes unrelated muscles receive the fibers that originally belonged to one muscle alone. The third factor is some inborn capacity of a given individual to master his limb, which may be witnessed in the normal individual by an ability to perform manual work, practice sports, draw, drive a car, or play a musical instrument. Some people are able or talented and others are not. This also depends on whether the dominant or nondominant extremity is affected and how much an individual is left- or right-handed. In order to reduce erroneous orientation of fascicular group sutures and grafting, attempts have been made by numerous researchers, including the author (Narakas, 1978), to establish a topography at the level of the brachial plexus similar to the one presented by Sunderland (1968) for peripheral nerves. Repeated studies on cadavers, together with clinical experience, have shown that a precise topography does not exist. However, there are some rules of thumb the surgeon must know in order to avoid errors. He can find solace, when he does so, in the fact that total inversion (e.g., suture of the proximal radial to the distal median, as the author's team did when replanting an arm amputated at the level of the shoulder) gives far better results than partial or multiple mixed erroneous orientations that produce undesired synkinesias between several functionally unrelated muscles. If this were not so, musculotendinous and nerve transfers would never function.

After 22 years of brachial plexus surgery, the author and many other plexus surgeons rely on the following assumptions:

1. The anterior (ventral) segments of the spinal nerves carry fibers that mostly go to the lateral and medial cords, i.e., from 11 to 6 o'clock.

2. The posterior (dorsal) half of the spinal nerves give fibers that will be innervating structures depending on the posterior cord, i.e., from 6 to 11 o'clock.

3. Nerve fibers for the suprascapular nerve are located in the region of 12 o'clock in C5.

4. Those for the axillary nerve are located near 9 o'clock in C5 and C6, while those for

Figure 111–13. The palmar carpal ligament. A thick fibrous ligament located distal to the transverse carpal ligament must also be released during decompression of the carpal tunnel. The recurrent motor branch is shown exiting from the median nerve distal to the palmar carpal ligament. The many anomalous origins and courses for this nerve make it necessary that the ligaments be released on their ulnar border adjacent to the hook of the hamate. Also to be noted is the location of the palmar cutaneous branch of the median nerve adjacent to the base of the third metacarpal.

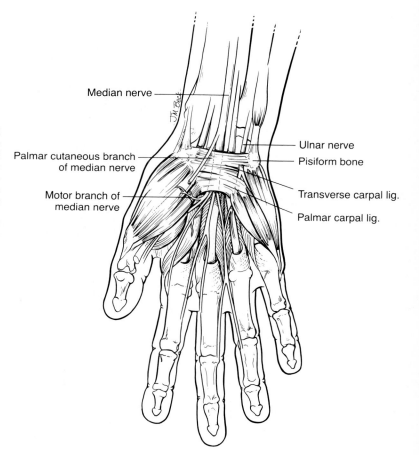

Median nerve

Palmar cutaneous branch of median nerve

Motor branch of median nerve

Ulnar nerve

Pisiform bone

Transverse carpal lig.

Palmar carpal lig.

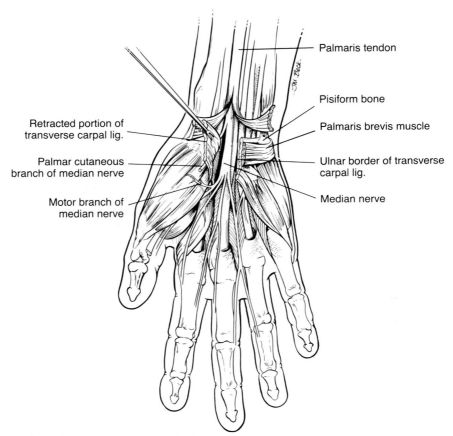

Palmaris tendon

Pisiform bone

Palmaris brevis muscle

Ulnar border of transverse
carpal lig.

Median nerve

Retracted portion of
transverse carpal lig.

Palmar cutaneous
branch of median nerve

Motor branch of
median nerve

Figure 111–14. Carpal tunnel. The ulnar border of the transverse carpal ligament and palmar carpal ligament are released. Note the relationship of the ulnar nerve to the palmaris brevis, pisiform, and hook of the hamate.

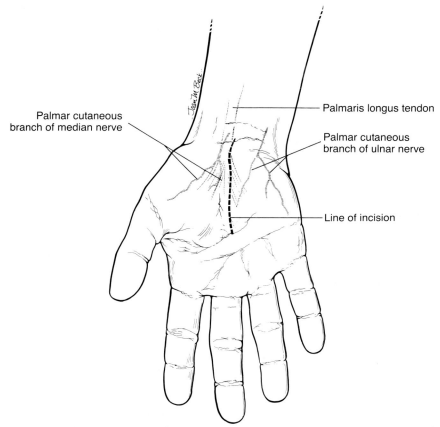

Palmar cutaneous
branch of median nerve

Palmaris longus tendon

Palmar cutaneous
branch of ulnar nerve

Line of incision

Figure 111–15. Surgical dissection of the hand. Note that the incision has been placed ulnar to the third metacarpal, and upon transection of the tranversed carpal ligament the most superficial structure is the median nerve. The ligament has been released so that the recurrent motor branch of the median nerve is readily identified. The palmaris tendon is not incised and should be located on the radial side of the incision.

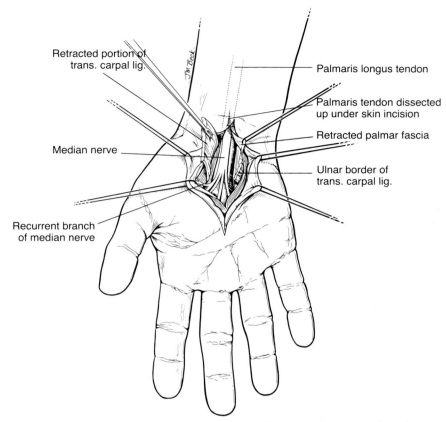

Figure 111–16. When a carpal tunnel incision is planned, the incision should not cross the wrist crease, and should be located ulnar to the ulnar side of the third metacarpal and ulnar to the palmaris longus tendon if present. Locating the incision radial to the palmaris longus risks injury to the palmar cutaneous branch of the median nerve. Placing the incision too ulnar in location risks injury to the palmar cutaneous branches of the ulnar nerve. The incision usually extends to the level of the midpalmar crease.

mors, ganglions, anomalous muscles, synovitis, or other causes of volume increase in the tunnel. In selected cases, synovium can be removed both for diagnostic purposes and in an attempt to decrease the volume of the carpal tunnel contents. However, Freshwater and Arons (1978) were unable to demonstrate any benefit from synovectomy.

The transverse carpal ligament is one of the important annular pulleys of the flexor mechanism. As such, it is important that the tendons be kept from herniating out of the tunnel during the postoperative period. Although rare, this complication has been reported by MacDonald and associates (1978). To prevent it, a Z-plasty of the ligament can be performed with the tips of the Z-flaps approximated to help prevent herniation and lengthen the ligament. Splinting the wrist in a slightly extended position for two to three weeks after surgery is essential to prevent this problem. It is helpful to approximate the hypothenar fat pad and components of the palmar fascia before skin closure to ensure a protective padding over the nerve.

Patients who undergo a carpal tunnel release should be warned that they will not be able to return to heavy manual work for approximately six weeks because of pain, and that they can expect deep tenderness or pain if they use their hands for vigorous activities before at least six months have elapsed. They should be advised of a flattening of the transverse arch of the palm following surgery.

After surgical release of the transverse carpal ligaments, if the patient returns to an occupational environment in which vibratory or rapidly repetitive activities are required, the symptoms may return. In that event, Ditmars (1986) advocated a change of occupation; this often represents a major problem in the vocational rehabilitation of some patients.

Management Summary

1. The patient should be carefully assessed for associated metabolic or nerve lesions.

2. When surgery is being contemplated, correlation between the electrophysiologic studies and the clinical findings is important, particularly in manual laborers.

3. The incisions must be kept ulnar to the palmar cutaneous branch of the median nerve and radial to the palmar cutaneous branch of the ulnar nerve.

4. Temporary immobilization of the wrist with a static wrist extension splint will prevent bowstringing or herniation of the flexor mechanisms out of the carpal tunnel. Splinting also helps to control pain.

5. The rehabilitation process after carpal tunnel release usually involves six weeks' absence from a labor-intensive occupation and six months before the hand is asymptomatic.

ANTERIOR INTEROSSEOUS NERVE SYNDROME

This syndrome was clearly defined by Kiloh and Nevin in 1952, and further reviewed by Bell and Goldner (1956), Stern and associates (1967), and Spinner (1978). The anterior interosseous nerve syndrome makes up only 1 per cent of compression syndromes (Nigst and Dick, 1979). Patients with an anterior interosseous nerve syndrome may present with only a history of weakness of pinch or an unusual posturing of the thumb when pinching. This occurs because of paralysis of the flexor profundus to the index finger or the flexor pollicis longus. Often, both muscles are partially paralyzed. There is often discomfort or pain over the flexor mass of the forearm, and symptoms are usually insidious in onset and slowly progressive. Nakano, Lundergran, and Okihiro (1977), Wiens and Lau (1978), and Saeed and Gatens (1983), advocated the need for positive electrodiagnostic studies to confirm the diagnosis.

When there is a history of pain in the proximal forearm, it is usually localized to the medial distal corner of the antecubital fossa. This approximates the anatomic location of the origin of the pronator muscle. Specific clinical tests are necessary to diagnose the anterior interosseous nerve syndrome. The flexor pollicis longus must be compared with the contralateral side for strength, as must the flexor profundi to the index fingers. Forced resisted pronation is considered a provocative test for reproducing or increasing symptoms.

Individuals with pain over the proximal arm adjacent to the anterior interosseous nerve combined with weakness of the flexor pollicis longus and the profundus to the index finger must be presumed to have an anterior interosseous nerve syndrome. A positive EMG result firmly establishes the diagnosis, and if there are denervation potentials in the skeletal muscle in the distribution of the anterior interosseous nerve, surgical exploration is recommended. In this syndrome, paralysis to the flexor profundus to the index and long fingers is often incomplete. This, in conjunction with the fact that there is no sensory deficit in this disorder, often delays detection of this compression syndrome.

The pronator quadratus may also be paralyzed in an anterior interosseous nerve syndrome. To test for pronator quadratus function, the effect of the pronator teres needs to be neutralized by maximally flexing the elbow and then asking the patient to pronate. If there is differential weakness of pronation with the elbows flexed, it is likely that the pronator quadratus is also paralyzed. There are several variations both in the clinical manifestations and in the anatomic etiology of the anterior interosseous nerve syndrome. The diagnosis must be entertained when there is an isolated loss of function in the flexion of the thumb or index finger, as anatomical variations may occur that can cause isolated paralysis. These deficits may also be difficult to detect by EMG if it is not possible to identify or locate the appropriate muscle. If this diagnosis is suspected, the anomalies of presentation should be reviewed; these have been described by Seddon (1975), Spinner (1978), Stern and Kutz (1980), and Hill, Howard, and Huffer (1985).

The anterior interosseous nerve syndrome can be differentiated from the pronator syndrome or other more proximal median nerve neuropathies in that sensibility is altered in more proximal lesions.

Etiology

Most anterior interosseous syndromes are thought to be compression related. Hovelius and Tuvesson (1980), Meya and Hacke (1983), and Collins and Weber (1983) described previous trauma, especially supracondylar fractures, as causes of these syndromes. Congenital constricting bands (Knight and Kozub, 1979), tumors, and soft tissue trauma (Saeed and Gatens, 1983) have also been associated factors.

Surgical Indications

Surgical exploration of the anterior interosseous nerve should be reserved for patients who have pain over the area of the anterior interosseous nerve, weakness or paralysis of the flexor pollicis longus and/or flexor digitorum profundus of the index finger, weakness of the flexor profundus to the middle finger, or weakness of the pronator quadratus. Confirmatory EMG's are important to exclude patients with a pain dysfunction syndrome. No studies are available regarding exploration of the patient when EMG results are normal.

The anterior interosseous nerve is explored through a linear incision made over the pronator. The median nerve is identified as it crosses the antecubital fossa and extends distally underneath the pronator teres (Fig. 111–17). The nerve is traced distally underneath the pronator, and the pronator, flexor carpi radialis, and flexor carpi ulnaris are retracted out of the way. Under the edge of the pronator the median nerve is further identified and the anterior interosseous nerve branch can be identified. Compression of the anterior interosseous nerve is usually associated with mechanical obstruction or tethering by the tendinous origin of the deep head of the pronator. This occurs just where the anterior interosseous nerve branches from the median nerve. After release of the deep head of the pronator and flexor fascia, the constricting band across the anterior interosseous nerve is usually relieved, and return of nerve function may be anticipated.

The deep head of the pronator is usually sutured to the origin of the superficial head (Fig. 111–18). After surgery the elbow is immobilized with a sugar tong splint, and the forearm is maintained in a position of slight supination for approximately 10 to 14 days. After this time, the arm is mobilized.

Most neuropathic conditions consist of first and second degree injuries to the nerve. Therefore, the recovery period is usually in two phases. In the first phase, the neurapraxia or first degree injury recovers quickly. However, axonotmesis or a second degree injury requires a longer time to recover.

Management Summary

1. The physician should look for direct pain over the anatomic origin of the interosseous nerve.

2. Paralysis of the flexor pollicis longus; paralysis of the flexor digitorum sublimis to

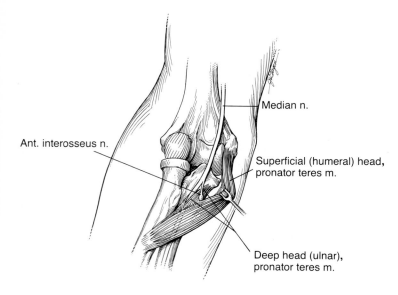

Ant. interosseus n.

Median n.

Superficial (humeral) head, pronator teres m.

Deep head (ulnar), pronator teres m.

Figure 111–17. In the anterior interosseous nerve syndrome, the deep head of the pronator and the superficial head serve to entrap the anterior interosseous nerve between them. In this syndrome the median nerve is not entrapped.

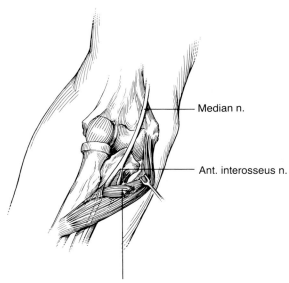

Median n.

Ant. interosseus n.

Ulnar head (deep) of pronator teres
excised and sutured to belly of
superficial pronator m.

Figure 111–18. Release of the deep head of the pronator from its origin off the ulna and attaching it to the superficial head relieve this site of entrapment.

the index finger; weakness of the middle finger profundus; or variations of weakness and paralysis are often hallmarks of the anterior interosseous nerve syndrome. Patients are frequently diagnosed as having ruptured tendons in these areas.

3. An abnormal EMG is an invariable part of the diagnosis.

4. The median nerve proximal to the pronator should be identified and traced distally until the deep head of the pronator is identified. The deep head of the pronator is usually the compressing mechanical problem.

5. Postoperative immobilization is helpful for pain control and may help to prevent a recurrent fibrous band.

PRONATOR SYNDROME

Compression neuropathy of the median nerve in the proximal forearm is referred to as the pronator syndrome. Seyffarth (1951) described a neuropathy of the median nerve associated with a primary myosis in the pronator teres. The role of the pronator teres in causing a compression neuropathy because of tight bands within the muscle was recognized by Solnitzky (1960). Subsequent reports by

Morris and Peters (1976), Johnson, Spinner, and Shrewsbury (1979), and Hartz and associates (1981) clearly delineated this compression neuropathy. Compression of the median nerve in the proximal forearm can have three causes. The most common is tendinous bands within the pronator muscle. The fibrous arch of the superficialis muscle through which the median nerve must pass can also compress the nerve. Of the three etiologies, the least common is lacertus fibrosis (Johnson, Spinner, and Shrewsbury, 1979). The clinical symptoms associated with the pronator syndrome (Omer and Spinner, 1980) are slow in onset and somewhat insidious. The patient usually has a history of one or two years of nonspecific pain in the flexor area of the forearm. This may be associated with athletic activity or repetitive manual labor, or may be post-traumatic (Loomer, 1982; King and Dunkerton, 1982). Clinical examination usually delineates a Tinel's sign or irritation over the nerve in the area of entrapment when tapping or pressing over the nerve. Resisted pronation of the forearm can also cause increased pain and sensitivity over the proximal border of the pronator, and resisted flexion of the flexor digitorum superficialis tendon of the middle finger may also aggravate the symptoms.

If a suspicious clinical history is obtained and the clinical examination supports this diagnosis, electrophysiologic studies are indicated. It was demonstrated by Goldner (1984), Hartz and associates (1981), and Morris and Peters (1976) that this syndrome is usually associated with abnormal EMG results. These usually demonstrate a decrease of conduction velocity across this segment of the nerve with a normal latency across the wrist.

Further clinical examination reveals some loss of sensibility in the distribution of the median nerve in more severe cases, as well as motor weakness in some of the flexor muscles of the hand in advanced cases.

The pronator syndrome can be differentiated from the anterior interosseous syndrome because of the associated decrease in sensibility associated with the pronator syndrome.

Treatment of the pronator syndrome consists of immobilization, the use of anti-inflammatory agents, or surgical exploration and decompression of the nerve.

Splinting of the forearm with a sugar tong

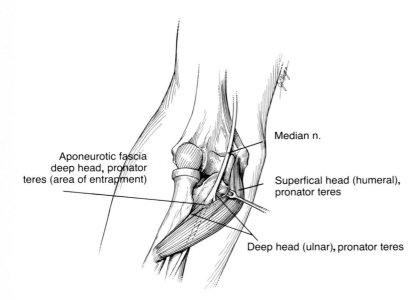

Aponeurotic fascia
deep head, pronator
teres (area of entrapment)

Median n.

Superfical head (humeral),
pronator teres

Deep head (ulnar), pronator teres

Figure 111–19. As the median nerve crosses the antecubital area, it positions itself deep within the muscles of the forearm. To reach this site, it runs underneath an aponeurotic arch formed by the pronator teres. This arch is formed by the confluence of the deep head of the pronator teres with the superficial head. Irritation of the nerve at this level can cause symptoms in both the median nerve and the anterior interosseous nerve.

splint to prevent pronation and supination can give substantial relief to patients who have repetitive trauma-induced symptoms, but this often interferes with work activities.

Injection of a corticosteroid into the pronator teres muscle itself also provides considerable relief to most patients, according to Morris and Peters (1976).

Surgical Technique

Using a linear incision, starting at the antecubital flexion crease and paralleling the proximal margin of the pronator, the pronator muscle is identified (Fig. 111–19). In addition, the lacertus fibrosis is identified and released. After identification of the median nerve it is traced along its course underneath the pronator muscle. If there are taut bands in the pronator muscle, these must be released within the muscular portion of the pronator. If the nerve appears to be compressed at the flexor superficialis fibrous epineuritic arch, the arch must be released and slit (Fig. 111–20); this will be just adjacent to the area of the anterior interosseous nerve. If a marked hourglass constriction is identified in the nerve, an external epineurotomy is performed with the operating microscope to ensure that there is no perineural fibrous constriction at the level of the hourglass deformity.

After surgery a long-acting steroid is instilled into the wound. The elbow is immobilized in neutral position, with a splint to prevent pronation and supination, for approximately two weeks.

Management Summary

1. A history of slow onset of weakness and numbness in the distribution of the median nerve, along with proximal forearm symptoms, is significant.

2. The resisted pronator test, the resisted flexor superficialis of the middle finger test, and the location of Tinel's sign in conjunction with proximal forearm pain, all support the diagnosis.

3. If the clinical diagnosis is of a pronator syndrome, confirmatory electrophysiologic studies are necessary.

4. Initial treatment should consist of immobilization and potentially the injection of cortisone into the pronator muscle.

5. Surgical exploration of the median nerve in the proximal forearm should involve release of the lacertus fibrosis, release of tendinous bands within the pronator if present, and release of the fibrous arcade of the superficialis muscle if compression of the nerve is confirmed.

POSTERIOR INTEROSSEOUS NERVE SYNDROME

The posterior interosseous nerve is a branch of the radial nerve that innervates the extensor indicis proprius, extensor digiti

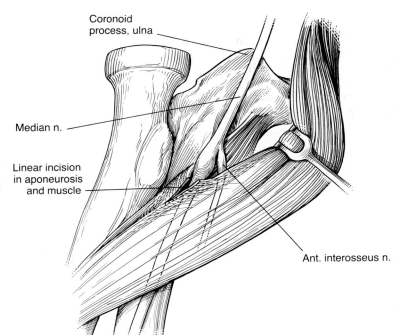

Coronoid
process, ulna

Median n.

Linear incision
in aponeurosis
and muscle

Ant. interosseus n.

Figure 111–20. Release of ligamentous bands in the pronator, if present, and release of a constraining fibrous aponeurosis.

quinti, extensor carpi ulnaris, abductor pollicis longus, extensor pollicis brevis, and extensor digitorum communis. Entrapment of the posterior interosseous nerve is usually noted at the proximal edge of the supinator. Distal to the proximal border of the supinator, the posterior interosseous nerve courses under the supinator and begins to arborize to the extensor muscles. The motor branches to the extensor carpi radialis longus and brachioradialis originate above this level and their function is usually preserved in this syndrome. The area where the posterior interosseous nerve penetrates the supinator is through a ligamentous arch referred to as the arcade of Frohse, described in 1908. Compression of the posterior interosseous nerve was recognized in 1905 by Guillain. Mulholland (1966), Spinner (1968), Nielsen (1976), and others have described the clinical and electrophysiologic sequence of the posterior interosseous syndrome. Patients on presentation usually have localized tenderness over the extensor muscle mass between the short and long extensor mass. This point of tenderness is located distal to the lateral epicondyle by 3 to 5 cm and can be differentiated from lateral epicondylitis on that basis. Point tenderness and weakness of some of the muscles innervated by the posterior interosseous nerve establishes the clinical diagnosis. Usually the muscle paralysis is incomplete, and is varied in presentation (Spinner, 1978). Possible causes include a post-traumatic condition (Lichter and Jacobsen, 1975), ganglions (Bowey and Stone, 1966), rheumatoid arthritis (Roth and associates, 1986), an intermuscular tumor (Pidgeon and associates, 1985), the Guillain-Barré syndrome (Sucher and Cavanaugh, 1982), and numerous others (Sunderland, 1978). Individuals who perform activities requiring prolonged, repetitive use of extensor muscles often develop this syndrome. This is common people who perform certain industrial tasks or sports activities, or who are keyboard musicians.

The clinical examination should check for point tenderness, weakness of the extensor muscles in comparison with the opposite side, and evidence of muscle atrophy. The clinical diagnosis should be confirmed by electrophysiologic studies, and if these study results are abnormal, surgical exploration is anticipated.

Individuals in whom the clinical history is strong and physical findings positive, but who show no changes electrophysiologically, should undergo a course of wrist immobilization and a period of observation. It is important to differentiate this syndrome from pain dysfunction or overuse syndromes.

Surgical Technique

With the use of tourniquet hemostasis, a linear incision is made over the extensor muscles mass paralleling the plane between the long and short extensor muscles of the forearm (Fig. 111–21). The incision, approximately 5 to 8 cm in length, starts 2 to 3 cm

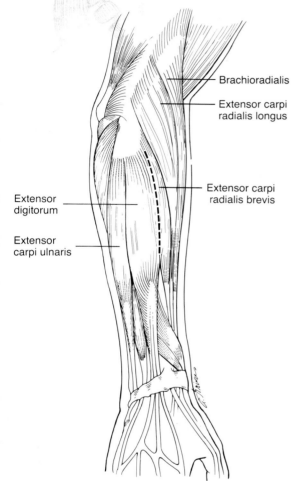

distal to the elbow crease. The cleavage plane between the long and short extensor muscles is identified and they are retracted medially and laterally. The radial nerve can be identified coursing just over the radial head bifurcating into superficial sensory and posterior interosseous nerve branches. This area is identified by a generous amount of adipose tissue surrounding the nerve (Fig. 111–22). The posterior interosseous nerve branch can then be traced distally and found to be coursing under the arcade of Frohse; it is in this area that irritation or compression of the nerve occurs.

During the surgical dissection, caution is required in order not to damage the radial nerve's efferent supply to the long extensor muscles. The superficial sensory branch of the radial nerve is in the immediate area of dissection. After identification and dissection of the nerve, the arcade of Frohse is released and a ligamentous segment of the arcade excised to prevent the supinator muscle from tightly encircling the nerve (Fig. 111–23).

Postoperatively the elbow and forearm are immobilized for two weeks with the forearm rotated into degrees of pronation.

Management Summary

1. It should be determined whether point tenderness is present over the extensor muscle mass distal to the lateral epicondyle.

2. The patient is examined to identify any weak extensors.

3. Positive electrodiagnostic studies are essential to establish a firm diagnosis.

4. The radial nerve is located by exploring between the cleavage plane of long and short components of the extensor muscle mass.

5. The arcade of Froshe is excised.

Figure 111–21. Note the mobile extensor muscles, the brachial radialis, and the extensor carpi radialis longus. The nonmobile extensor muscles, the extensor carpi radialis brevis, the extensor digiti, and the extensor carpi ulnaris. The incision to approach the posterior interosseous nerve should be made between the cleavage plane of the mobile and immobile extensor muscles. Dissection in the muscle plane between these two extensor groups allows access to the area of the radial head; it is in this area that the radial nerve will be identified. The distal branches of the radial collateral artery accompany the nerve. This then branches into the superficial radial nerve and the posterior interosseous nerve. The latter immediately courses through the arcade of Frohse and goes under the supinator muscle. It is in this fibrous arcade of the proximal border of the supinator muscle that the posterior interosseous nerve is entrapped.

Labels on figure:
- Brachioradialis
- Extensor carpi radialis longus
- Extensor carpi radialis brevis
- Extensor digitorum
- Extensor carpi ulnaris

THORACIC OUTLET SYNDROME

The term "thoracic outlet syndrome" is applied to many potentially compressive structures in the area of the thoracic outlet. Historically, this syndrome has been attributed to various causes such as anatomic cervical rib (Figs. 111–24 to 111–26) (Willshire, 1860; Murphy, 1906; Adson, 1927); first rib (Morley, 1913; Wright, 1945); scalene muscle (Ochsner, Gage, and Debakey, 1935); and trauma (Moore, 1986). The first recognition of a thoracic outlet syndrome that merited surgical intervention seemed to be a successful oper-

with associated neuroma incontinuity, and pseudoneuromas are common problems.

Some neuromas always form after a nerve injury, but not all neuromas become painful. Devor (1983) and Nathan (1983) reviewed the mechanism of neuroma pain and the potential associated etiologies. Neuromas and associated problems are also well described by Snyder and Knowles (1965); Poth, Bravo Fernandez, and Drager (1945); Frackelton, Teasley, and Tauras (1971); Spencer (1974); Herndon, Eaton, and Littler (1976); Tupper and Booth (1976); and Fisher and Boswick (1983).

Painful neuromas may also be found in other areas such as the foot (Kenzora, 1986), oral cavity (Shira, 1980), and abdomen (Prinz, Greenlee, and Caporale, 1979).

When evaluating patients with localized pain, a careful review of the history, psychologic stability, work status, and previous work record must be combined with a careful and thorough evaluation of the peripheral nerve status. It is important to determine the following (Fig. 111–35):

1. Is the neuroma located within the extremity stump dermal scar?

2. Is the neuroma stump directly under a prehensile surface?

3. Is the neuroma attached to a gliding tendon that could cause traction on the neuroma?

4. Is the neuroma surrounded by dense scar associated with the zone of injury?

5. Is the neuroma in an ischemic environment?

6. Is there pain directly over the neuroma?

7. Is there pain in the surface area innervated by the injured nerve?

8. Is phantom pain or perception present?

The answers to these questions will help differentiate the mechanism of pain that may be causing a sensitive painful neuroma.

Huber and Lewis (1920), Snyder and Knowles (1965), and Fisher and Boswick (1983) documented the histology of neuromas. The histology of a neuroma is characterized by disorganized nerve fibers surrounded by large masses of fibroblast. Myelinated and

Locations causing painful neuromas
Prehensile areas
Skin closure
Zone of injury

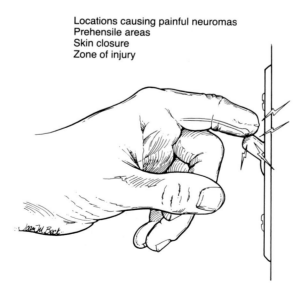

Figure 111–35. Painful stump neuromas can often be avoided if a planned nerve resection is performed at the time of residual digit closure. The regenerated neuroma when it occurs should not be located in a prehensile area, within the skin closure, within the zone of injury, adjacent to a flexor crease, or in an area adjacent to a mobile joint. Prevention of a painful neuroma is another important surgical factor when closing amputation sites.

unmyelinated nerve fibers are present within the neuroma and may form minifascicles. Schwann cells are also increased in numbers within neuromas. Established neuromas produce spontaneous volleys of afferent impulses, as documented by Seltzer and Devor (1979) and Devor (1983). These impulses are associated with nociceptor fibers, and the frequency of afferent impulses is increased by ischemia, mechanical stimulation, and compression. Gluck (1980) demonstrated that nerve fiber compression was a cause of pain from neuromas.

Formation of a neuroma is closely linked to the nerve regeneration process. After nerve injury the inflammatory process begins immediately at the site of injury. Van Beek and Zook (1982) demonstrated that within three to five days axon sprouts begin to enter the inflammatory gap between the nerve's cut and repaired ends. Schwann cells also proliferate immediately, and fibroblast proliferation begins seven to ten days after injury. The inflammatory granulation reaction is soon replaced by proliferating and regenerating nerve fibers, Schwann cells, and fibroblasts. If masses of receptive neurotubules

are not present, this process becomes disorganized and forms a neuroma. Plans should be made to alter this early phase of neuroma formation. Appropriate management of the injured nerve at this phase may prevent some of the factors contributing to painful neuromas.

When taking the history of someone with neuroma pain, it is important to classify the type of pain the patient describes. Is the injured area painless or painful, is the pain annoying, does it interfere with some or most of the patient's activities, or is the patient completely incapacitated with pain? As recommended by Sunderland (1978), generally these types of pain can be rated from P1 to P4.

The most common site of painful neuromas is an amputation stump, but stump-type neuromas also occur when sensory cutaneous nerves are severed. The two ends of the nerve retract, and the proximal stump is unable to join the distal glioma and thus forms a neuroma. This type of neuroma lends itself to reconstruction of nerve continuity, a form of treatment that is not possible for digit or extremity amputation stumps.

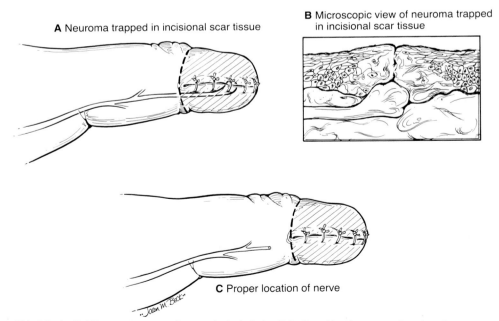

A Neuroma trapped in incisional scar tissue

B Microscopic view of neuroma trapped in incisional scar tissue

C Proper location of nerve

Figure 111–36. *A, B,* When a transected nerve is included within the skin closure at the site of an amputation, an exquisitely painful stump can occur. The neuroma trapped within the dermis sends nerve fibers almost to the surface of the skin, where they can be triggered with just the slightest of mechanical stimulation. At the time of stump closure, the nerve should be resected out of the zone of injury and well away from the skin closure.

Painful Stump Neuromas

If a neuroma is apparently away from a fibrous bed, not in a prehensile area, the neuroma should be managed nonsurgically before an operation is considered. It is important to try to desensitize, compress, or protect the sensitive area. Transcutaneous electrical nerve stimulation or repeated long-acting local anesthetic nerve blocks may be useful in breaking the cycle of pain.

The most exquisitely painful stump neuromas are usually produced when the nerve stump is unknowingly sutured into the skin closure at the injury site (Fig. 111–36). When this occurs it is usually in an area of prehensile touching of the amputation stump. This produces an exquisitely tender finger that often prevents the patient from using any portions of the hand for fear of touching the exquisitely sensitive area (Fig. 111–36). Resection of the neuroma well away from any anticipated suture lines or digital tactile areas is advisable and usually curative.

When the neuroma lies under an important prehensile surface and in an area where mechanical stimulation is likely, the neuroma should be displaced to a less significant area or into an area where mechanical stimulation is minimized (Figs. 111–37, 111–38).

In the author's practice the most common cause of painful stump neuromas is related to inadequate nerve resection at the time amputation stump closure was performed. This allows neuromas to form within the zone of injury (Fig. 111–39A) and this area is usually a prehensile surface. This combination produces a painful stump neuroma. Nerve resection at the time of closing an amputation site usually ensures that the neuroma is outside the zone of injury, away from the dermis, and away from a prehensile area (Fig. 111–39B). Locating a digital stump neuroma in a muscle mass, as in the intrinsic muscle or lumbrical muscle, has been advocated as a successful method of management. Digital amputation stump neuromas have been successfully treated by the central union technique (Kon and Bloere, 1987) (Fig. 111–40) or by burying the neuroma within the skeletal confinements of a phalanx or metacarpal (Fig. 111–41). Generally these techniques are used after neuroma resection has failed (Mass and associates, 1984). Some guidelines for the surgical management of residual extremity neuroma are:

1. Use the old cutaneous incision.

2. Extend the incision proximally to allow identification of the involved nerve and its neuroma.

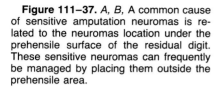

Figure 111–37. *A, B,* A common cause of sensitive amputation neuromas is related to the neuromas location under the prehensile surface of the residual digit. These sensitive neuromas can frequently be managed by placing them outside the prehensile area.

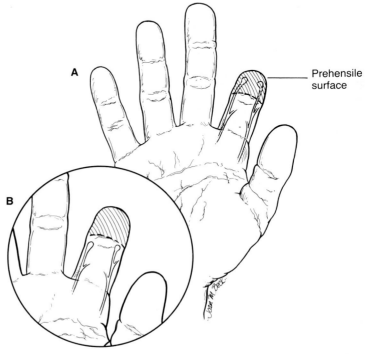

Prehensile surface

Dorsal translocation of neuroma

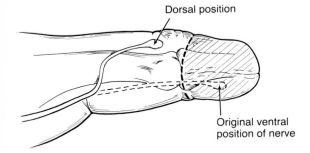

Dorsal position

Original ventral
position of nerve

Figure 111–38. When an injury is extensive, an alternative to neuroma resection out of the prehensile area and zone of injury is to translocate the neuroma dorsally. The patient is informed that the neuroma will be located dorsally, the reason being to avoid mechanical stimulation of the neuroma during touch activities on the palmar surfaces.

Figure 111–39. *A, B,* Frequently the zone of injury is also the area of prehension. However, in some instances the zone of injury can extend proximal to the prehensile touch surface. It is advisable to resect nerves out of the zone of injury when possible because of the fibrosis associated with the injury. This resection is most applicable when closing an amputation acutely.

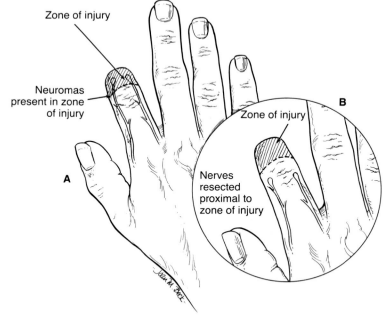

Zone of injury

Neuromas
present in zone
of injury

Zone of injury

B

Nerves
resected
proximal to
zone of injury

A

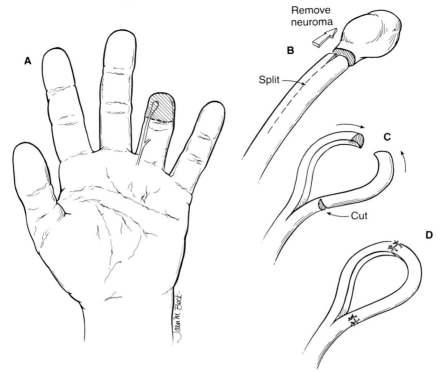

Figure 111–40. *A* to *D,* The central union technique of neuroma management is applicable when neuroma resection or translocation is not feasible. Using the central union technique, a portion of the peripheral nerve and its circulation is preserved by maintaining the epineurium. A microneurorrhaphy is then performed between the split components of the nerve, and a denervated segment is created by a second nerve incision. It is important to maintain the epineurium when creating the second cut, to ensure nerve viability. A second microneurorrhaphy is then performed, and the denervated segment of nerve is then a receiving conduit for active fibers that previously would have formed a neuroma.

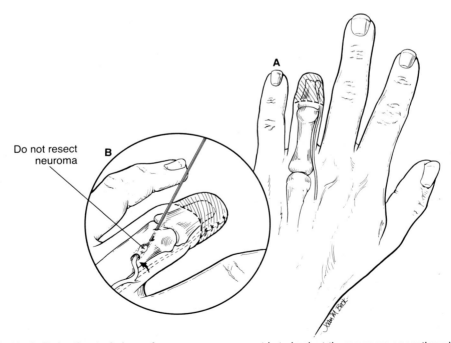

Figure 111–41. *A, B,* Another technique of neuroma management is to implant the neuroma or sectioned nerve within the skeletal portions of the extremity in an attempt to prevent mechanical stimulation. This technique is generally used after a failed resection or displacement procedure.

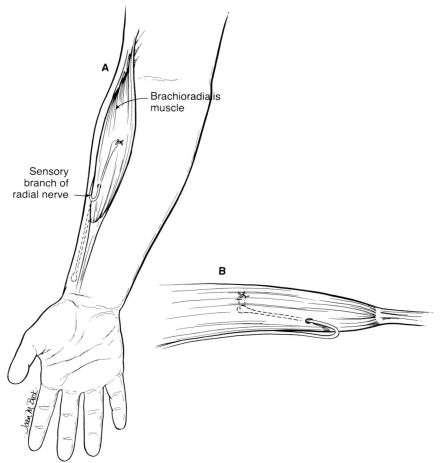

A

Brachioradialis
muscle

Sensory
branch of
radial nerve

B

Figure 111–42. *A, B,* Painful cutaneous neuromas can be managed by resection out of a zone of injury, as the initial management of the cutaneous neuroma can be mobilized and translocated away from the surface of the skin into a muscle. A muscle with a short amplitude of excursion should be chosen for implantation. To prevent perineural fibrosis, a small tunnel can be made within the muscle and a traction suture used to pull the neuroma into the skeletal muscle bed.

3. Mobilize the neuroma along with its attached proximal nerve, and resect the neuroma and nerve until the newly formed neuroma is out of the zone of injury (Fig. 111–42). If this is not possible, move the neuroma to a more dorsal location away from prehensile areas or areas where it could be mechanically stimulated.

4. If the nerve is in a nonfibrotic bed away from the prehensile area but is still painful, resect the neuroma and suture the nerve into a dorsal nonfibrotic bed; suture the nerve into an opening made in the skeletal phalanx; or use the central union technique.

5. Postoperative management should consist of immediate massage, desensitization, work rehabilitation, and if necessary the continued use of a transcutaneous electrical nerve stimulator. Avoid narcotic and other medications that have a tendency to produce dependence.

Painful Neuromas with Associated Glioma

In some painful neuromas the distal nerve trunk can be found, and is referred to as the gliomatous stump. When the distal nerve stump can be identified, a decision must be made regarding management. Should the neuroma be mobilized and displaced to a new bed, or should the nerve be repaired using nerve grafts or nerve conduits to span the gap that has resulted?

If the distal glioma cannot be identified or

the tissue adjacent to the nerve stump is fibrotic, displacement of the neuroma to a more favorable location is desirable. This has been well described by several authors (Mitchell, 1874; Poth, Bravo Fernandez, and Drager, 1945; Munro and Mallory, 1959; Petropoulos and Stefanko, 1961; Herndon, Eaton, and Littler, 1976; Tupper and Booth, 1976; Gorkisch, Boese-Landgraf, and Uaubel, 1984; Mass and associates, 1974; Dellon and MacKinnon, 1986). The most common and preferred procedure seems to be to insert the mobilized nerve stump into a nonmobile muscle mass (Fig. 111–42). An ideal muscle is the distal portion of the brachioradialis, pronator quadratus, and other muscles in which the amplitude of excursion is not excessive. Capping or covering neuroma stumps has been advocated by Swanson, Boeue, and Lumsden (1977) and Snow, Switzer, and DeMarco (1980). However, pain may recur after capping. The silicone cap may cause a technical problem because of its size in some areas such as the digit stump. If the adjacent tissue is well vascularized without dense fibrosis and the glioma is identifiable, nerve repair by direct repair or nerve grafting techniques is preferred (Fig. 111–43). The technique of nerve grafting is beyond the scope of this chapter and is thoroughly discussed elsewhere. Some guidelines for the management of painful neuromas with associated glioma follow:

1. A careful preoperative clinical examination helps determine where the proximal neuroma stump is located.

2. Careful surgical dissection allows identification of the gliomatous stump.

3. A suitable bed must be present to allow nerve grafting.

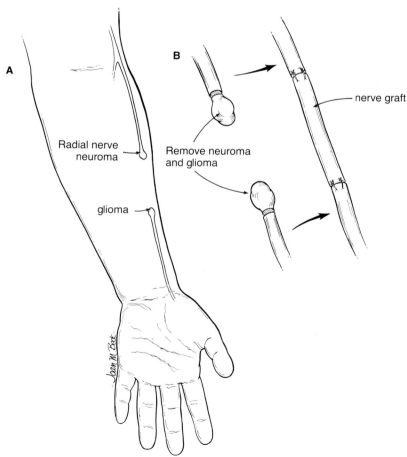

Figure 111–43. *A, B,* When a glioma is present in conjunction with a sensitive cutaneous nerve neuroma, the author prefers to reconstruct the nerve with a nerve graft if there is a suitable recipient bed.

4. Suitable nerve graft material must be present to permit nerve grafting.

5. If a nerve graft is undesirable or impossible, implantation of the neuroma with muscle or bone may also alleviate symptoms.

6. The patient must understand that the nerve reconstruction will provide an incomplete recovery and produce a new sensory deficit caused by harvesting the nerve graft.

7. Microsurgical neurorrhaphy is the preferred technique.

8. Painful cutaneous neuromas involving nerves with a diameter of less than 1.5 mm are most effectively treated by burying the proximal neuroma rather than by attempts at nerve repair, even when a glioma is available.

9. Careful postoperative management is required to facilitate rehabilitation, a return to work, and the control of pain symptoms.

Individuals with long-term pain from neuromas may not respond to correction of the peripheral cause of the pain. Central mechanisms of pain are a major factor in producing pain and usually are not amenable to peripheral surgery. MacKinnon and Dellon (1985) demonstrated that in some instances injury to branches of two different nerves may mean a failure of management if the neuroma of only one nerve is identified. Thus, more than one sensitive trigger point must be sought in all patients who present with painful neuromas. In patients who do not respond to desensitization and in whom surgery is not indicated, local blocks and cortisone injections have shown some beneficial effects. If after multiple attempts at neuroma resection or implantation the patient continues to have chronic unrelenting pain, the problem should probably be managed as a central pain mechanism. In that instance, supportive care, work rehabilitation, and alteration of the working environment may be necessary.

The best treatment for painful neuromas is prevention. This is most appropriately accomplished when the surgeon observes the following principles:

1. Make sure that the neuroma is not located near or within the suture line or area of soft tissue injury.

2. Educate the patient immediately after surgery as to the nature of the Tinel's sign and sensitivity associated with a neuroma.

3. Keep neuromas away from prehensile areas and from areas where mechanical stimulation will be frequent.

4. Teach patients about desensitization activities so that they understand and accept some of the discomfort that may be associated with the neuroma.

5. Early intervention when a progressive pain syndrome is developing is essential. Treatment may include sympathetic blocks, point tenderness blocks, and transcutaneous electrical nerve stimulation (TENS).

6. Closely coordinated work and physical rehabilitation is essential.

7. Be sure to support the patient and if necessary modify the environment or occupation to allow a return to meaningful employment.

8. Expect with time that the neuroma sensitivity will abate, so that multiple and repetitive operations will not be necessary for persistent and painful neuromas.

Acknowledgements: The author would like to thank microsurgical fellows Etienne Massac, M. D., and Pamela Rosen, M. D., for their help and suggestions.

REFERENCES

Adelaar, R. S., Foster, W. C., and McDowell, C.: The treatment of the cubital tunnel syndrome. J. Hand Surg., *9A*:90, 1984.

Adson, A. W.: The classical surgical treatment for symptoms produced by cervical ribs and the scalenus anticus muscle. Clin. Ortho., *207*:3, 1986.

Adson, A. W., and Coffey, J. R.: Cervical rib. Ann. Surg., *85*:839, 1927.

Battista, A. F., Cravioto, H. M., and Budzilovich, G. N.: Painful neuroma: Changes produced in peripheral nerves after fascicle ligation. Neurosurgery, *9*:589, 1981.

Bell, G. E., and Goldner, J. L.: Compression neuropathy of the median nerve. South. Med. J., *49*:966, 1956.

Benedeich, G. J.: Ulnar nerve compression in the wrist and hand. J. Bone Joint Surg., *55B*:227, 1973.

Bowey, T. L., and Stone, K. H.: Posterior interosseous nerve paralysis caused by a ganglion at the elbow. J. Bone Joint Surg., *48B*:774, 1966.

Britt, L. P.: Nonoperative treatment of the thoracic outlet syndrome symptoms. Clin. Orthop., *51*:45, 1967.

Brown, H., and Flynn, J. E.: Abdominal pedicle flap for hand neuromas and entrapped nerves. J. Bone Joint Surg., *55A*:575, 1973.

Brown, W. F., Yates, S. K., and Ferguson, G. G.: Cubital tunnel syndrome and ulnar neuropathy. Ann. Neurol., *7*:289, 1980.

Carroll, R. E., and Green, D. P.: The significance of the palmar cutaneous nerve at the wrist. Clin. Orthop., *83*:24, 1972.

Cherington, M.: Proximal pain in carpal tunnel syndrome. Arch. Surg., *108*:69, 1974.

Cherington, M.: Surgery for thoracic outlet syndrome? N. Engl. J. Med., *314*:322, 1986.

Cherington, M., Happer, I., Machanic, B., and Parry, L.: Surgery for thoracic outlet syndrome may be hazardous to your health. Muscle Nerve, 9:632, 1986.

Clark, C. B.: Cubital tunnel syndrome. J.A.M.A., 241:801, 1979.

Coccia, M. R., and Satiani, B.: Thoracic outlet syndrome. Am. Fam. Physician, 29:121, 1984a.

Coccia, M. R., and Satiani, B.: A systematic approach to thoracic outlet syndrome. Curr. Surg., 41:10, 1984b.

Cohen, B. E., and Cukier, J.: Simultaneous posterior and anterior interosseous nerve syndromes. J. Hand Surg., 7:398, 1982.

Collins, D. N., and Weber, E. R.: Anterior interosseous nerve syndrome. South. Med. J., 76:1533, 1983.

Craven, P. R., Jr., and Green, D. P.: Cubital tunnel syndrome. Treatment by medial epicondylectomy. J. Bone Joint Surg., 62:986, 1980.

Curtis, R. M., and Eversmann, W. W.: Internal neurolysis as an adjunct to the treatment of the carpal tunnel syndrome. J. Bone Joint Surg., 55A:733, 1973.

Dawson, D. M., Hallett, M., and Millender, L. H.: Entrapment Neuropathies. Boston: Little, Brown & Company, 1983.

Dellon, A. L., and MacKinnon, S. E.: Treatment of the painful neuroma by neuroma resection and muscle implantation. Plast. Reconstr. Surg., 77:427, 1986.

Devor, M.: Nerve pathophysiology and mechanism of pain in causalgia. J. Auton. Nerv. Sys., 7:371, 1983.

Ditmars, D. M., Jr., and Dorwart, B. B.: Carpal tunnel syndrome: a review. Semin. Arthritis Rheum., 14:134, 1984.

Ditmars, D. M., Jr., and Houin, H. P.: Carpal tunnel syndrome. Hand Clin., 2:525, 1986.

Eason, S. Y., Belsole, R. J., and Greene, T. L.: Carpal tunnel release: analysis of suboptimal results. J. Hand Surg., 10B:365, 1985.

Eboh, N., and Wilson, D. H.: Surgery of the carpal tunnel. Technical note. J. Neurosurg., 49:316, 1978.

Eisen, A., Schomer, D., and Melmed, C.: The application of F-wave measurements in the differentiation of proximal and distal upper limb entrapments. J. Neurol., 27:662, 1977.

Ellis, J., Folkers, K., Levy, M., Takemura, K., Shizukuishi, S., et al.: Therapy with vitamin B₆ with and without surgery for treatment of patients having the idiopathic carpal tunnel syndrome. Res. Commun. Chem. Pathol. Pharmacol., 33:331, 1981.

Farquhar Buzzard, E.: Some varieties of traumatic and toxic ulnar neuritis. Cancer, 1:317, 1922.

Farrell, H. F.: Pain and the pronator teres syndrome. Bull. Hosp. Joint Dis., 37:59, 1976.

Fields, W. S., Lemak, N. A., and Ben Menachem, Y.: Thoracic outlet syndrome: review and reference to stroke in a major league pitcher. A.J.R., 146:809, 1986.

Fisher, G. T., and Boswick, J. A.: Neuroma formation following digital amputation. J. Trauma, 23:136, 1983.

Ford, D. J., and Ali, M. S.: Acute carpal tunnel syndrome. Complications of delayed decompression. J. Bone Joint Surg., 68B:758, 1986.

Frackelton, W. F., Teasley, J. L., and Tauras, A.: Neuromas of the hand treated by transplantation and silicone capping. J. Bone Joint Surg., 53A:813, 1971.

Freshwater, M. F., and Arons, M. S.: The effect of various adjuncts on the surgical treatment of carpal tunnel syndrome secondary to chronic tenosynovitis. Plast. Reconstr. Surg., 61:93, 1978.

Frohse, F., and Frankel, M.: Die Muskeln des Men-

schlechen Armes. Bardeleben's Handbuch der Anatomie des Meuschliden. Jena Fisher, 1908.

Fullerton, D. M.: The effect of ischemia on nerve conduction in the carpal tunnel syndrome. J. Neurol. Neurosurg. Psychiat., 26:385, 1963.

Gluck, T.: Ueber Neuroplaskik auf dem Wege der Transplantation. Arch. Klin. Chir., 25:606, 1980.

Goldner, J. L.: Median nerve compression evaluation. Bull. Hosp. Joint Dis. Orthop. Inst., 44:199, 1984.

Gorkisch, K., Boese-Landgraf, J., and Uaubel, E.: Treatment and prevention of amputation neuromas in hand surgery. Plast. Reconstr. Surg., 73:293, 1984.

Grundberg, A. B.: Ulnar tunnel syndrome. J. Hand Surg., 9:72, 1984.

Guillain, G.: Guillain-Barré syndrome with secondary bilateral posterior interosseous nerve syndrome. Arch. Phys. Med. Rehab., 63:184, 1982.

Guillain, G., Courtellermont: L'Action du muscle court supinator dans la paralysie du nerf radial. Presse Med., 13:50, 1905.

Harris, C. M., Tanner, E., Goldstein, M. N., and Pettee, D. S.: The surgical treatment of the carpal tunnel syndrome correlated with preoperative nerve conduction studies. J. Bone Joint Surg., 61A:93, 1979.

Hartz, C. R., Linscheid, R. L., Gramse, R. R., and Daube, J. R.: The pronator teres syndrome: compressive neuropathy of the median nerve. J. Bone Joint Surg., 63A:885, 1981.

Helmholtz, H.: Vorlaufiger Bericht über die Fort Planzungsgeschwindigkeit der Nerven Reizung. Arch. Anat. Physiol. Wiss. Med., 71, 1850.

Herndon, J. H., Eaton, R. G., and Littler, J. W.: Management of painful neuromas in the hand. J. Bone Joint Surg., 58A:212, 1976.

Hill, N. A., Howard, F. M., and Huffer, B. R.: The incomplete anterior interosseous nerve syndrome. J. Hand Surg., 10:4, 1985.

Hodes, R., Larrabee, M. G., and German, W.: The human electromyogram in response to nerve stimulation and the conduction velocity of motor axons. Arch. Neurol. Psychiat., 60:340, 1948.

Hovelius, L., and Tuvesson, T.: Anterior interosseous nerve paralysis as a complication of supracondylar fractures of the humerus in children. A report of two cases. Arch. Orthop. Trauma Surg., 96:59, 1980.

Hubbard, J. H.: The quality of nerve regeneration: factors independent of the most skillful repair. Surg. Clin. North Am., 52:1099, 1972.

Huber, C. G., and Lewis, D.: Amputation neuromas. Arch. Surg., 1:85, 1920.

Huet, E., and Guillain, G.: Neurite cubitale professionelle chez un boulanger. Rev. Neurol., 8:266, 1900.

Hunt, J. R.: Occupational neuritis of the deep palmar branch of the ulnar nerve. J. Nerv. Ment. Dis., 35:673, 1908.

Hunt, J. R.: Described thenar atrophy and numbness (carpal tunnel syndrome). Trans. Am. Neurol. Assoc., 35:184, 1909.

Hunt, J. R.: The thenar and hypothenar types of neural atrophy of the hand. Am. J. Med. Sci., 141:224, 1911.

Inbal, R., Rousso, M., Ashur, H., Wall, P. D., and Devor, M.: Collateral sprouting in skin and sensory recovery after nerve injury in man. Pain, 28:141, 1987.

Jamieson, W. G., and Merskey, H.: Representation of the thoracic outlet syndrome as a problem in chronic pain and psychiatric management. Pain, 22:195, 1985.

Johnson, R. K., Spinner, M., and Shrewsbury, M. M.:

Median nerve entrapment syndrome in the proximal forearm. J. Hand Surg., 4:48, 1979.

Judy, K. L., and Heymann, R. L.: Vascular complications of thoracic outlet syndrome. Am. J. Surg., 123:521, 1972.

Kenzora, J. E.: Sensory nerve neuroma—leading to failed foot surgery. Foot Ankle, 7:110, 1986.

Kiloh, L. G., and Nevin, S.: Isolated neuritis of the anterior interosseous nerve. Br. Med. J., 1:850, 1952.

Kimura, J. N.: Electrodiagnosis in Diseases of Nerve and Muscle: Principles and Practice. Philadelphia, F. A. Davis, 1983.

King, R. J., and Dunkerton, M.: The pronator syndrome. J. R. Coll. Surg. Edinb., 27:142, 1982.

Kleinert, H. E., and Hayes, J. E.: The ulnar tunnel syndrome. Plast. Reconstr. Surg., 47:21, 1971.

Kline, D. G., Hackett, E. R., and May, P. Z.: Evaluation of nerve injuries by evoked potentials and electromyography. J. Neurosurg., 31:128, 1969.

Knight, C. R., and Kozub, P.: Anterior interosseous syndrome. Ann. Plast. Surg., 3:72, 1979.

Kon, M., and Bloere, J. J.: The treatment of amputation neuromas in fingers with a centrocentral nerve union. Ann. Plast. Surg., 1:506, 1987.

Lanz, U.: Anatomical variations of the median nerve in the carpal tunnel. J. Hand Surg., 2:44, 1977.

Learmouth, J. R.: The principles of decompression in the treatment of certain diseases of the peripheral nerve. Surg. Clin. North Am., 13:905, 1933.

Leffert, R. D.: Brachial Plexus Injuries. New York, Churchill Livingstone, 1985.

Lichter, R. L., and Jacobsen, T.: Tardy palsy of the posterior interosseous nerve with a Monteggia fracture. J. Bone Joint Surg., 57A:124, 1975.

Linscheid, R. L.: Injuries to the radial nerve at the wrist. Arch. Surg., 91:942, 1965.

Loomer, R. L.: Elbow injuries in athletes. Can. J. Appl. Sport Sci., 7:164, 1982.

Louis, D. S., Hunter, L. V., and Keating, T. M.: Painful neuromas in long below-elbow amputees. Arch. Surg., 115:742, 1980.

MacDonald, R. I., Lichtman, D. M., Hanlon, J. J., and Wilson, J. N.: Complications of surgical release for carpal tunnel syndrome. J. Hand Surg., 3:70, 1978.

MacKinnon, S. E., and Dellon, A. L.: Overlap of lateral antebrachial cutaneous nerve and superficial branch of the radial nerve. J. Hand Surg., 10A:522, 1985.

Mahring, M., Semple, C., and Gray, I. C.: Attritional flexor tendon rupture due to a scaphoid nonunion imitating an anterior interosseous nerve syndrome: a case report. J. Hand Surg., 10:62, 1985.

Mame, P., and Foix, C.: Atrophie isolée de l'eminence thenar d'origine neuritique. Rev. Neurol., 26:647, 1913.

Martinelli, P., Gabellini, A. S., Poppi, M., Gallassi, R., and Pozzati, E.: Pronator syndrome due to thickened bicipital aponeurosis. J. Neurol. Neurosurg. Psychiat., 45:181, 1982.

Masear, V. R., and Hayes, J. M.: An industrial cause of carpal tunnel syndrome. J. Hand Surg., 11A:222, 1986.

Mass, D. P., Ciano, M. C., Tortossa, R., Newmeyer, W. L., and Kilgore, E. S.: Treatment of painful hand neuromas by their transfer into bone. Plast. Reconstr. Surg., 74:182, 1984.

Mass, D. P., and Silverberg, B.: Cubital tunnel syndrome: anterior transposition with epicondylar osteotomy. Orthopedics, 9:711, 1986.

Medical Research Council of the United Kingdom: Aids to the Examination of the Peripheral Nervous System.

Memorandum 4J. Palo Alto, CA, Pendragon House, 1978.

Meya, U., and Hacke, W.: Anterior interosseous nerve syndrome following supracondylar lesions of the median nerve: clinical findings and electrophysiological investigations. J. Neurol., 229:91, 1983.

Miller, R. G.: The cubital tunnel syndrome: diagnosis and precise localization. Ann. Neurol., 6:56, 1979.

Miller, R. G., and Hummel, E. E.: The cubital tunnel syndrome: treatment with simple decompression. Ann. Neurol., 7:567, 1980.

Mitchell, S. W.: Traumatic neuralgia: section of the median nerve. Am. J. Med. Sci., 67:2, 1874.

Moore, M., Jr.: Thoracic outlet syndrome experience in a metropolitan hospital. Clin. Orthop., 207:29, 1986.

Morley, J.: Brachial pressure neuritis due to a normal first thoracic rib. Clin. J., 42:461, 1913.

Morris, H. H., and Peters, B. H.: Pronator syndrome: clinical and electrophysiological features in seven cases. J. Neurol. Neurosurg. Psychiat., 39:461, 1976.

Mulholland, R. C.: Non-traumatic progressive paralysis of the posterior interosseous nerve. J. Bone Joint Surg., 48B:781, 1966.

Munro, D., and Mallory, G. K.: Elimination of the so-called amputation neuromas of divided peripheral nerves. N. Engl. J. Med., 260:358, 1959.

Murphy, J. B.: The clinical significance of cervical ribs. Surg. Gynecol. Obstet., 3:515, 1906.

Naffziger, H. C., and Grant, W. T.: Neuritis of the brachial plexus mechanical in origin. The scalenus syndrome. Surg. Gynecol. Obstet., 67:722, 1938.

Nakano, K. K., Lundergran, C., and Okihiro, M. M.: Anterior interosseous nerve syndromes. Diagnostic methods and alternative treatments. Arch. Neurol., 34:477, 1977.

Nathan, P. W.: Pain and the sympathetic system. J. Auton. Nerv. Syst., 7:363, 1983.

Neundorfer, B., and Kroger, M.: The anterior interosseous nerve syndrome. J. Neurol., 213:347, 1976.

Nielsen, H. O.: Posterior interosseous nerve paralysis caused by fibrous band compression at the supinator muscle. A report of four cases. Acta Orthop. Scand., 47:304, 1976.

Nielsen, V. K., Osgaard, O., and Trojaborg, W.: Interfascicular neurolysis in chronic ulnar nerve lesions elbow: an electrophysiological study. J. Neurol. Neurosurg. Psychiat., 43:272, 1980.

Nigst, H., and Dick, W.: Syndromes of compression of the median nerve in the proximal forearm (pronator teres syndrome; anterior interosseous nerve syndrome). Arch. Orthop. Trauma Surg., 93:307, 1979.

Ochsner, A., Gage, M., and Debakey, M.: Scalenus anticus syndrome. Am. J. Surg., 28:669, 1935.

Odier, L.: Manual de médicine pratique. Geneva, 1811.

Odusote, K., and Eisen, A.: An electrophysiological quantitation of the cubital tunnel syndrome. Can. J. Neurol. Sci., 6:403, 1979.

Omer, G. E.: Injuries to nerves of the upper extremity. J. Bone Joint Surg., 56A:1615, 1974.

Omer, G. E., and Spinner, M.: Management of Peripheral Nerve Problems. Philadelphia, W. B. Saunders Company, 1980.

Osborne, G. V.: The surgical treatment of tardy ulnar palsy. J. Bone Joint Surg., 39B:782, 1957.

Osborne, G. V.: Acroparaesthesia and the carpal tunnel. Br. Med. J., 1:98, 1959.

Pechan, J., and Kredba, J.: Treatment of cubital tunnel syndrome by means of local administration of corticosteroids. I. Short-term follow-up. Acta Univ. Carol., *26*:125, 1980a.

Pechan, J., and Kredba, J.: Treatment of cubital tunnel syndrome by means of local administration of cortisonoids. II. Long term follow-up. Acta Univ. Carol., *26*:135, 1980b.

Pechan, J., and Kredba, J.: Cubital tunnel syndrome. II. Clinical aspects. Acta Univ. Carol., *27*:321, 1981.

Peet, R. M., Henriksen, J. P., Anderson, T. P., and Martin, G. M.: Thoracic outlet syndrome: evaluation of a therapeutic exercise program. Mayo Clin. Proc., *31*:281, 1956.

Pernkopf, E.: Atlas of Topographical and Applied Human Anatomy. 2nd Ed. Philadelphia, W. B. Saunders Company, 1980.

Petropoulos, P. C., and Stefanko, S.: Experimental observations on the prevention of neuroma formations. J. Surg. Res., *1*:241, 1961.

Phalen, G. S.: Spontaneous compression of the median nerve at the wrist. J.A.M.A., *145*:1128, 1951.

Phalen, G. S.: The carpal tunnel syndrome. Seventeen years experience in diagnosis and treatment of 644 hands. J. Bone Joint Surg., *48A*:211, 1966.

Phalen, G. S.: Reflections on 21 years experience with the carpal tunnel syndrome. J.A.M.A., *212*:1365, 1970.

Pidgeon, K. J., Abadee, P., Kanakamedala, R., and Uchizono, M.: Posterior interosseous nerve syndrome caused by an intermuscular lipoma. Arch. Phys. Med. Rehabil., *66*:468, 1985.

Platt, H.: The pathogenesis and treatment of traumatic neuritis of the ulnar nerve in the post-condylar groove. Br. J. Surg., *13*:409, 1926.

Poth, E. J., Bravo Fernandez, E., and Drager, G. A.: Prevention of formation of end-bulb neuromata. Proc. Soc. Exp. Biol. Med., *60*:200, 1945.

Prinz, R. A., Greenlee, H. B., and Caporale, F. S.: Amputation neuroma of the cystic duct: a treatable cause of post cholecystectomy pain. Am. J. Surg., *45*:543, 1979.

Qvarfordt, P. G., Ehrenfeld, W. K., and Stoney, R. J.: Supraclavicular radical scalenectomy and transaxillary first rib section for the thoracic outlet syndrome. A combined approach. Am. J. Surg., *148*:111, 1984.

Roos, D. B.: Thoracic outlet syndrome. Arch. Surg., *93*:71, 1966.

Roth, A. I., Stulberg, B. N., Fleegler, E. J., and Belhobek, G. H.: Elbow arthrography in the evaluation of posterior interosseous nerve compression in rheumatoid arthritis. J. Hand Surg., *11B*:120, 1986.

Saeed, M. A., and Gatens, P. F.: Anterior interosseous nerve syndrome: unusual etiologies. Arch. Phys. Med. Rehabil., *64*:182, 1983.

Sällström, J., and Gjöres, J. E.: Surgical treatment of the thoracic outlet syndrome. Acta Chir. Scand., *149*:555, 1983.

Schaumburg, H. H., Spencer, P. S., and Thomas, P. K.: Disorders of peripheral nerves. Philadelphia, F. A. Davis, 1984.

Scherokmarr, B., Husain, F., Cuetter, A., Jabbari, B., and Maniglia, E.: Peripheral dystonia. Arch. Neurol., *43*:830, 1986.

Seddon, H.: Surgical Disorders of the Peripheral Nerves. Edinburgh, Churchill Livingstone, 1975.

Seltzer, Z., and Devor, M.: Ephaptic transmission in chronically damaged peripheral nerves. Neurology, *29*:1061, 1979.

Sendzischew, H., and Hempel, G. K.: Anterior approach for resection of the first rib and total scalenotomy. Surg. Gynecol. Obstet., *160*:275, 1985.

Seyffarth, H.: Primary myoses in the pronator teres as cause of lesion of the nerve medianus (the pronator syndrome). Acta Psychiat. Neurol. Suppl., 74, 1951.

Shalimov, A. A., Driuk, N. F., Polyshchuk, YuE., Oleynick, L. I., and Lisajchuk, YuS.: Pathophysiology and selection of method for surgical management of thoracic outlet syndrome. Int. Angiol., *4*:147, 1985.

Shea, J. D., and McClain, E. J.: Ulnar nerve compression syndromes at and below the wrist. J. Bone Joint Surg., *51A*:1095, 1969.

Shenkin, H. A.: Scalenotomy in patients with and without cervical ribs. Analysis of surgical results. Arch. Surg., *87*:892, 1963.

Shira, R. B.: Painful traumatic neuromas in the oral cavity. Oral Surg., *49*:191, 1980.

Siivola, J., Pokela, R., and Sulg, I.: Somatosensory evoked responses as a diagnostic aid in thoracic outlet syndrome. A post-operative study. Acta Chir. Scand., *149*:147, 1983.

Simonet, W. T., Gannon, P. G., Lindberg, E. F., and Satterfield, J. R., Jr.: Diagnosis and treatment of thoracic outlet syndrome. Minn. Med., *66*:19, 1983.

Smith, K. F.: The thoracic outlet syndrome: a protocol of treatments. J. Orthop. Sports Phys. Ther., *18*:89, 1979.

Smith, R. J.: Anomalous muscle belly of the flexor digitorum superficialis causing carpal tunnel syndrome. Report of a case. J. Bone Joint Surg., *53A*:1215, 1971.

Snider, H. C., and King, G. D.: Minnesota Multiphasic Personality Inventory as a predictor of operative results in thoracic outlet syndrome. South. Med. J., *79*:1527, 1986.

Snow, J. W., Switzer, H. E., and DeMarco, J. A.: Silastic overlay in the treatment of painful neuromata. J. Fla. Med. Assoc., *67*:1079, 1980.

Snyder, C. C., and Knowles, R. P.: Traumatic neuromas. J. Bone Joint Surg., *47A*:641, 1965.

Solnitzky, O.: Pronator syndrome: compression neuropathy of the median nerve at the level of pronator teres muscle. Georgetown Med. Bull., *13*:232, 1960.

Spencer, P. S.: The traumatic neuroma and proximal stump. Bull. Hosp. Joint Dis., *35*:85, 1974.

Spinner, M.: The arcade of Frohse and its relationship to posterior interosseous nerve paralysis. J. Bone Joint Surg., *50B*:809, 1968.

Spinner, M.: Injuries to the Major Branches of Peripheral Nerves of the Forearm. 2nd Ed. Philadelphia, W. B. Saunders Company, 1978.

Spinner, M., Freundlich, B. D., and Tercher, J.: Posterior interosseous nerve paralysis as a complication of Monteggia fracture in children. Clin. Orthop., *58*:141, 1968.

Stallworth, J. M., and Horne, J. B.: Diagnosis and management of thoracic outlet syndrome. Arch. Surg., *119*:1149, 1984.

Stern, M. B.: The anterior interosseous nerve syndrome (the Kiloh-Nevin syndrome). Report and follow-up study of three cases. Clin. Orthop., *187*:223, 1984.

Stern, M. B., Rosner, L. J., Blinderman, E. E.: Kiloh-Nevin syndrome. Report of a case and review of the literature. Clin. Orthop., *53*:95, 1967.

Stern, P. J., and Kutz, J. E.: An unusual variant of the anterior interosseous nerve syndrome: a case report and review of the literature. J. Hand Surg., *5*:32, 1980.

Sucher, B. M., and Cavanaugh, J. A.: Guillain-Barré syndrome with secondary bilateral posterior interosseous nerve syndrome. Arch. Phys. Med. Rehabil., *63*:184, 1982.

Sumner, A. J.: The Physiology of Peripheral Nerve Disease. Philadelphia, W. B. Saunders Company, 1980.

Sunderland, S. S.: Nerves and nerve injuries. Edinburgh, Churchill Livingstone, 1978.

Swanson, A. B., Boeue, N. R., and Lumsden, R. M.: The prevention and treatment of amputation neuromas by silicone capping. J. Hand Surg., *2*:70, 1977.

Tobin, S. M.: Carpal tunnel syndrome in pregnancy. Am. J. Obstet. Gynecol., *97*:493, 1967.

Tountas, C. P., MacDonald, C. J., Meyerhoff, J. D., and Bihrle, D. M.: Carpal tunnel syndrome. A review of 507 patients. Minn. Med., *66*:479, 1983.

Tupper, J. W., and Booth, D. M.: Treatment of painful neuromas of sensory nerves in the hand: a comparison of traditional and newer methods. J. Hand Surg., *1*:144, 1976.

Urschel, H. C., Jr., and Razzuk, M. A.: The failed operation for thoracic outlet syndrome: the difficulty of diagnosis and management. Ann. Thorac. Surg., *42*:523, 1986.

Van Beek, A. L., Hubble, B., Kinkead, L., Torros, S., and Suchy, H.: Clinical use of nerve stimulation and recording techniques. Plast. Reconstr. Surg., *71*:225, 1983.

Van Beek, A. L., Massac, E., and Smith, D. O.: The use of signal averaging computer for evaluation of peripheral nerve problems. Clin. Plast. Surg., *13*:407, 1986.

Van Beek, A. L., and Zook, E. G.: Nerve regeneration—evidence for early sprout formation. J. Hand Surg., *7*:79, 1982.

Vanderpool, D. W., Chalmers, J., Lamb, D. W., and Whiston, T. R.: Peripheral compression lesions of the ulnar nerve. J. Bone Joint Surg., *50B*:792, 1968.

Wadsworth, T. G.: The external compression syndrome of the ulnar nerve at the cubital tunnel. Clin. Orthop., *124*:189, 1977.

Wallace, D.: Disc compression of the eighth cervical nerve: pseudo ulnar palsy. Surg. Neurol., *18*:295, 1982.

Werner, C. O., Rosen, I., and Thorngren, K. G.: Clinical and neurophysiologic characteristics of the pronator syndrome. Clin. Orthop., *197*:231, 1985.

Wiens, E., and Lau, S. C.: The anterior interosseous nerve syndrome. Can. J. Surg., *21*:354, 1978.

Willshire, W. H.: Supernumerary first rib. Lancet, *2*:633, 1860.

Wood, W.: Observations of neuromas with cures and histories of the disease. Trauma Med. Chir. Soc. Edinb., *3*:68, 1829.

Wright, I. S.: Neurovascular syndrome produced by hyperabduction of the arms. Am. Heart J., *29*:119, 1945.

Yamada, T., Kimura, J., and Nitz, D. M.: Short latency somatosensory evoked potentials following median nerve stimulation in man. Electroencephalogr. Clin. Neurophysiol., *48*:367, 1980.

Zamora, J. L., Rose, J. E., Rosario, V., and Noon, G. P.: Hemodialysis-associated carpal tunnel syndrome. A clinical review. Nephron, *41*:70, 1985.

Michael G. Orgel

Innervated Free Flaps and Free Vascularized Nerve Grafts in the Hand

INNERVATED FREE TISSUE TRANSFERS

The loss of sensation from an injury to the glabrous skin of the hand can limit the capacity to appraise environmental stimuli critically. Recovery of functional sensation is dependent on the reestablishment of precise anatomic pathways from the periphery to the central nervous system. The ability of regenerating axons to "cross innervate" another like or unlike type of sensory nerve ending provides the physiologic basis for sensory replacement procedures. The most desirable tissues for restoration of sensation in the hand would contain a significant concentration of similar nerve terminals. Therefore, when possible, glabrous skin should replace glabrous skin loss (Dellon, 1981).

Basis for Sensory Perception

An understanding of the anatomic-physiologic basis for sensory perception and the pathophysiology associated with injury to this system allows the most appropriate tissue for its replacement to be chosen. Normal sensory perception depends on a unique pattern of impulses initiated by cutaneous receptors and transmitted via sensory nerve fibers to the central nervous system (Fig. 112–1) (Melzack and Wall, 1962). There are three different anatomic groups of cutaneous receptors in the glabrous skin of the hands and feet that are responsible for the transduction of specific stimuli (Dellon, 1981). The skin of the remainder of the body also contains sensory nerve endings, but their concentration and specificity are less developed than in the glabrous tissues.

The cutaneous receptors of the skin and the group A-beta fibers of a peripheral nerve constitute two separately functioning systems dependent on the stimulus applied to the skin. These two systems allow for the perception of constant touch and pressure (slowly adapting fiber-receptor system) and of moving touch (quickly adapting fiber-receptor system), and can be measured by the static two-point discrimination test (Fig. 112–2*A*) or the moving two-point discrimination test (Fig. 112–2*B*) respectively (Dellon, 1981). While other sensory stimuli are perceived and transmitted by the hand (protective sensation), tactile gnosis is mainly determined by the slowly and quickly adapting fiber-receptor systems.

After a sensory nerve transection, deterioration of sensory nerve endings occurs at varying rates (Dellon, 1981). Once fully degenerated, these nerve terminals probably cannot regenerate de novo in the adult mammal (Ridley, 1970; Orgel, Aguayo, and Williams, 1972; Dellon, 1976, 1981). Additionally, a regenerating sensory nerve population

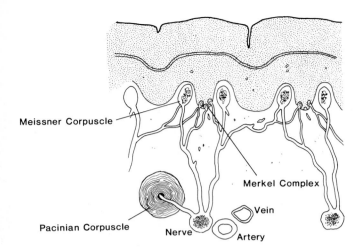

Figure 112–1. Sensory perception is dependent on patterns of impulses initiated by three anatomic groups of cutaneous receptors and transmitted to the central nervous system by sensory nerve fibers.

imbalance with a decrease of the group A-beta fibers, accompanied by a conduction velocity impairment, have been reported (Orgel, Aguayo, and Williams, 1972; Terzis, 1976). All these events contribute to the decreased and distorted sensory function seen after nerve and soft tissue injuries in the hand.

Restoration of Sensation in the Hand

A brief overview of traditional methods used for the treatment of sensory loss in the hand (see Chap. 109) helps to define the place for innervated free tissue transfers. Consideration of all these techniques from simple to complex leads to a "best choice" for each patient.

The use of local flaps (Kutler, 1947; Atasoy and associates, 1970; Berger, 1977; Biddulph, 1979), has the potential for providing innervated skin of similar characteristics to that

which is missing. In principle they involve advancing tissue by release of the fibrous septa surrounding the terminal neurovascular units. Their use is therefore limited to small defects of the finger pulp.

Neurovascular island flaps can cover larger but still limited tissue defects. They have been in use for over three decades (Littler, 1953) and are still advocated for the restoration of critical sensation to the index finger and thumb (Markley, 1977). These flaps have been reported to lose sensibility over time, possibly owing to tension or inattention to anatomic details during transfer (Markley, 1977). Additionally, their transfer leads to misrepresentation at the cortical level that may persist indefinitely. The latter problem has been avoided by the use of neurovascular island flaps from the injured finger itself (Moberg, 1961; O'Brien, 1968).

Correct cortical representation and larger amounts of tissue can be supplied to the damaged hand by innervated full-thickness skin grafts from the great toe when the vas-

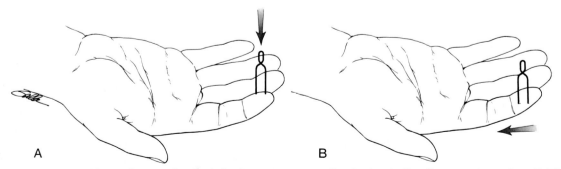

Figure 112–2. *A,* The static two-point discrimination test measures the slowly adapting fiber-receptor system. *B,* The moving two-point discrimination test measures the quickly adapting fiber-receptor system.

cular bed of the injury is adequate (Maquieira, 1974; Berger, 1977). The use of these grafts involves a difficult dissection to preserve neural supply, but good results have been reported (Maquieira, 1974). A defect the size of the full pulp of the fingertip can be covered with one-half of the pulp of the great toe.

Innervated palmar flaps have been used to cover larger proximal defects in severe degloving injuries of the hand with preservation of palmar sensory function (Nicolle and Woolhouse, 1966). Additionally, directly innervated conventional flaps have provided good protective sensation in severe injuries (Dolich, Olshansky, and Babar, 1978; Sommerlad and Boorman, 1981). The use of these flaps is dependent on an adequate vascular bed; as noted below, the choice of a donor site may prove critical to the final sensory recovery of the hand.

The Place of Innervated Free Tissue Transfers in Restoration of Sensation in the Hand. Innervated free flaps play a role in sensory restoration to the hand only in patients with no functional alternative (Morrison and associates, 1978a,b). This principle was demonstrated in the first successful great toe to hand transfer in 1968 (Cobbett, 1969) after Buncke had shown this to be possible in monkeys (Lumley, 1981). Eight months after surgery the patient was using the transfer as a normal thumb even though only protective sensation was present and two-point discrimination measured more than 20 mm. If an innervated transfer is critically needed to provide normal prehensile function it will be fully used by the patient, even if the return of sensory function is suboptimal. The corollary to this principle is that the patient usually bypasses a sensory transfer if an adjacent normal substitute is available, even though the return of function can be measured as normal or near-normal in the transferred tissue. The severely mutilated sensory deprived hand (see Fig. 112–5A) and a hand with severe damage and sensory loss to the thumb, therefore, constitute the major indications for use of these flaps. However, before an innervated free flap is considered, two other requisites should be present in the injured hand: a large amount of soft tissue loss that cannot be supplied locally, and the need for an augmented blood supply. These latter requisites are, of course, identical considerations to those for noninnervated free

tissue transfers. It therefore becomes apparent that the indications for use of an innervated free flap are quite limited and specific.

Donor Tissue for Neurovascular Free Flaps

Since McCraw and Furlow (1975) first described the dorsalis pedis arterialized flap and its accompanying nerve supply, interest has focused on the foot as a major donor site for sensate free tissue transfers. Three separate microsurgical units independently reported the use of this flap for the supply of sensation to anesthetic extremities (Daniel, Terzis, and Midgely, 1976; Ohmori and Harii, 1976; Robinson, 1976). Furthermore, Daniel, Terzis, and Midgely (1976) described an intricate method for mapping the "neural boundaries" of this flap to demonstrate the pattern of innervation of the superficial peroneal nerve. Follow-up time in these preliminary reports was short, but sensory recovery was progressive if not complete.

Since these original accounts, a large number of papers have discussed the subject of neurosensory free flaps for coverage problems in the hand. The qualities of the ideal neurosensory free flap can now be stated, and a survey of available donor sites and their potential for meeting these criteria can be given. The perfect neurosensory free flap for use in the hand should possess the following qualities (Strauch and Greenstein, 1985): its skin-subcutaneous tissue thickness should approximate that of the normal hand; it should have a consistent blood supply with good-sized vessels for ease of anastomosis; its nerve supply should be constant and should preferably course axially with the blood supply (Taylor and Daniel, 1975) (flaps with multiple or overlapping neural supply should probably be avoided unless careful study reveals a dominant nerve (Daniel, Terzis, and Schwarz, 1975); the number and quality of sensory nerve endings in the skin should approximate that of the glabrous skin of the hand (Dellon, 1981); and lastly, donor site morbidity should be minimal. This ideal free neurovascular flap should supply the damaged hand with a large area of tissue, new blood supply, and useful sensation (Morrison, 1978a,b).

Dorsalis Pedis Flap. The dorsalis pedis (DP) flap continues to play a role in sensory reconstruction of the damaged hand (Takami, Takahashi, and Ando, 1983; Strauch and Greenstein, 1985). It meets all the requisites noted above, with the exception that it does not replace glabrous skin and therefore cannot supply exquisite sensory recognition to the recipient area. This flap can provide an area of coverage as large as 14 × 12 cm (Strauch and Greenstein, 1985) and include underlying tendon and/or bone. When this combination of reconstructive needs exists, the DP flap should be considered.

The DP flap is based on the dorsalis pedis artery, the terminal branch of the anterior tibial artery. Its use therefore mandates an intact posterior tibial arterial supply to the foot. Venous return from this area can be via the superficial saphenous system or the deep venae comitantes that form interconnections (Fig. 112–3A) (McCraw and Furlow, 1975). The nerve supply to the DP flap is the multifascicular superficial peroneal nerve, which supplies all the skin of the dorsal foot except the first web space (Fig. 112–3B). While accurate sensory mapping of each of these fascicles (Daniel, Terzis, and Midgely, 1976) can direct more appropriate connections of donor and recipient nerves, most centers are not equipped or motivated to perform these extensive examinations.

Two-point discrimination of the dorsum of the foot in the superficial peroneal nerve distribution has been variously reported as ranging from 10 to 20 mm (Daniel, Terzis, and Midgely, 1976) to an average of 32 mm (May and associates, 1977) or 34 mm (Morrison and associates, 1978a,b). Since this is generally greater than acceptable for normal tactile gnosis, only protective sensation can be expected after transfer of this tissue to the hand. Detailed results of the return of sensory function after transfer of the DP sensory flap are limited. "Nearly normal" sensory recovery (Ohmori and Harii, 1976) and "successful reinnervation" (Daniel, Terzis, and Midgely, 1976) have been challenged by others (Morrison, 1978a,b; Strauch and Greenstein, 1985). The point that a DP flap transferred to a hand may develop better two-point discrimination than seen in situ (Takami, Takahashi, and Ando, 1983) is controversial and is addressed in more detail later in this chapter. A significant drawback to the use of the DP flap is the frequent slow healing of the obligatory skin graft in the donor site (McCraw and Furlow, 1975).

First Web Space Flap. Following the use of the DP flap as a neurosensory entity, it became desirable to improve the results of sensory functional return while retaining the other desirable characteristics of the original flap. Extension of the DP territory into the first web space of the foot as a neurovascular free flap has been well documented in the literature, and its anatomy, neurophysiology, indications, and results have been clearly elucidated (Gilbert, 1976; May and associates, 1977; Morrison and associates, 1978a,b, 1980; Strauch and Tsur, 1978; Baumeister and Wilhelm, 1979; Hamilton and Morrison, 1980; Leung and Ma, 1982).

The first web space of the foot supplies a stellate flap of tissue whose transverse dimension includes the lateral portion of the great toe and the medial portion of the second toe, and measures 12 to 14 cm in the adult (Morrison, 1978a,b; Strauch and Tsur, 1978). The longitudinal dimension of this flap can extend as far proximally on the dorsum of the foot as needed (7 to 8 cm or further) (Morrison, 1978a,b).

The arterial supply of the first web space flap is via the first dorsal metatarsal (FDMA) and the first plantar metatarsal (FPMA) arteries, both of which branch from the DP artery (Fig. 112–4A) (Gilbert, 1976; May and associates, 1977; Strauch and Tsur, 1978). In most cases (78 per cent) the FDMA branches from the DP artery just at the point where the latter dives between the first and second metatarsals, and courses superficially to terminate as the first and second dorsal digital arteries. The FDMA, however, may arise deeply from the descending DP artery or the plantar arch (22 per cent) and it then ascends into the first metatarsal space. In both of these variations the FDMA then passes dorsal to the transverse metatarsal ligament and turns as the distal communicating artery to join the FPMA. The plantar digital arteries arise near this junction (May and associates, 1977). Because of the ease of dissection, length, and large diameter of the DP-FDMA system, the dorsal approach is the method of choice for this flap (Morrison, 1978a,b). However, in approximately one out of four instances the plantar arterial system needs to be used.

The veins of the first web space drain deeply into the venae comitantes of the FDMA and FPMA, and superficially into one or more dorsal veins that join as a large vessel

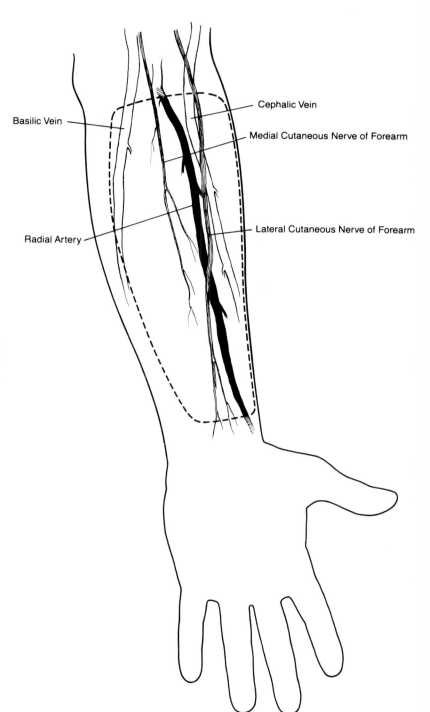

Figure 112–7. A forearm flap based on the radial artery and cephalic or basilic veins. Sensory innervation of this area is via the lateral and medial cutaneous nerves of the forearm.

1984). Proximal and/or distal use of the radial artery adds to the reconstructive possibilities of the flap (Strauch and Greenstein, 1985). However, the disadvantages probably outweigh the advantages, when this flap is considered primarily for its sensory potential. The donor site is quite visible and almost always requires a skin graft for closure. The radial artery must be taken with the flap (but can be reconstructed with a reverse vein graft) (Strauch and Greenstein, 1985). The greatest deficiency, however, is that like the DP flap, this flap can supply only minimal sensation to the hand. In this respect, its shortcomings may be greater than the DP flap because of its side by side overlapping nerve supply. Without nerve block studies or extensive mapping (Daniel, Terzis, and Schwarz, 1975), confusion will prevail concerning the most appropriate nerve to use.

Two other flaps situated in the lower extremity can be considered as potential neurovascular donors for hand coverage (Acland and associates, 1981; Walton and Bunkis, 1984; Walton and Petry, 1985).

Saphenous Flap (Fig. 112–8). The skin over the medial aspect of the knee, especially that below the knee joint, is quite thin but usually hair bearing. A large flap (29 × 8 cm has been reported) (Acland and associates, 1981) based on the saphenous artery (which branches from the descending genicular

branch of the femoral artery) can be harvested from this area. Venous drainage can be either via venae comitantes of the saphenous artery or the closely proximate long saphenous vein. The nerve supply of this area of skin is dual but serial, i.e., not side by side, and this, theoretically, is less bothersome than that of the forearm flap mentioned above. Above the knee the sensory nerve supply is the medial femoral cutaneous nerve; below the knee the flap is supplied by the saphenous nerve. These nerves travel in close proximity to either the arterial supply above or the venous drainage below. Two-point discrimination in the area of the saphenous nerve distribution has been reported as 6 to 8 mm in normal subjects (Acland and associates, 1981), which suggests that this area has the most exquisite sensation recorded for the nonglabrous skin of the body. Sensory recovery in the only saphenous free flap reported for hand coverage was 9 to 14 mm 18 weeks after surgery (Acland and associates, 1981). This flap has the advantages of providing a large amount of thin skin, a long and constant pedicle, and good potential for reasonable sensory recovery. Disadvantages include a donor site that requires skin grafting when flap width is greater than 7 cm, and a sensory deficit in the frequently injured proximal one-half to two-thirds of the anteromedial leg. It remains to be shown whether these

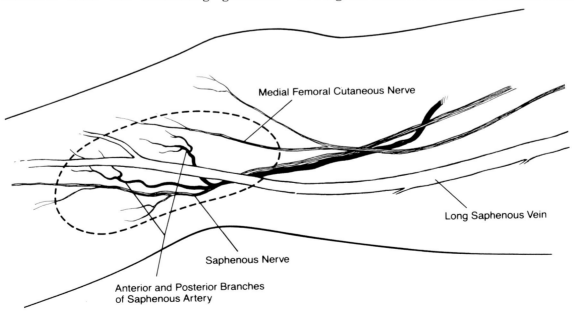

Figure 112–8. The saphenous neurosensory free flap is based on the saphenous artery and its venae comitantes or the long saphenous vein. Sensory nerve supply to this area is the medial femoral cutaneous nerve above the knee and the saphenous nerve below the knee.

deficiencies can be overshadowed by superior sensory recovery in selected instances.

Posterior Calf Flap. The posterior calf fasciocutaneous free flap (Fig. 112–9) has been used more often to provide sensation to the anesthetic hand (Walton and Bunkis, 1984; Walton and Petry, 1985). The skin of the posterior calf is thin but usually hair bearing. This flap can extend from lateral to medial midaxial lines of the leg, and from the lower border of the popliteal fossa to the juncture of the middle and lower one-third of the leg. The largest clinical flap reported has been 11×19 cm. The arterial supply to this

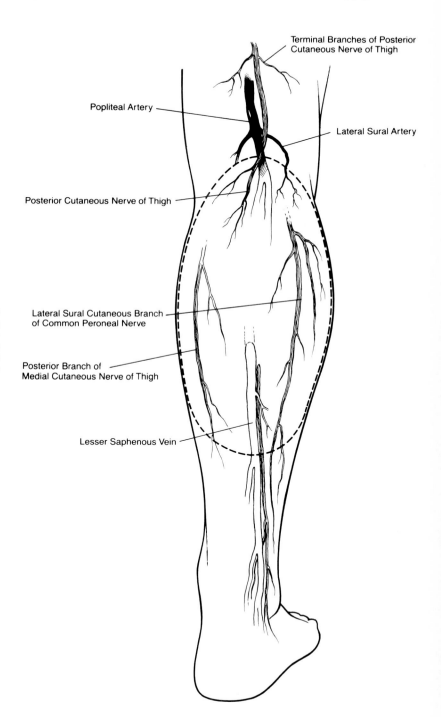

Figure 112–9. The posterior calf neurosensory free flap is based on a vascular supply arising from the popliteal artery or the lateral sural artery and their venae comitantes. Sensory nerve supply to this area is multiple (see text).

Terminal Branches of Posterior Cutaneous Nerve of Thigh

Popliteal Artery

Lateral Sural Artery

Posterior Cutaneous Nerve of Thigh

Lateral Sural Cutaneous Branch of Common Peroneal Nerve

Posterior Branch of Medial Cutaneous Nerve of Thigh

Lesser Saphenous Vein

area is axial via an artery that arises from either the popliteal artery or the lateral sural artery. In 95 per cent of dissections, the vessels are found in the "interval between the posterior midline of the calf and the fibular head" (Walton and Petry, 1985). Venous drainage of this flap is via the venae comitantes of the artery, which empty into the popliteal or sural vessels. The lesser saphenous vein has been a less reliable source of venous drainage. The sensory nerve supply to the posterior calf is multiple, theoretically making this flap less desirable for hand reconstruction, but several clinical cases have shown promising results. Terminal branches of the posterior cutaneous nerve of the thigh supply the upper part of the posterior calf. The middle and lower parts of this flap are supplied medially by the posterior branch of the medial cutaneous nerve of the thigh, and laterally by the lateral sural cutaneous branch of the common peroneal nerve (Walton and Bunkis, 1984).

In situ measurement of two-point discrimination in the posterior calf has been reported as 9 to 14 mm (Walton and Bunkis, 1984). In four out of 12 posterior calf fasciocutaneous flaps used for reconstruction of the upper extremity, two-point discrimination was less than 12 mm. The other flaps have remained insensate (Walton and Petry, 1985). Advantages of this flap include the availability of a large area of thin skin and fair potential for restoration of meaningful sensation. Disadvantages include variable vascular anatomy, vessels of small caliber, and a multiple sensory nerve supply, making it difficult to determine which branches will dominantly supply the flap being used for the most precise restoration of sensation.

Summary

The perception of cutaneous sensation is a complex phenomenon based on specialized nerve endings and terminal nerve branches that are best developed in the glabrous skin on the volar aspect of the hand and the plantar surface of the feet (Cauna, 1954; Weddell, 1955; Winkelmann, 1960; Jabaley and Dellon, 1980). After a destructive injury to the skin and underlying neural elements of the hand, reconstructive efforts should attempt to restore these relationships with sim-

ilar tissue. Whenever possible, use of local neurosensory flaps should be the method of choice. However, when this is not possible, and critical sensation is needed for thumb or distal hand reconstruction, an innervated free tissue transfer should be considered. The first web space of the foot provides a large area of glabrous skin, with well-defined neural and vascular anatomy, all or part of which can be used for restoring sensation to the hand. Although numerous other areas of the body have been advocated for use as neurosensory free flaps, the first web space flap provides the standard against which these must be analyzed. Results after the use of innervated free tissue transfers have been inconsistent. Usually, only protective sensation has been restored, but several studies have reported normal or near-normal sensory function. Indeed, it has been claimed that two-point discrimination in the recipient site can surpass that of the donor site (Strauch and Tsur, 1978; Buncke and Rose, 1979). If this proves to be a consistent finding, it most likely will be found to be related to an increased cortical representation of the recipient nerves and/or to sensory reeducation (Dellon, 1981). As a general rule, an innervated free flap should be used only when critical sensory function is lacking from one side of the prehensile unit, since only then will it be fully utilized by the patient.

FREE VASCULARIZED NERVE GRAFTS

The use of free vascularized nerve grafts for reconstruction in the upper extremity is a logical combination of solving the problem of nerve grafting in a poorly vascularized bed, with the technical potential associated with microsurgery (Taylor and Ham, 1976).

The treatment of a nerve gap with nerve grafts was reported over 100 years ago (Phillipeaux and Vulpian, 1870; Albert, 1885). However, technical failures in a large percentage of cases (Platt, 1919) helped to promote the common practices of extensive mobilization of proximal and distal nerve stumps, nerve transposition, and joint positioning to close gaps of up to 17 cm (Babcock, 1927; Seddon, 1972). The extensive scarring found in nerves treated in this fashion was thought to be responsible for the high rate of failure of this technique. Successful results from nerve grafts of short length rekindled interest in this method of repair (Vallance and Duel, 1932; Bunnell and Boyes, 1939). However, longer nerve grafts continued to fail clinically (Spurling and associates, 1945). The concept of the cable graft was introduced for clinical use by Bunnell and Boyes in 1939. It was then shown experimentally that large nerve trunk grafts undergo central necrosis and scarring owing to a lack of blood supply to their core (Sanders and Young, 1942; Tarlov and Epstein, 1945). These studies focused concentration on the blood supply to peripheral nerves and nerve grafts, and led to current clinical refinements defining conventional nerve grafting techniques (Millesi, Meissl, and Berger, 1972).

In 1947 St. Claire Strange introduced the concept of the pedicled nerve graft to solve the problem of central necrosis of large trunk grafts (St. Claire Strange, 1947, 1950). Since this procedure required the use of an adjacent major nerve, its indications were limited. Further clinical evidence of superior results with pedicled nerve grafts (Seddon, 1963; Edgerton, 1968; Alpar and Brookes, 1978) and the advent of microsurgery prompted the introduction of the free vascularized nerve graft by Taylor and Ham in 1976.

Blood Supply

The extrinsic blood supply to a peripheral nerve develops coaxially with the nerve (Taylor and Ham, 1976). Nutrient vessels connecting the extrinsic and intrinsic vascular systems course through a connective tissue sheath at various points along the length of the nerve (Fig. 112–10*A*). Vessels do not enter or leave the nerve at other points around its circumference (Smith, 1966a,b). This mesoneurium is variable in terms of its

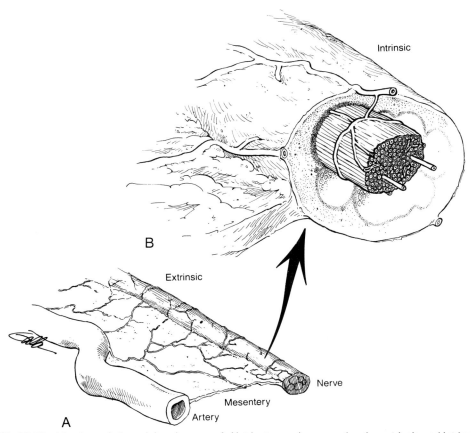

Figure 112–10. The blood supply to peripheral nerves. *A,* Nutrient vessels connecting the extrinsic and intrinsic vascular systems through a mesoneurium. *B,* The intrinsic system is composed of longitudinally oriented epineural, perineural, and endoneural vessels that freely anastomose.

extension along the length of a peripheral nerve; thus, long lengths of nerve may be devoid of an extrinsic blood supply (Smith, 1966a,b). The intrinsic vascular system of a nerve consists of longitudinal epineurial, perineurial, and endoneurial vessels that anastomose at frequent intervals (Fig. 112–10*B*). Only part of this system is functional at any specific time, and the amount and direction of flow can be varied as needed (Lundborg, 1970, 1975). It has been shown that the intrinsic and extrinsic vessels of a peripheral nerve are partially independent, and that the intrinsic system alone can support the nerve over limited distances (Lundborg and Branemark, 1968; Lundborg and Rydevik, 1973). Microdissection studies of various peripheral nerves have revealed several different patterns of blood supply from a single dominant vessel, to multiple vessels, to no dominant supply at all (Breidenbach and Terzis, 1984).

Experimental Studies

Laboratory Studies. The ideal intervening conduit between proximal and distal nerve stumps should direct axonal growth, remyelinate regenerating axons, limit tension, and protect regenerating fibers from connective tissue ingrowth. Additionally, it should be well vascularized to prevent central necrosis and scarring.

Theoretically, free vascularized nerve grafts offer the advantage of an increased chance of graft survival, especially in a poorly vascularized recipient bed (Taylor, 1978). Furthermore, a vascularized graft has been advocated as the best conduit for achieving accurate axonal growth and realignment between the proximal and distal nerve stumps. However, experimental evidence for these proposed advantages has not been uniformly convincing. A free vascularized nerve graft undergoes wallerian degeneration in the same manner as do free nonvascularized grafts. It has been proposed, however, that more rapid degeneration and clearance of neural elements and better preservation of Schwann cells and funicular architecture occurs with vascularized grafts (Townsend and Taylor, 1984). The Schwann cells in the graft would ideally then be available earlier in the regeneration sequence to remyelinate and direct the axons growing from the proximal nerve stump. While it has been convincingly

demonstrated that the Schwann cells of a nerve graft (and not those from the proximal nerve stump) are responsible for remyelination of regenerating axons (Aguayo and associates, 1979), dynamic disruptive phenomena have been shown to occur at each suture line of a nerve graft, making it relatively impossible for individual axons to enter "correct" distal endoneurial tubes except in random fashion (Morris, 1972a,b). Recent experimental evidence showing successful axonal regeneration through autogenous veins has questioned the need for Schwann cell elements in the intervening conduit (Chiu and associates, 1982; Rice and Berstein, 1984). These studies need to be repeated with conventional and vascularized nerve graft controls.

Several studies comparing vascularized and nonvascularized nerve grafts have produced conflicting results. In well-vascularized beds, nonvascularized cable grafts were compared with vascularized counterparts in the greyhound dog (Townsend and Taylor, 1984). In almost all instances the vascularized nerve was "associated with more rapid axonal regeneration and remyelination than the nonvascularized cable grafts." Similarly, poorly vascularized beds in rats were used to compare vascularized and nonvascularized grafts (Koshima and Harii, 1985). Greater density and generally larger diameters of myelinated fibers were found distal to the vascularized nerve grafts. Nerve action potentials and conduction velocities were also greater. However, recent blood flow studies of vascularized and nonvascularized nerve grafts have not corroborated these studies. A canine model using the saphenous nerve based on the femoral vessels was used, and blood flow was determined at four to six days by microsphere injection (Settergren and Wood, 1984; Daly and Wood, 1985). Results showed significantly greater blood flow in the nonvascularized grafts. This experiment was repeated measuring blood flow in both isolated fascicular and epineural tissues, and demonstrated superior flow rates in the conventional grafts at all levels. Although these results are discrepant, no functional results were reported for any of these studies, and further work is needed before firm conclusions can be made.

Clinical Studies. Relatively few case reports of free vascularized nerve grafts have appeared in the literature since the first in

1976 (Taylor and Ham, 1976; Taylor, 1978; Doi and associates, 1984; Townsend and Taylor, 1984; Rose and Kowalski, 1985). The patients treated have usually sustained severe trauma to the upper extremity ranging from electrical burns to crush, avulsion, or amputation injuries that have resulted in severely scarred, relatively avascular extremities with motor and/or sensory nerve deficits. Although the return of sensory function has not been optimal in most of the cases presented, protective sensation has been achieved, whereas previous attempts with nonvascularized grafts had provided none. In addition, selected cases have shown remarkable results with rapid rates of neural regeneration (Townsend and Taylor, 1984; Rose and Kowalski, 1985) and sensory recovery to accepted levels for accurate tactile gnosis (Rose and Kowalski, 1985). Motor nerve regeneration has also been seen in several cases in which specific attempts were made to achieve this end (Taylor, 1978; Townsend and Taylor, 1984). However, because of the associated extensive muscle injuries, no significant functional return has been reported for these few cases.

Indications

In view of the sparse literature on this subject, a discussion of the indications for free vascularized nerve grafts must be limited at this time. As further data become available the place for this procedure will be more easily stated. The proposed indications for free vascularized nerve grafts include a severely scarred recipient bed (often in patients with failed conventional grafts (Taylor and Ham, 1976; Taylor, 1978; Breidenbach and Terzis, 1984; Doi and associates, 1984; Rose and Kowalski, 1985); the need for long or thick grafts between proximal and distal nerve stumps (Taylor and Ham, 1976; Taylor, 1978; Breidenbach and Terzis, 1984; Doi and associates, 1984); supplementation of blood supply to the involved limb (Taylor and Ham, 1976; Rose and Kowalski, 1985); the need for a vascular "carrier" for nonvascularized grafts (Taylor and Ham, 1976; Breidenbach and Terzis, 1984); and proximal nerve lesions (Breidenbach and Terzis, 1984).

Analysis of the existing information, including both experimental and clinical studies, leads to the conclusion that the major

indication for free vascularized nerve grafts in the upper extremity is the need for an augmented blood supply in the recipient bed. The experimental evidence seems to indicate that the vascularized graft per se is not responsible for the improved nerve regeneration seen clinically. In fact, conventional grafts may be more advantageous in well-vascularized recipient beds (Settergren and Wood, 1984; Daly and Wood, 1985). Rather, a vascularized graft should be used only in instances in which the bed is so poor that regeneration could not be expected through a nonvascularized graft, or in which the latter has previously failed. It has not been proved that the nerve graft is the only or best conduit for axonal regeneration through a nerve gap; it may be that any well-vascularized conduit will produce the same or better results. This subject should prove to be fertile ground for further experimental work.

Donor Sources

To serve as a free vascularized graft, the ideal donor nerve should have a single dominant vascular supply that accompanies the nerve for most of its length (Breidenbach and Terzis, 1984). Constant anatomy, ease of accessibility, large diameter, long conducting length, high axonal to connective tissue ratio, large donor vessels, and minimal donor site morbidity are also important considerations in the choice of an ideal donor nerve (Taylor, 1978).

The major mixed nerves of the limbs have been shown to have adequate blood supply, but are indicated for use as free vascularized grafts only when nonreplantable amputation stumps are available (Taylor, 1978; Breidenbach and Terzis, 1984). Donor nerves that have proven clinical records of desirable anatomic prerequisites include the superficial radial nerve (Taylor and Ham, 1976; Taylor, 1978; Breidenbach and Terzis, 1984); the sural nerve (Frachinelli and associates, 1981; Breidenbach and Terzis, 1984; Doi and associates, 1984; Townsend and Taylor, 1984); the saphenous nerve (Breidenbach and Terzis, 1984); the superficial peroneal nerve (Breidenbach and Terzis, 1984); and the deep peroneal nerve (Rose, 1985). The anterior tibial neurovascular bundle represents another possible donor site that has been used clinically (Townsend and Taylor, 1984), but its small diameter, the tedious dissection procedure, and the mandatory sacrifice of a major lower extremity vessel combine to make it an unlikely choice (Breidenbach and Terzis, 1984). As experience with free vascularized grafts has accumulated, attempts have been made to meet the needs of the recipient area without sacrifice of major vascular or neural supply at the donor site (Breidenbach and Terzis, 1984; Townsend and Taylor, 1984; Rose, 1986).

Superficial Radial Nerve. The superficial radial nerve is easily accessible, and has a consistent vascular supply from the radial artery and its venae comitantes via a mesentery to the middle one-third of the nerve (Fig. 112–11) (Taylor and Ham, 1976; Taylor, 1978; Breidenbach and Terzis, 1984). A vascular pedicle can be developed for 2 to 5 cm between the brachial vessels and the mesentery, and the diverging vessels continue distally for the full length of the nerve (Taylor, 1976). The vessels are of large diameter throughout their course. The superficial radial nerve will supply 17 to 28 cm of a nonbranching graft from elbow to wrist. Its length can be extended proximally for several centimeters by intraneural dissection, and its primary divisions can be included distally (Taylor and Ham, 1976). The nerve is smaller in cross section proximally (1.5 to 2.5 mm) than distally (2.5 to 3.5 mm) and has a high axon to connective tissue ratio. As with most donor nerves, its diameter is smaller than the median or ulnar nerves, but supplemental sural nerve cable grafts may be "carried" by it. Donor site morbidity includes loss of sensation in the radial nerve distribution and a potential sensory neuroma (neither of which has proved significant in reported cases). The major disadvantage of the free vascularized radial nerve lies in the necessary sacrifice of the radial artery.

Sural Nerve. The sural nerve based on the superficial sural artery and vein does not have sufficiently consistent vascular anatomy for reliable use as a free vascularized graft (Frachinelli and associates, 1981; Breidenbach and Terzis, 1984). However, two nuances in technique have been reported and have renewed interest in its use (Doi and associates, 1984; Townsend and Taylor, 1984). Doi and associates (1984) demonstrated that the blood supply to the distal two-thirds of the sural nerve is derived through a "fascial vascular plexus" supplied by the cutaneous branch of the peroneal artery or the muscular perforating branch of the posterior tibial artery (Fig. 112–12*A*). A nerve graft up to 25 cm in length and vessels between 1 and 3 mm in diameter can be obtained. By careful protection of the fascia and segmental blood supply, the nerve can be bi- or trisected to form cables that satisfy the cross sectional dimensions of the recipient nerve. Donor site morbidity from loss of the sural nerve or neuroma formation is negligible. Sacrifice of a major blood supply to the limb is not inherent in this technique.

Townsend and Taylor (1984) have reported the use of a composite sural neurovenous graft (Fig. 112–12*B*). This system is based on the reversed short saphenous vein being perfused by a recipient artery. Cadaver studies demonstrated good flow into the capillary bed of the nerve by this retrograde perfusion. Additionally, in all dissections the vein stayed adjacent to the nerve from the lateral malleolus to the point at which the nerve penetrates the deep fascia. Experimental work confirmed flow through these reversed neurovenous grafts. While venous drainage was obtained via a reversed artery segment in this study, clinical cases have done well without formal venous drainage as long as a distal vein to artery anastomosis is also done. In most cases a neurovenous graft of approximately 40 cm in length can be obtained with a vessel that averages 2 mm in diameter distally and 2.5 mm proximally. This composite graft is superficial and easy to dissect, and donor site morbidity is minimal. Furthermore, it has been shown that changing the polarity of a nerve graft does not affect functional nerve regeneration (Stromberg, Vlastou, and Earle, 1979).

Saphenous Nerve. The saphenous nerve has been touted as the "nerve of choice" for upper extremity peripheral nerve reconstruction (Breidenbach and Terzis, 1984). Its anterior access is advantageous, and as a free vascularized graft it is based on the saphenous artery and vein (Fig. 112–13). These vessels are of suitable diameter (average 2.0 and 2.1 mm, respectively) and a proximal pedicle 2 to 6 cm in length can be provided. The vessels accompany the nerve only in its middle section. The rest of the nerve is vascularized by intrinsic blood supply alone. A saphenous nerve graft approximately 40 cm from groin to knee can be obtained. Cross sectional diameter measurements and axon

of this condition, and the author would prefer that it be recognized far earlier, especially in patients who have not had major nerve injury.

Listening carefully to the patient's description and observing his or her behavior provides the best opportunity for early diagnosis. Patients will frequently describe a constant diffuse "deep ache," or "tearing," "burning," "shooting" or "sharp, cutting" pain that spontaneously varies in intensity and is aggravated by motion and work and may interfere with sleep. Although the pain often radiates to nonanatomic distributions along peripheral nerves, it usually remains within a confined region, as would be expected in cortical midbrain representation. Evidence for "mirror image" advancement of changes in the opposite extremity is reported in as many as 25 per cent of patients (Schott, 1986; Kozin, 1986), although it has never been observed by this author.

Observation of the patient's response is as important as the pain description in making an early diagnosis. Patients with reflex sympathetic dystrophy seem less able to cope than other hand-injured patients. They are more depressed, angry, and anxious about their dilemma and will quickly feel rejected and resentful when a well-meaning but impatient surgeon points out their relative lack of physical findings. The examining physician will sense a lack of trust and a mood of desperation. These patients want explanations. They often repeat questions in a strained, anxious fashion. Many times they appear to seek a magical operation or cure. Patients with established cases often indict all previous treatment efforts and former physicians and therapists. Although they already have chronic, constant discomfort, the pain is predictably aggravated by active or passive motion, especially work, and seems worsened by their emotional state. Because these patients express greater distress and frustration over their plight than do others, they demand greater attention, but they are quick to anger and to experience feelings of rejection. Unless the diagnosis is made early, gaining their confidence takes great patience.

Although on examination the extremity may appear anatomically capable, pain initially stops functional activity. The patient quickly develops avoidance patterns. Whereas other patients with hand wounds will readily permit the injured hand to be examined, the patient with reflex sympathetic dystrophy withdraws the involved hand and wards away the examiner with the other hand. This disproportionate withdrawal response in any hand-injured patient should alert the physician to the need to provide additional support to prevent a painful dystrophy. Although there may be numerous autonomic abnormalities, the dominant factor limiting function remains pain until the later dystrophic changes such as stiffness and osteoporosis develop. This pain usually starts out well localized but, if uncontrolled, will advance proximally, with numerous myofascial trigger points identifiable, until the entire upper extremity and, rarely, the entire side of the body may become involved. A careful history and meticulous characterization of the pain along with observation of the patient's emotional response remain the best diagnostic tools for early recognition.

Physical Findings and Stages of Disease

The most common early physical manifestations of reflex dystrophy are those of low-grade inflammation or of autonomic nervous system dysfunction. Pain usually precedes these changes, which most often start with edema that may be pitting or nonpitting; color change, which usually starts with mottled redness; temperature abnormality with either warmth or coolness; and an increase in sweating or dryness. Early decrease in joint motion due to pain is usually seen. The pattern generally is one of low-grade inflammatory change with disproportionate pain. Indeed, biopsy of synovial tissue has revealed mild inflammatory changes in comparison with control tissue (Kozin, 1976b; Genant and associates, 1975), but the subjective pain seems out of proportion to these mild changes. Betcher and Casten (1955) pointed out that most of these signs and symptoms, in their mild form, are universal following trauma. However, patients without reflex sympathetic dystrophy will show diminution of these signs and symptoms with time, whereas patients with the condition may go on to have greater autonomic and later trophic changes.

Most workers agree with Betcher's (1955) classification of the clinical features of reflex sympathetic dystrophy into three progressive stages (Table 113–3); however, patients ac-

Table 113–3. Stages of Reflex Sympathetic Dystrophy

Stage I Acute
Lasts approximately 3 months (variable)
Constant burning or throbbing pain (intensity varies)
Allodynia and hyperpathia
Trigger points may develop
Variable vasomotor changes such as edema (pitting or nonpitting); color change (usually redness, sometimes cyanosis); temperature change (usually warmth, sometimes coolness); increased sweating; sometimes dryness
Decreased joint range of motion due to pain, sometimes swollen
Fingernail ridging (occasional)
Increased hair growth or pigmentation (occasional)

Stage II Subacute
Lasts approximately 9 to 12 months (variable)
Constant aggravating pain (intensity varies)
Atrophy of skin and subcutaneous tissue
Loss of fingertip pads ("pencil pointing")
Glossy, thin skin
Decreased hair growth
Cyanosis
Brawny edema
Joint ankylosis
Palmar fasciitis and Dupuytren's nodules (occasional)
Myofascial trigger points (usual)
Subchondral patchy osteoporosis (usual)

Stage III Chronic
Chronic intractable pain
Pale, cool, dry extremity
Thin, stretched skin
Muscle atrophy
Fixed flexion or extension contractures
Diminished hair growth (usual)
Patchy to generalized osteoporosis
Patient is chronically depressed and may contemplate suicide

tually exhibit very wide variation in the onset, duration, and mixture of characteristics in each stage. Some unfortunate patients will rapidly progress to late (chronic) disease in three to six months, whereas others have features of the first stage literally for many years. Because of this variation, these stages hold no great clinical value except for communication and prognostication. Identifying the stage of a particular patient's disease is helpful if we recognize that the more advanced the disease process, the more limited the expected functional return, and anticipate the greater difficulty in treatment. One must recognize that the terms acute, subacute, and chronic refer to the amount of autonomic and trophic change and not necessarily to chronology. The stages may be summarized as acute (stage I), with mild inflammatory change; subacute (stage II), with marked autonomic change; and chronic (stage III), with predominantly dystrophic change. In all three stages, pain is the preeminent feature.

The *acute or stage I* symptoms of reflex dystrophy are dominated by a constant burning or aching pain that varies in intensity and may radiate. This pain is inexplicably intense and interferes with function or even motion. Aggravation by non-noxious stimuli (allodynia) is evident, and the patient may seek to avoid the examiner's soft touch. Physical signs in this stage are variable, but as they become visible they are largely vasomotor, with swelling and edema, redness or other color changes, increased warmth or coolness, and increased sweating or possibly dryness (Lankford, 1982) (Fig. 113–1). Limited joint motion, present in over half the patients, is largely due to pain. Blood flow in the extremity may be increased. Some early trophic changes may occur, such as ridging of the nails, increased hair growth, pigmentation change, and obliteration of fat planes. Bone scintigraphic studies have revealed

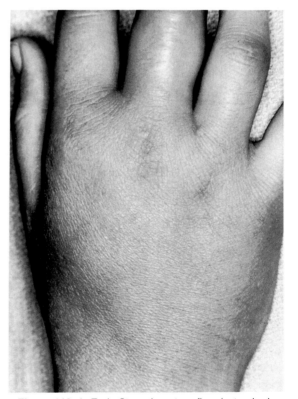

Figure 113–1. Early Stage I acute reflex dystrophy in a young man after minor trauma at work. He had intense pain, edema, and increased temperature. He responded to hand therapy and anti-inflammatory medication.

changes as early as six weeks, and Kozin (1976a) has demonstrated synovial inflammatory cells on biopsy during this phase. The acute stage usually lasts around three months, and the findings are sufficiently subtle that affected patients are commonly misdiagnosed until the second stage changes appear (Thompson, 1979).

The *subacute stage (stage II)* of reflex dystrophy may characteristically last nine to 12 months, and the symptoms are still dominated by constant pain that reaches maximum intensity and causes great agitation (Lankford, 1982). The diagnosis is more obvious, because now trophic changes become evident, with atrophy of skin and subcutaneous tissue causing glossy, thin skin, decreased hair growth, and loss of wrinkling and of fingertip pads ("pencil-pointing" of involved digits). As this syndrome progresses, Raynaud's phenomenon may develop, with previous redness now giving way to a cyanotic, cold-intolerant extremity that maintains a reduced resting temperature. Brawny edema may be present, and the restriction in joint motion that was previously a voluntary response to pain now becomes physically necessary owing to capsular remodeling and ankylosis (Fig. 113–2). A curious association is the development of palmar fascitis, thickening of palmar fascia, and Dupuytren's nodules in many patients (Steinbrocker, 1968). Mottled, patchy subchondral osteoporosis may be evident on routine radiographs, and muscle atrophy may become measurable. When carefully sought, over half these patients will have palpable trigger points over muscles proximal to the primary area of discomfort, and signs and symptoms may progressively spread to adjacent areas if not brought under control during this stage (Evans, 1947).

In *chronic or stage III* reflex dystrophy the dominant symptom is still chronic intractable pain. However, now the physical appearance better corresponds to the symptoms, with a pale, cool, dry extremity that has thinly stretched skin and progressive muscle atrophy. Often there is fixed flexion or extension joint contracture with fibrous ankylosis and loss of the thumb web (Fig. 113–3). Hair growth is diminished. Osteoporosis may change from spotty to a generalized demineralization, and at this stage patients may persuade surgeons to perform amputation to control the pain in their functionless extremity. Although it may appear to be a reasona-

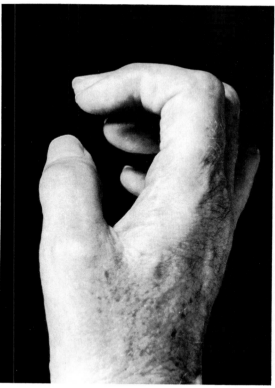

Figure 113–2. Stage II (subacute) reflex dystrophy with joint stiffness, decreased hair growth, thumb web contracture, and loss of skin wrinkles in a woman one year after a Colles fracture.

ble request, amputation should be avoided. In the late stage of reflex dystrophy, the intractable pain likely involves reflex patterns at the cortical level; therefore, amputation may lead only to phantom pain and pleas for additional, higher amputations. Individuals with stage III disease are chronically depressed and may well become suicidal (Horowitz, 1984).

Clinical Forms

Many of the different terms for reflex sympathetic dystrophy arise from workers' focusing attention on different precipitating causes, symptoms, severity, and anatomic locations in what is likely the same phenomenon (see Table 113–1). Lankford (1982) identified five clinical forms of the disease according to severity: (1) minor causalgia following minor injury to a purely sensory nerve; (2) minor traumatic dystrophy follow-

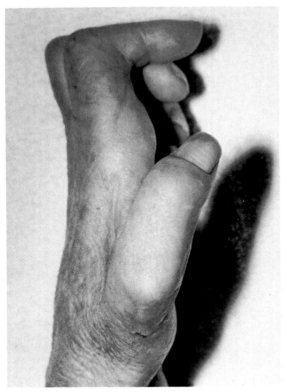

Figure 113–3. Stage III late reflex dystrophy in a patient with causalgia from proximal electrical nerve injury.

ing minor non-nerve trauma such as a sprain, fracture, or laceration; (3) shoulder-hand syndrome, which may be caused by either proximal trauma or a visceral lesion; (4) major traumatic dystrophy, which usually follows a significant traumatic incident without major nerve involvement, such as a crush injury or Colles' fracture; and (5) major causalgia, which classically involves a high-velocity wound to proximal mixed major nerves and responds to sympathectomy.

Because virtually any inciting injury, or even no apparent injury at all, may lead to reflex dystrophy, and because the severity and duration have no correlation with the site or nature of onset, these classifications are of questionable value and do not imply different outcomes, origins, or treatment techniques. However, three clinical forms do seem so distinct that their use facilitates describing the individual patient's symptoms, and they warrant separate discussion: causalgia, shoulder-hand syndrome, and Sudeck's osteoporosis.

CAUSALGIA

Major causalgia is the most distinct form of reflex dystrophy, if indeed we should even place it in this category. As originally described, first by Denmark in the War of 1812 and then by Mitchell in the American Civil War, this disorder has a specific onset associated with penetrating wounds adjacent to major nerves. Thus, it is distinguished from other forms of reflex dystrophy by a specific known nerve injury. The International Association for the Study of Pain Subcommittee on Taxonomy defines causalgia as "a syndrome of sustained burning pain after a traumatic nerve lesion combined with vasomotor and pseudomotor dysfunction and later trophic change" (Bonica, 1979b). Of all the hand pain dystrophic syndromes, causalgia has the most obvious peripheral irritation to the nervous system. Sunderland (1976) points out that "with few exceptions, causalgia is confined to those nerve lesions which are situated above the elbow and knee." These are usually mixed nerve lesions caused by high-velocity missile wounds in which the nerve is known to have been subjected to rapid and violent deformation. In the upper extremity, the median nerve is most commonly involved, and most patients report the onset of pain immediately after or within hours of being wounded; it then becomes a continuous burning pain (Sunderland, 1976; Turf and Bacardi, 1986). In one series of war casualties in Beirut, Lebanon, the incidence of causalgia was 5.8 per cent with onset of symptoms in less than six hours in 75 per cent of the patients. Sympathectomy corrected all of the cases in this series (Jebara and Saade, 1987).

Although the injury is usually above the elbow or knee, causalgia pain remains confined to the distal part of the extremity more often than other types of reflex dystrophy, but it does not remain restricted to the skin distribution of the involved nerve (Kirklin, Chenoweth, and Murphy, 1947). Trophic changes in causalgia appear early, and because of the associated nerve injury, they are more severe and more likely to result in irreversible change than are other forms of reflex dystrophy.

Mitchell, Moorehouse, and Keen (1864), Sunderland (1976), Echlin, Owens, and Wells (1949), and others have pointed out that in most patients the neurologic deficit and pain gradually improve to a variable degree,

not genuine (Pulvertaft, 1975). Rather, it is important to clearly document that the patient's symptoms are not understood and that the findings are inconsistent for unknown reasons. Let others pass the judgment.

Factitious wounding, especially when there is no apparent secondary gain, is a serious psychiatric disorder that can be most troublesome to diagnose. In the true factitial disorder, the patient seems unaware that the injury is self-inflicted and often has supportive family members who share in the denial (Pulvertaft, 1975). Such a case can be most difficult to diagnose, even after one suspects its presence, because the patient will always deny the possibility and has to be shown by use of cast, direct observation on an in-patient basis, or some other means to ever acknowledge that the edema, nonhealing ulcer, or other manifestation is self-inflicted. Sometimes, self-inflicted injury causes apparent peritendinous fibrosis on the hand dorsum, as described by Secretan in 1901. Unfortunately, simple confrontation does little or nothing to help patients with factitious disorders, who will simply take their symptoms elsewhere unless they can be persuaded to undergo intensive psychotherapy.

Conversion disorders, or hysteric neuroses, are signs and symptoms of physical disorders that originate from psychologic conflict. These are not deliberate, conscious, or understood by the patient and have no explicable physical disorder associated with them (Pulvertaft, 1975). Two examples are hysterical paralysis and clenched fist syndrome. Physical examination will reveal the sincerity of the patient as well as the absence of findings appropriate for the bizarre symptoms. Complete loss of sensation will often follow non-anatomic patterns, such as stocking-glove anesthesia, and the patient does not seem terribly concerned about these dramatic findings. Simmons and Vasile (1980) suggested that the "clenched fist syndrome" may be symbolic of the patient's suppressed anger. These patients usually respond favorably to psychotherapeutic intervention.

Myofascial Dysfunction

Myofascial dysfunction may be one of the conditions most commonly mistaken for reflex sympathetic dystrophy. Indeed, the finding of myofascial dysfunction in over half the pa-

tients with reflex dystrophy makes one wonder whether the two disorders have common features in etiology and mechanisms of persistence. Like that in reflex dystrophy, the pain in myofascial dysfunction seems disproportionate, with no obvious apparent cause until the trigger point is identified. The diagnosis becomes evident once trigger points are found that clearly precipitate the referred pain.

When myofascial dysfunction is associated with reflex dystrophy, the latter's symptoms predominate. In treatment, however, it becomes important to inactivate the proximal trigger points as part of effective therapy for the distal sites of reflex sympathetic dystrophy.

Volkmann's Ischemic Contracture

Volkmann's ischemic contracture (see also Chap. 120) is a response to partial vascular compromise, such as displaced supracondylar humeral fracture compression of the brachial artery. Volkmann himself (1881) attributed the cause to ischemia from tight bandaging. It is still debated whether the condition is due to arterial spasm, small vessel occlusion, venous congestion, compartment syndrome, or all of the above (Tsuge, 1982). This condition may cause ischemic contracture of the forearm flexors or the intrinsic muscles following trauma, especially if a cast becomes too tight. The ultimate result—progressive fibrosis, contracture, and ankylosis—looks like late stages of reflex sympathetic dystrophy. Legal advisors may therefore misinterpret the reflex dystrophy patient as having had a cast too tight, confusing these two disorders. However, the onset and findings are quite distinct, even though either condition often may arise as a sequel to trauma and immobilization.

The classic symptoms and progression of Volkmann's ischemic contracture are the "five P's": paresthesia, pallor, pulselessness, pain with finger extension, and paralysis (Boyes, 1970). Their presence indicates immediate need for release of dressings or cast, better stabilization of fractures, escharotomy, fasciotomy, or whatever it takes to correct the vascular compromise. If the condition progresses, contracture and necrosis of the involved muscles develop, usually in the finger flexors of the forearm or intrinsic muscles of the hand. The resultant fibrotic process has been shown to have myofibroblast formation (Madden, Carlson, and Hines, 1975). When the process is in the forearm, the progressive neurologic loss can be stopped, and sometimes sensation improved, by extensive neurolysis, placing the median and ulnar nerves in a subcutaneous position (Peacock, 1984). There is no fully satisfactory treatment for established Volkmann's ischemic contracture of the forearm muscles, but flexor slide procedures (Tsuge, 1982) and free microvascular muscle replacement (Mankeltow and McKee, 1976) have been used to correct contracture and replace the lost flexors.

Volkmann's ischemic contracture of the intrinsic muscles is not as easily recognized and may occur in injuries confined to the hand and look much like reflex dystrophy. The early manifestations include intrinsic tightness and pain when the "intrinsic test" is performed—placing the metacarpophalangeal joint in extension and assessing whether tight intrinsic muscles now cause the interphalangeal joints to remain extended or to resist flexion. Early intrinsic contracture is best handled by intrinsic fasciotomy.

Although the late dystrophic hand of Volkmann's ischemic contracture is similar in appearance to the hand in the late stages of reflex sympathetic dystrophy, the pain characteristics are quite distinct. The reflex sympathetic dystrophy patient complains bitterly of persistent pain, whereas the patient with Volkmann's ischemic contracture develops progressive anesthesia and paralysis of the hand. In late stages, the patient with Volkmann's ischemic contracture of forearm muscles will characteristically have flexed metacorpophalangeal and interphalangeal joints, and the patient with intrinsic muscle contracture will have swan-neck deformities (Fig. 113–7). These changes are rarely seen with reflex sympathetic dystrophy. Although both reflex dystrophy and Volkmann's ischemic contracture begin with symptoms of pain and may benefit from loosening dressings, it is important to distinguish between them. Fasciotomy can be of great benefit in Volkmann's ischemic contracture but is usually contraindicated in reflex dystrophy, in which any operation may further aggravate and complicate the pain syndrome.

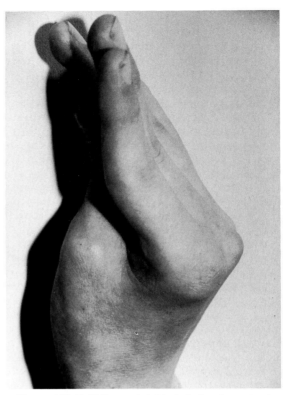

Figure 113–7. Volkmann's intrinsic ischemic contracture subsequent to a self-inflicted radial artery injury (through a drug injection) in a young woman. It resembles reflex sympathetic dystrophy, but there are swan-neck deformities from intrinsic contractures.

Local Nerve Irritation

Certain persistent nerve irritation or inflammation, such as occurs with atypical carpal tunnel syndrome or painful neuroma, appears to either mimic or precipitate reflex sympathetic dystrophy. Patients with acute carpal tunnel syndrome, incomplete carpal tunnel release, or neuroma formation from severance of the palmar sensory branch of the median nerve may demonstrate exaggerated pain, edema, and vasomotor instability, often with proximal trigger points and pain in the entire upper extremity. In the author's experience, preoperative control of these diffuse inappropriate manifestations of pain allows a smoother course after surgery for neurolysis of residual compression or resection of painful neuromas. Early surgery in the midst of a pain syndrome may accelerate these manifestations.

TREATMENT

Treatment of reflex dystrophy, which is as varied as the myriad of names given the disorder, should be directed toward interrupting the existing cycle of reflex pain (Lankford, 1982). This statement is true whether the reflex cycle is at the midbrain level, at the dorsal horn of the spinal cord, or in an injury site of a major peripheral nerve. Although proponents enthusiastically endorse each of their own reported treatment techniques, the mere fact so many different methods still exist is testimony to the fact that none is universally successful.

Without doubt, whenever it is possible, the best treatment for advanced reflex dystrophy is prevention (Markoff and Farole, 1986). It can be achieved only by prompt diagnosis of the earliest possible manifestations to prevent the later autonomic and trpohic changes. Any patient who appears to have an undue response to injury or surgery, such as exaggerated pain on suture removal or excessive and irrelevant, anxious questions, should be followed carefully and given whatever additional support and encouragement he or she needs to resume active use of the hand. Hand therapists can be very helpful because they can provide the additional time and reassurance so often needed for functional use in these more anxious patients.

Patients with established reflex dystrophy cases also need support, but by this stage they often are suspicious, depressed, resentful, and pessimistic. A variety of different treatment options may now be necessary. The surgeon must remain optimistic and positive in outlook with these late cases, but realistic about the knowledge that no magical cure is available. The goal will be to help the patient cope and live with the condition, with gradual improvement expected from treatment. A strenuous effort must be made in each case (1) to gain the confidence of the patient, (2) to make the patient understand the surgeon's sincere desire to help and (3) to communicate the belief that with the patient's cooperation, satisfactory rehabilitation can be a realistic goal (Shumacker, 1985). Treatment may run the spectrum from psychotherapy to sympathectomy, but every worker agrees that the earlier any treatment is instituted, the better the prognosis. The principal generalization in treatment should be the willing individualization of management to fit each patient's different manifestations, needs, and clinical course. The following treatment methods vary greatly, but in most patients it is advisable to start with the least invasive and morbid techniques and gradually add new methods until a regimen succeeds, maintaining a positive, constructive outlook throughout these efforts.

Sympathetic Block

Sympathetic nerve block has remained the most widely accepted form of treatment for reflex sympathetic dystrophy since Leriche first reported its successful use in 1930. In fact, some clinicians even feel that successful nerve block should be a prerequisite for diagnosis (Betcher and Casten, 1955; Linson, Leffert, and Todd, 1983). However, blocks are not uniformly successful, as shown in the literature and in the author's personal experience. Therefore, sympathetic nerve interruption should be recognized as only one of the many treatment possibilities and should not be used as the sole criterion of diagnosis and treatment. Sympathetic nerve block is most successful (temporarily—for the block's duration) in the nerve-injured causalgia form of reflex dystrophy (Shumacker, 1985; Abram, 1986). The procedure may fail in as many as one-third of patients with other clinical forms of reflex dystrophy (Wang, Johnson, and Ilstrup, 1985; Shumacker, 1985).

If the sympathetic nervous system malfunction in reflex dystrophy is sympathetic modification of afferent pain fibers to lower pain thresholds and release neurotransmitter pro-inflammatory substances, it is understandable how blocking this modification may be beneficial in some patients. In other patients, however, it is possible to hypothesize central neurotransmitter activity at the mesencephalon level that will not be impressed by sympathetic block and its peripheral control activity. Reflex pain at this central level might better respond to the endogenous opioid internal pain control system, which is known to interfere with neurotransmitter (substance P) production (Leeman and associates, 1981). This endogenous control might explain why "placebo blocks" are reported to be successful in as many as 30 per cent of cases (Bonica, 1953; Beecher, 1959), as well as the reported successes with transcutaneous electrical neural stimulation (TENS) (Richlin and associates, 1978), acupuncture (Chan and Chow, 1981), hypnosis (Merskey, 1978), and other methods that instill and require patient confidence.

Permanent relief has been noted following repeated sympathetic nerve blocks (Kleinert and associates, 1973; Bonica, 1979a), and a few patients have experienced complete relief after a single nerve block combined with a program of active exercise (Shumacker, 1985; Abram, 1986). Bonica (1979a) estimated a success rate of 80 per cent in his review of reports on use of sympathetic nerve block, noting that the worst results occurred when the disorder had been present a long time. Most workers recommend that when this method is used as the primary form of treatment, daily or alternate-day blocks be attempted for a series of three to five days (Abram, 1986). When this technique is successful, pain relief should outlast the duration of the local anesthetic, whether short-acting or long-acting, and as long as the duration of analgesia increases and the severity of the recurrent pain decreases, blocks should be repeated. While the pain is at bay, the patient should be persuaded to do those things that formerly hurt, and the importance of making frequent, active, vigorous use of the extremity as the condition improves must be stressed and encouraged.

When repeated blocks do not offer relief any longer than the duration of the anesthetic, sympathectomy or other alternative forms of treatment should be considered (Abram, 1986). Lankford (1982) clearly describes techniques for percutaneous intermittent sympathetic nerve block and points out that the stellate and upper two or three dorsal sympathetic ganglia must be involved for a successful block that does not interfere with somatic or motor function. This technique generally produces warming, drying, and loss of piliary action in the hairs of the extremity. If complete block of the upper portion of the stellate ganglion is achieved, a Horner's syndrome will be noted including ptosis (eyelid drooping), miosis (pupil constriction), enophthalmos, and dilatation of conjunctival vessels.

Wang, Johnson, and Ilstrup (1985) studied three-year follow-up results of sympathetic nerve block and found that 40 per cent of the patients had good to excellent results, 22 per cent had pain relief, and 38 per cent had a poor outcome. This is in contrast to other reports with more optimistic findings but shorter follow-up. These researchers did note, however, that in patients who were treated within six months of onset of their disease, there was a 70 per cent success at three years, indicating that this treatment, as all others, is most successful when instituted early. Use of continuous infusion block has been described but requires hospitalization to be done safely (Omer and Thomas, 1971; Linson, Leffert, and Todd, 1983). Reports of enkephalin and endorphin in sympathetic ganglia (DiGuilio, 1978; Schultzberg and associates, 1979) led Mays, North, and Schnapp (1981) to use morphine for stellate ganglion block. They produced relief in eight of their ten patients so treated, leading to speculation whether this technique activated the endogenous pain control system.

Although sympathetic nerve block remains the most widely accepted treatment and diagnostic test for reflex dystrophy, its primary use seems most appropriate for patients whose manifestations include marked autonomic change. Patients with minimal sympathetic abnormality but characteristic pain often respond to an active program of hand therapy alone, nerve blocks being reserved for use if the hand therapy fails (Pak and associates, 1970; Abram, 1986). Recent studies suggest that sympathetic nerve block by pharmacologic agents may also prove equally promising (Glynn, Basedow, and Walsh, 1981; Bonelli and associates, 1983; Duncan and associates, 1988).

Sympathectomy

Most surgical techniques for reflex dystrophy, such as periarterial sympathectomy (Jebara and Saade, 1987), posterior rhizotomy (dorsal root section) (Sunderland, 1976), chordotomy (spinothalamic tract section), neurolysis, and neurectomy (Greenberg, Price, and Becker, 1983; Abram, 1986), have proved to be of little value. Sympathectomy, however, has remained useful ever since Leriche introduced the concept in 1916 and Spurling popularized the operation for reflex dystrophy in 1930. This operation is of greatest value in cases with pronounced peripheral irritation from proximal nerve injury such as causalgia (Jebara and Saade, 1987), and may be less useful in the slowly developing dystrophy from minor trauma or from central nervous system origin such as stroke. When the pain reflex arc originates more centrally, the peripheral modulation by sympathectomy may be less meaningful.

The patient who is most likely to benefit from sympathectomy is one who obtains repeated dramatic temporary relief from sympathetic blocks, but for whom the relief never lasts longer than the duration of the anesthetic, and for whom there is no placebo effect using saline for the block. Patients who have no response to sympathetic blocks are not likely to respond to sympathectomy, and another treatment should be attempted (Evans, 1947; Abram, 1986). Failure of sympathectomy to relieve reflex dystrophy symptoms may be due to technical problems (Mayfield and Devine, 1951; Jebara and Saade, 1987); however, the fact that some patients with successful sympathectomy have developed recurrent symptoms which occasionally advance to involve the other extremity (the "mirror effect") suggests central phenomena that cannot be explained on a technical basis. Adequate sympathectomy usually includes resection of the lower half of the stellate ganglion and the first four thoracic ganglia (Manart and associates, 1985). Lankford (1982) has suggested that such a goal may be achieved by means of the arthroscope. Shumacker (1985) points out the importance of an active hand therapy program when using nerve blocks and sympathectomy and believes failures are sometimes due to lack of such a therapy program.

Although sympathectomies are useful, they do have significant morbidity and should usually be done only after adequate trial of nonsurgical management. In fact, sympathectomy itself is known to precipitate localized dystrophic pain (Schott, 1986). Also, Horner's syndrome occurs in approximately 14 per cent of patients undergoing sympathectomy. The complication rate of this procedure seems greater with the transaxillary approach than the anterior thoracic approach, but the morbidity less (Manart and associates, 1985). Causalgia is the one form of reflex dystrophy most consistently improved by sympathectomy, although an initial trial of serial nerve blocks, with either anesthetic or pharmacologic agents, is still warranted. Bonica's review (1979a) of 500 patients treated with surgical sympathectomy for causalgia found that 84 per cent experienced excellent pain relief, 12 per cent fair relief, and only 4 per cent no improvement. Sympathectomy for other forms of reflex dystrophy does not have such an encouraging rate of success (Evans, 1947).

Pharmacologic Agents

Drugs used for reflex dystrophy generally fall into one of three categories: neurologic blocking agents, anti-inflammatory drugs, and psychotrophic medication.

SYMPATHOLYTIC AGENTS

Pharmacologic sympathetic block is an attractive consideration for reflex dystrophy. In particular, intravenous guanethidine and similar drugs seem the most promising. Guanethidine is infused into the involved arm, which is isolated by arterial tourniquet (Hannington-Kiff, 1974) after venous evacuation. Guanethidine blocks the sympathetic nervous system by displacing norepinephrine in the postganglionic system and preventing its re-uptake (Glynn, Basedow, and Walsh, 1981); this agent then may reduce pain by interfering with the efferent sympathetic modification of the afferent somatic pain receptors. The performance time of this Bier (1908) type intravenous block is only 15 to 20 minutes, but the duration of response seems to last even better than that to stellate ganglion block (Bonelli and associates, 1983). This may be because of the five-day half-life of guanethidine (Woosley and Niews, 1976). Controlled studies clearly show guanethidine to give significantly better pain relief and blood flow than placebo in reflex dystrophy extremities (Glynn, Basedow, and Walsh, 1981). It has been effective even in late cases of reflex dystrophy when combined with lidocaine and methylprednisolone, and a hand therapy program (Duncan and associates, 1988). Unfortunately, parenteral guanethidine is not yet approved in the United States. It has had limited use as an oral agent (guanethidine sulfate) for reflex dystrophy, but orthostatic hypotension has been a limiting complication (Tabira, Shibasaki, and Kuroiwa, 1983). Intravenous reserpine has been similarly used in the United States, but the results were not as satisfactory (Hannington-Kiff, 1982; Abram, 1986), and it is no longer available for parenteral use. The author has recently used intravenous blocks of bretylium tosylate, which is available in the United States in parenteral form for cardiac ventricular arrhythmias. This drug has inhibitory action on norepinephrine release and uptake similar to guanethidine, and the early results encourage one to hope it may prove as useful.

Phenoxybenzamine (Dibenzyline), an alpha blocker, proved effective in one group of causalgia patients after six weeks of treatment, none of whom required later sympathectomy (Ghostine and associates, 1984). A starting dose of 10 mg per day was used, and gradually increased by 10 mg per day every two to three days until either pain relief or postural hypotension occurred, with average dosage of 80 mg per day. Although this drug blocks the alpha adrenergic vasoconstrictors in the upper extremity, it also blocks vasoconstriction in the rest of the body and frequently causes dizziness with change of body posture, and reflex tachycardia. Other side effects are nasal stuffiness, miosis, and inhibition of ejaculation (Goodman and Gilman, 1980).

Propranolol (Inderal), a beta-adrenergic receptor blocker, has also been successfully used for reflex dystrophy (Simson, 1974; Visitsunthorn and Prete, 1981), probably by means of its known ability to reduce human peripheral vein and artery response to sympathetic stimulation (Stjarne and Brundin, 1978). The usual oral dose is 40 mg three or four times a day, but this drug must be used cautiously in any patient with impaired myocardial function, and it is contraindicated in patients with asthma (Goodman and Gilman, 1980).

Nifedipine, a calcium channel blocker often used for Raynaud's phenomenon, has been effective in reflex dystrophy (Prough and associates, 1985). It may be especially useful in patients who have cardiac disease or who cannot tolerate the side effects of alpha or beta adrenergic blockers. The usual starting dose is 10 mg three times a day, which is gradually increased until the drug is effective, an average maximum of 40 to 50 mg per day (Neumann, 1988).

ANTI-INFLAMMATORY AGENTS

Nonsteroidal anti-inflammatory drugs can provide good analgesia, reducing inflammation through prostaglandin inhibition, and pain through direct desensitization of nociceptors (Neumann, 1988). Ibuprofen (Motrin, Advil) in a dosage of 600 mg three times a

day has been effective in the earliest stage of reflex dystrophy, while patients are undergoing hand therapy, but this medication does not seem useful in the more symptomatic or advanced cases.

Corticosteroids have proved quite useful for reflex sympathetic dystrophy either using a short-term, high dosage method as proposed by Kozin (1976a,b) or with long-term use as proposed by Glick and Helal (1976). Controlled comparison of steroid and placebo treatments confirmed the efficacy of this drug for reflex dystrophy (Christensen, Jensen, and Noer, 1982). If neurotransmitter peptides are indeed released at afferent pain terminals and stimulate an inflammatory response, steroids may directly reduce the onset and subsequent inflammation in this disorder. Kozin (1986) observed that the response to steroids in reflex dystrophy patients who predominantly have pain without many inflammatory findings is not as good as in those who have characteristic autonomic and dystrophic features. This difference may be explained by the secretion, in the former group, of fewer neuropeptide inflammatory mediators at the peripheral nerve terminals for steroids to oppose.

Kozin (1986) recommends a "burst" use of systemic corticosteroids, starting with 15 mg of prednisone four times a day for three to four days; then using 10 mg four times a day for another three to four days; and then tapering the dosage by giving morning doses only of 30 mg, 20 mg, 15 mg, 10 mg, and 5 mg for three days each. His success has been comparable to that reported for other medications and blocks. Others have described use of intravenous steroids with an arterial tourniquet, having success in as many as 75% of patients (Poplawski, Wiley, and Murry, 1983). Biopsies of synovium in patients with reflex sympathetic dystrophy have shown mild inflammatory changes (Genant and associates, 1975; Kozin and associates, 1976a,b), and steroids seem most useful in those patients with marked edema, redness, joint swelling, stiffness, and other symptoms of inflammatory or autonomic response.

Calcitonin has been used successfully in reflex dystrophy patients who have the bone resorption of Sudeck's osteoporosis. Calcitonin has relieved edema, pain, vasomotor disturbance, and osteoporosis by means of animal (DeBastiani, Nogarin, and Lechi, 1974), human (Vattimo and associates, 1982), and synthetic preparations of this medication (Nuti and associates, 1987). However, in a randomized therapeutic trial comparing results of thyrocalcitonin, beta blockers, and the combination of griseofulvin and penthonium, approximately half of the patients had a positive response to the medications within a month, and there was no significant difference in the results with these three very different drugs (Cherot and Amor, 1983). The authors of this study stressed the importance of a rehabilitation program and the need for a long term of therapy.

PSYCHOTROPIC MEDICATIONS

Psychotropic drugs for reflex sympathetic dystrophy fall into categories of medications for depression, anxiety, pain, and for sleep disturbance. Psychiatric testing indicates significant depression and anxiety among patients with this disorder, and it is often difficult to determine which of the two is predominant and needs treatment. The psychiatric literature clearly points out difficulties in distinguishing anxiety and depression and suggests that response to antidepressant medication may be the best diagnostic indicator (Roth and Mountjoy, 1982). Usually the best drugs for depression are the tricyclic antidepressants, often combined with phenothiazine when dystrophic pain is present (Taub and Collins, 1974; Kocher, 1976). In particular, amitriptyline (Elavil) is the most potent of these, and its pharmacologic effect is attributed to inhibition of neurotransmitter re-uptake at nerve terminals, especially serotonin and norepinephrine. This action may conceivably reduce pain transmission and inflammatory response as well as depression (Hollister, 1978). A relatively small amount of amitriptyline (25 to 50 mg) often is effective (Neumann, 1988); it is usually given in the evening because of its sedative effect. However, it usually takes two to three weeks for a complete therapeutic effect to be seen (Mindham, 1982). This delay is thought to be due to a gradual change in the synthesis of amine transmitter substances in the nerve cell. Severe depression requires a much higher dosage, up to 300 mg per day, and patients must be persuaded to continue the drug for two to three weeks to realize its effect.

Diazepam (Valium) has been recommended for reflex dystrophy (Kleinert and associates, 1973; Lankford, 1982), and although useful for anxiety, this agent is not particularly effective for depression. The patient may develop an antianalgesic response and physical dependence after long-term use (Neumann, 1988). It is necessary to identify depression and specifically treat it with antidepressant drugs. Other tranquilizers such as barbiturates and meprobamate have antianalgesic properties and should not be used in patients with reflex sympathetic dystrophy (Neumann, 1988).

When the patient complains of difficulty going to sleep, a mild sleep medication such as the antihistamine hydroxyzine in an average 50 mg to 100 mg dosage (Halpern, 1984) should be considered a better choice than diazepam (Neumann, 1988). Poor rest is well known to create hyperirritable muscular response, and reflex dystrophy patients need rest to avoid developing trigger points of hyperirritable muscular foci. For those patients whose sleep is chronically disturbed because of awakening in the early hours of the morning, the probable diagnosis is depression, and antidepressants will be more effective than sleep medication.

Narcotics for this chronic pain condition are usually counterproductive. They merely reinforce pain behavior and offer the distinct possibility of drug addiction (Neumann, 1988). Nonsteroidal anti-inflammatory analgesics, such as ibuprofen, are much preferable, although they may be of minimal benefit in established cases. Hand therapy, steroids, nerve blocks, and other treatment methods apart from narcotics must be used to help these patients cope with their pain.

Transcutaneous Electrical Nerve Stimulation (TENS)

Transcutaneous electrical nerve stimulation has been effectively used in reflex sympathetic dystrophy (Meyer and Fields, 1972; Wall and Sweet, 1977; Stilz, Carron, and Saunders, 1977; Richlin and associates, 1978). Its mechanism is thought to be activation of the endogenous opioid analgesic system to release endorphin (Peets and Pomeranz, 1985), which inhibits pain at the level of the spinothalamic tract (Lee, 1985). Certainly animal and human studies using high intensity, low frequency TENS suggest such a mechanism (Frederickson and Geary, 1982).

Although this technique has been reported as a sole effective treatment for reflex dystrophy, the author has generally used it as adjunctive therapy to assist with pain control. Transcutaneous electrical nerve stimulation may be particularly useful when there are minimal inflammatory or autonomic changes. Like all methods of treatment in this disorder, TENS is most effective when initiated soon after the onset of symptoms and may be of minimal value, or valuable only as adjunctive therapy, after the pain reflex is established.

Acupuncture

Chan and Chow (1981) reported excellent results using electroacupuncture for reflex dystrophy in patients who did not respond to hand therapy and analgesic treatment. Their technique varied from the standard use of loci in Chinese acupuncture texts, in that they chose loci in the region of maximum discomfort in the affected limb and followed known innervation patterns. Chan and Chow reported excellent results in 70 per cent and improvement in 90 per cent of their patients but pointed out that these were Chinese patients, whose expectations of relief may have played a role in activating the release of endorphin pain inhibitors from the central nervous system. In experimental subjects, acupuncture analgesia can be blocked by naloxone, a morphine antagonist, indicating the importance of the endogenous pain control system in this technique (Mayer, Price, and Rafii, 1977). This technique has usually been employed as an adjunctive measure in Western usage but without as much success, possibly because patients' lack of confidence in the method leads to less activation of the endogenous pain control system.

Surgical Control of Peripheral Nerve Irritants

Many patients with reflex dystrophy have a peripheral nerve irritant that seems unduly painful but can be corrected surgically. Examples of peripheral irritants are painful neuromas, stiff joints, fracture malunions or non-unions, stenosing tenosynovitis, and incomplete carpal tunnel release. The wary surgeon will gain control of the inappropriate

symptom complex *prior* to elective surgery, so that the continuous pain, edema, withdrawal, and hyperesthesia are all well controlled and the patient's symptoms have narrowed to an appropriate level for the problem. This is usually accomplished by a goal-oriented hand therapy program using desensitization techniques (Hardy, Moran, and Merritt, 1982). Modalities such as ultrasound and phonophoresis as well as nonsteroidal anti-inflammatory agents are often helpful. Premature surgery in these patients with disproportionate pain can lead to full-blown reflex sympathetic dystrophy.

When resecting painful neuromas the author has used cyanoacrylic tissue adhesive (Histocryl) on nerve stumps following resection, because it appears to provide a seal that prohibits recurrent neuroma formation. Control of the pain seems a separate entity, however, and desensitization and pain control (Hardy, Moran, and Merritt, 1982) need to be gained prior to resection of annoying neuromas or other peripheral irritants.

For the preoperative carpal tunnel patients who have continuous unrelieved pain that radiates to the shoulder and neck, multiple trigger points in the forearm, and loss of significant hand function due to pain, the inappropriate degree of symptoms should be controlled before carpal tunnel release is performed. Otherwise, the patients may become included among the 2 per cent (MacDonald and associates, 1978) to 5 per cent (Lichtman, Florio, and Mack, 1979) known to develop reflex dystrophy following carpal tunnel release.

Hand Therapy

Regardless of the method chosen to manage reflex sympathetic dystrophy, a knowledgable hand therapist can be of invaluable assistance. Busy hand surgeons usually find reflex dystrophy patients a burden because of their excessive demand for time and understanding as well as the commitment for long-term treatment of this usually nonsurgical problem. Hand therapists can supply this demand. For this author, hand therapy itself is the chosen method of treatment for most patients with reflex sympathetic dystrophy, with transcutaneous electrical neural stimulation, medication, psychotherapy, and nerve blocks used as adjunctive measures.

Whatever the method of treatment, it is important to establish baseline measurement criteria by either the therapist or surgeon, which should include ninhydrin sweat testing, sensory testing with Semmes-Weinstein monofilaments and moving or two-point discrimination, vibratory sense, volumetric measurement of edema, resting temperature measurement, the response to cold stimulation (cold recovery time), grip strength, pinch strength, range of motion, and a hand function test such as the Purdue pegboard, Jebsen, or Moberg test. The therapists may often become the ideal compromise between surgeon and psychiatrist, as an acceptable support individual who will offer much-needed attention and has sufficient knowledge to be credible in reassuring the patient.

The knowledgable hand therapist individualizes treatment according to each patient's status and needs, choosing measured criteria as goals for improvement with therapy. For example, if temperature change and weakness are the major findings, temperature biofeedback therapy and strengthening exercises may be the chosen program, and if objective improvement cannot be documented, the program is altered. Splinting is often needed to protect wrist extension and restore range of motion. Heat can be valuable to relax muscle spasm and improve motion; however, heat with dependency in a whirlpool should be avoided because this will likely aggravate swelling (Lankford, 1982).

Desensitization is often needed for reflex dystrophy patients who have hypersensitivity and have developed disuse patterns. A graded program organized on the basis of objective measurements and a series of objective goals is utilized and must be administered by a supportive therapist working closely with the patient. The program starts with tuning-fork stimulation and works through battery and electrical vibratory stimulation, identification of textures, object identification, and, finally, work simulation (Hardy, Moran, and Merritt, 1982). It is surprising how quickly many patients with chronic pain take pride in achieving these objectives and returning to healthy functional use, even though many times they still acknowledge pain on a visual analog scale. The program seems to help them better adjust or cope with the discomfort. In certain patients, such as those with unduly painful amputation neuromas, desensitization should precede surgical correction to avoid activating a pain syndrome (Merritt, 1984).

Ultrasound for reflex dystrophy, using treatment over the stellate ganglion (Goodman, 1971), or over peripheral nerves in the involved area (Portwood, Lieberman, and Taylor, 1987), has been successful even when pharmacologic nerve blocks and therapy measures fail. However, daily treatments (0.5 watts/cm^2 for 5 minutes) were required for six to eight weeks when ultrasound was the sole treatment; most clinicians prefer to use it as an adjunct to other programs of therapy.

A novel method to carry out a *simple goal-oriented therapy* program was introduced by Watson and Carlson (1987), who initially proposed use of a scrub brush, then altered the concept by developing a graded device that measures resistance to scrubbing-type activity, so that the patient can score the improvement. No single modality or method succeeds in all patients, and individualization and flexibility of therapy is essential to success. Psychologic support and encouragement cannot be overemphasized, and it is valuable to try to have the same therapist work with a particular patient once a good rapport is established.

Myofascial dysfunction with proximal trigger points will be found in approximately half the patients diagnosed as having reflex dystrophy (Evans, 1947; Howell, Roseman, and Merritt, 1988). Indeed, this disorder may be mistaken for reflex dystrophy, especially when autonomic response as well as pain is associated with stimulation of the proximal trigger point. Direct treatment of myofascial trigger points by methods such as ice massage, cold spray, and injection should be done while treatment is directed to the other reflex sympathetic dystrophy manifestations such as edema, decreased range of motion, and temperature change.

Biofeedback therapy has proved very useful for reflex dystrophy (Blanchard, 1979; Blacker, 1980). In the author's experience, it has been most beneficial in those patients with temperature abnormalities. It appears that if patients can control their autonomic temperature function by temperature biofeedback methods, they gain control of other autonomic parameters and even their pain. Hardy and Merritt (1982) acknowledged, however, that the personal support given with such treatment (average of 12 sessions) may be an essential feature in its success.

Work simulation can be an exceedingly important component of any reflex sympathetic dystrophy treatment program, especially for worker's compensation cases. For unknown reasons, the anxiety and activity of work return seem to precipitate recurrent symptoms in many patients. The reassurance of having successfully completed work activity while being encouraged and supported in an understanding therapy environment will do much to allay a patient's fear and permit smooth transition returning to work.

Gradual return to work has been proposed as an ideal method for individuals who particularly have had difficulty with "flashback" associated with job injury (Grunert and associates, 1987). This concept entails a program involving initial observation of the job, followed by gradually increased participation starting with one hour of work. Unfortunately, few employers permit such a program.

Psychotherapy

Psychiatric literature identifies reflex dystrophy as a medical problem that may be mistakenly diagnosed as psychogenic and should be referred to the surgeon (Ecker, 1984), whereas many surgeons believe that reflex dystrophy patients need psychotherapy and should be referred for evaluation by a psychiatrist (Holden, 1948; Hartley, 1955; Bonica and Butler, 1978; Omer, 1978). This irony, in fact, acknowledges that neither specialty is comfortable with the disorder, which fits into neither discipline well. Most cases of reflex dystrophy are not surgical, but the patients do not regard their symptoms as emotional and do not easily accept psychotherapy as a sole method of treatment. The author has found that the best solution is to use a psychiatric consultant in the hand therapy arena, who is introduced as a supportive person there to help the patient deal with the emotional impact of losing hand function. Most patients are comfortable with this explanation and cooperate with the psychiatrist, who can explore etiologic patterns as well as assist with current conflicts involving the patient's personal and family life circumstances. The psychiatrist may then assist the hand therapist and surgeon in understanding major conflicts in these patients. Pre-existing psychologic disturbance is well known to contribute to the maintenance of a chronic pain syndrome (Jaeger and associates, 1986b), and previous, unresolved conflicts may require attention to permit recovery. It is interesting to note that the incidence of anxiety states in the general population is 2 to 5 per cent (Lader and Marks, 1971), which corresponds to estimates of the incidence reflex sympathetic dystrophy after trauma (Hartley, 1955).

Because most of these patients are resistant to the "central" psychoanalytic approach and because they do have an apparent peripheral problem, a more "peripheral" form of psychotherapeutic intervention is possible. This is accomplished with standard hand therapy techniques, biofeedback, and muscle relaxation, and also with "cognitive behavioral therapy," which provides the patient with skills in pacing activities and minimizing pain (Sternbach, 1984). The patient learns to extinguish pain behavior (even if he or she still experiences some pain) and develops a personal sense of control over the pain rather than feeling like its victim (Neumann, 1988). The psychiatrist is helpful in deciding whether tranquilizers or antidepressant drugs might benefit a particular patient. In most cases, low doses of amitriptyline (25 to 50 mg per day) are given for sleep disturbance, but some patients will require higher therapeutic doses for depression.

The few isolated reports of successful treatment of reflex dystrophy by psychotherapy alone (Lidz and Payne, 1945; Shumacker, 1948) have stressed the importance of helping the patients feel responsible and in control (Alioto, 1981). Whether the psychiatrist, psychologist, surgeon, internist, or hand therapist proves to be the major provider of therapy, the importance of consistent psychologic support, sympathy, reassurance, and encouragement for these patients cannot be underestimated. Any support from a psychiatrist or psychologist will likely be beneficial, provided that the surgeon continues to give support as well.

SUMMARY: PREVENTION OF REFLEX SYMPATHETIC DYSTROPHY, STIFF HANDS, AND LITIGATION

In many instances, reflex sympathetic dystrophy may prove to be a preventable disorder. This author quizzed several well-known hand surgeons who acknowledged that they cannot recall a single patient upon whom they operated who developed full-blown reflex sympathetic dystrophy, although they recalled many whom they thought might develop the disorder. At the same time, they had many patients with reflex dystrophy referred to them from a variety of sources, especially attorneys and insurance companies. Why is this? If one accepts that the disorder may sometimes arise in the biased central nervous system of susceptible patients, it becomes feasible that patients of a specific personality type or in some situational anxiety may respond to minor injury or elective surgery with a centrally stimulated outpouring of neurotramsmitter inflammatory substances that leads to the changes of reflex dystrophy. Early support, authoritative reassurance, and encouragement for these patients, which instill a sense of confidence and expectation of relief, may activate the endorphin central pain control system, which is known to inhibit neuropeptide neurotransmitter release (Leeman and Gamse, 1981), thus preventing further changes of reflex dystrophy.

The author has seen one of his postoperative patients suddenly develop profound reflex dystrophy four years after successful carpal tunnel surgery. At that time the patient's mother was hospitalized with metastatic carcinoma. The patient had symptoms of allodynia and hyperpathia, with edema and temperature change in the operated hand, and she responded to supportive hand therapy, which completely relieved her symptoms within a month from onset.

In a situation in which physicians have so little control and understanding of the internal mechanisms that initiate and exacerbate these symptoms, and indeed the patient has little or no conscious control or understanding, it seems unfair that litigation alleging negligence as a cause of reflex dystrophy has been brought against physicians (Horowitz, 1984). If our observations concerning suppressed anger in these patients are accurate, we cannot be surprised by the frequency with which they embrace litigation. For many reasons, it behooves us to try to understand the complex and abstruse psychologic make-up in each patient and support him or her as best we may while providing the objective goals for improvement in this disorder. Cer-

tainly, one can anticipate that improvement is usually slow and requires considerable personal attention. To this extent, hand therapy can be a major advantage. Whatever mode of therapy the individual physician prefers, the patient must be given consistent psychologic support and encouragement, and to whatever extent possible, such aggravating factors as pending litigation and adverse employee-employer relationships need to be resolved. Unrealistic unconscious expectations of dramatic cure, wealth from litigation settlement, or revenge against an employer or spouse will create additional progressive disappointment, resentment, and depression unless these expectations are recognized and gently eliminated. The patient must perceive that although the physician is "on his side," the physician can only help him cope with this disorder and encourage the gradual resumption of function.

Possible methods to reduce the incidence of this disorder are immediate psychologic support for patients who appear to be unduly anxious or depressed, or to have low pain thresholds, and early resumption of active motion following injury or surgery. Techniques to reduce time of immobilization, such as extensor tendon splinting, which permits early active motion following repair (Merritt, 1984), and mini-plate fracture fixation with early motion (Freeland and associates, 1986) are certainly desirable, although they will not universally prevent the disorder. Any time a patient complains of excessive pain following immobilization, some measure must be taken to relieve the pain, and it is imperative that the physician show concern about the patient's anxiety. Early recognition of symptoms of reflex sympathetic dystrophy offers the best opportunity to prevent it, along with the improved surgical and postoperative management techniques that permit early motion and minimize disruption of the patient's normal activities.

The importance of reflex sympathetic dystrophy lies in our inability to explain or fully understand what we see. This disorder stands as a landmark to our ignorance of the mechanisms involved in the interrelationship of central nervous system physiology and hand function. No other disorder brings into sharper focus our knowledge of the large amount of cerebral cortex known to be dedicated to hand activity, and the phenomenon of reflex sympathetic dystrophy remains a challenge to our capacities and endurance. Pulvertaft's (1975) belief that the hand is the "mirror of man's emotion" may well be literally expressed by neurotransmitter substances in reflex sympathetic dystrophy.

REFERENCES

Abram, S. E.: Pain of sympathetic origin. *In* Raj, P. (Ed.): Practical Management of Pain. New York, Yearbook Medical, 1986, p. 451.

Alioto, J. T.: Behavioral treatment of reflex sympathetic dystrophy. Psychosomatics, *22*:539, 1981.

Arnstein, A.: Regional osteoporosis. Orthop. Clin. North Am., *3*:585, 1972.

Basbaum, A. I., and Fields, H. L.: Endogenous pain control mechanisms: review and hypothesis. Ann. Neurol., *4*:451, 1978.

Beecher, H. K.: Measurement of Subjective Responses. New York, Oxford University Press, 1959.

Benson, H.: The Mind-Body Effect. New York, Simon & Schuster, 1979.

Berges, P. U.: Myofascial pain syndromes. Postgrad. Med., *53*:161, 1973.

Bernstein, B. H.: Reflex neurovascular dystrophy in childhood. J. Pediatr., *93*:211, 1978.

Bernstein, B. H., Singsen, B. H., Kent, J. T., Kornriech, H., King, K., et al.: Reflex neurovascular dystrophy in childhood. J. Pediatr., *90*:417, 1977.

Betcher, A. M., Bean, G., and Casten, D. F.: Continuous procaine blocks of paravertebral sympathetic ganglions. J.A.M.A., *151*:288, 1953.

Betcher, A. M., and Casten, D.: Reflex sympathetic dystrophy: criteria for diagnosis and treatment. Anesthesiology, *16*:994, 1955.

Bier, A.: Ueber einen neunen Weg Lokalanasthesie an den Giedmassen zu Erzeugen. Verh. Dtsch. Ges. Chir., *37*:204, 1908.

Biggs, J. T., and Miranda, F. J.: Dental causalgia: a chronic oral pain syndrome. Quintessence Int., *14*:595, 1983.

Bill, A., Stjernschantz, J., Mandahla, et al.: Substance P: release on trigeminal stimulation; effects in the eye. Acta Physiol. Scand., *101*:371, 1979.

Blacker, H. M.: Volitional sympathetic control. Anesth. Analg., *59*:785, 1980.

Blanchard, E. B.: The use of temperature biofeedback in the treatment of chronic pain due to causalgia. Biofeedback Self Regul., *4*:183, 1979.

Bonelli, S., Conoscente, F., Movilia, P. G., Restelli, L., Francucci, B., and Grossi, E.: Regional intravenous guanethidine vs. stellate ganglion block in reflex sympathetic dystrophies: a randomized trial. Pain, *16*:297, 1983.

Bonica, J. J.: Pain. Philadelphia, Lea & Febiger, 1953, p. 913.

Bonica, J. J.: Causalgia and other reflex sympathetic dystrophies. Postgrad. Med., *53*:143, 1973.

Bonica, J. J.: The need of a taxonomy. Pain, *6*:247–252, 1979.

Bonica, J. J., and Butler, S. H.: The management and function of pain centers. *In* Swerdlow, M. (Ed.): Relief of Intractable Pain. New York, Excerpta Medica Foundation, 1978, p. 49.

Boyes, J. H.: Bunnell's Surgery of the Hand. 5th Ed. Philadelphia, J. B. Lippincott Company, 1970.

Brain, S. D., William, T. J., Tippins, J. R., et al.: Calcitonin gene-related peptide is a potent vasodilator. Nature, *313*:54, 1986.

Branch, C.: Aspects of Anxiety. Philadelphia, J. B. Lippincott Company, 1965.

Brody, G.: Personal communication, 1988.

Bunnell, S.: Trophic and vascular conditions. *In* Boyes, J. H. (Ed.): Bunnell's Surgery of the Hand. 5th ed. Philadelphia, J. B. Lippincott Company, 1978.

Burch, G. E.: Of cardiac causalgia, Horner's syndrome, and the cardiac dermatome. Am. Heart J., *100*:938, 1980.

Burch, G. E., and Giles, T. D.: Cardiac causalgia. Arch. Intern. Med., *125*:809, 1970.

Calof, A. L., Jones, R. B., and Roberts, W. J.: Sympathetic modulation of mechanoreceptor sensitivity in frog skin. J. Physiol. (Lond.), *310*:481, 1981.

Carlson, D. H., Simon, H., and Wegner, W.: Bone scanning in diagnosis of reflex sympathetic dystrophy secondary to herniated lumbar discs. Neurology, *27*:791, 1977.

Carron, H., and Weller, R.: Treatment of post-traumatic sympathetic dystrophy. Adv. Neurol., *4*:485, 1974.

Chan, C. S., and Chow, S. P.: Electroacupuncture in the treatment of post-traumatic sympathetic dystrophy (Sudeck's atrophy). Br. J. Anaesth., *53*:899, 1981.

Cherot, A., and Amor, B.: Treatment of algodystrophy. A randomized study of ninety-five cases with three treatments: thyrocalcitonin, beta-blockers, and griseofulvin and penthonium. Rev. Rhum. Mal. Osteoartic., *50*:95, 1983.

Christensen, K., Jensen, E. M., and Noer, I.: The reflex dystrophy syndrome: response to treatment with systemic corticosteroids. Acta Chir. Scand., *148*:653, 1982.

Clark, G.: Causalgia: a discussion of the chronic pain syndromes in the upper limb. *In* Hunter, J. M. (Ed.): Rehabilitation of the Hand. St. Louis, C. V. Mosby Company, 1978.

Cronin, K. D., and Kirsner, R. L. G.: Diagnosis of reflex sympathetic dysfunction. Use of skin potential response. Anaesthesia, *37*:848, 1982.

Davis, S. W., Petrillo, C. R., Eichberg, R. D., and Chu, D. S.: Shoulder-hand syndrome in hemiplegic population: five-year retrospective study. Arch. Phys. Med. Rehabil., *58*:353, 1977.

DeBastiani, G., Nogarin, L., and Lechi, C.: La calcintonina nel trattamento della osteoporosi post-traumatica. *In* DeBastiani, G., and Sirtori, C. (Eds.): Atti del Simposio Internazionale, Un nuovo ormone: la Calcitonina e il suo impiego terapeutico. Milano, Fondazione Carlo Erba, 1974, p. 112.

Denmark, A.: An example of symptoms resembling tic douloureux, produced by a wound in the radial nerve. Med. Chir. Trans., *4*:48, 1813.

De Takats, G.: Sympathetic reflex dystrophy. Med. Clin. North Am., *49*:117, 1965.

Devor, M.: Nerve pathophysiology in mechanisms of pain in causalgia. J. Auton. Nerv. Syst., *7*:371, 1983.

Devor, M., and Janig, W.: Activation of myelinated afferents ending in a neuroma by stimulation of the sympathethic supply in the rat. Neurosci. Let., *24*:43, 1981.

DiGuilio, A. M.: Characterization of enkephalin-like material extracted from sympathetic ganglia. Neuropharmacology, *17*:989, 1978.

Doupe, J., Cullen, C. H., and Chance, G. Q.: Post-traumatic pain in causalgia syndrome. J. Neurol Psych., *7*:33, 1944.

Doury, P.: Reflex sympathetic dystrophy (algodystrophy). Int. Med. Special. 6:67, 1985.

Drucker, W., Hubay, C., Holden, W., and Bukovnic, J.: Pathogenesis of post-traumatic sympathetic dystrophy. Am. J. Surg., 97:454, 1959.

Duncan, K. H., Lewis, R. C., Jr., Raez, G., and Nordyke, M. D.: Treatment of upper extremity reflex dystrophy with joint stiffness using sympatholytic Bier blocks and manipulation. Orthopedics 11:883, 1988.

Echlin, F., Owens, F. M., Jr., and Wells, W. L.: Observations on major and minor causalgia. Arch. Neurol. Psychol., 62:183, 1949.

Ecker, Arthur: Reflex sympathetic dystrophy. Thermography in diagnosis: psychiatric considerations. Psych. Ann., 14:787, 1984.

Edeiken, J.: Shoulder-hand syndrome following myocardial infarction with special reference to prognosis. Circulation, 41:14, 1957.

Enelow, A.: Depression in Medical Practice. West Point, PA, Merck, Sharp, & Dohme, 1970.

Evans, J.: Sympathetic dystrophy: report of fifty-seven cases. Ann. Intern. Med., 26:417, 1947.

Fermaglich, D.: Reflex sympathetic dystrophy in children. Pediatrics 60:6:881, 1977.

Fields, H. L., and Levine, J. D.: Placebo analgesia—a role for endorphins? Trends Neurosci., 1:271, 1984.

Foreman, J. C., Jordan, C. C., and Piotrowski, W.: Interaction of neurotensin with the substance P receptor mediating histamine release from rat mast cells and the flare in human skin. Br. J. Pharmacol., 77:531, 1982.

Frederickson, R. C. A., and Geary, L. E.: Endogenous opioid peptides; review of physiological, pharmacological, and clinical aspects. Prog. Neurobiol., 19:19, 1982.

Freeland, A. E., et al.: Stable Fixation of the Hand and Wrist. New York, Springer-Verlag, 1986.

Frost, F. A., Jessen, B., and Siggard-Anderson, J.: A control, double blind comparison of mepivacaine injection versus saline injection for myofascial pain. Lancet, 1:499, 1980.

Frykman, G.: Complications of wrist fractures. In Hunter, J. M. (Ed.): Rehabilitation of the Hand. St. Louis, C. V. Mosby Company, 1978.

Genant, H., Kozin, F., Bekerman, C., McCarty, D., and Sims, J.: The reflex sympathetic dystrophy syndrome. Radiology, 117:21, 1975.

Ghostine, S. Y., Comair, Y. G., Turner, D. M., Kassell, N. F., and Azar, C. G.: Phenoxybenzamine in the treatment of causalgia. J. Neurosurg., 60:263, 1984.

Glick, E. N., and Helal, B.: Post-traumatic neurodystrophy: treatment by corticosteroids. Hand, 8:45, 1976.

Glynn, C. J., Basedow, R. W., and Walsh, J. A.: Pain relief following post-ganglionic sympathetic blockade with I.V. guanethidine. Br. J. Anaesth., 53:297, 1981.

Goodman, A. G., Goodman, L. S., and Gilman, A.: The Pharmacological Basis of Therapeutics. 6th Ed. New York, Macmillan Publishing Company, 1980.

Goodman, C. R.: Treatment of shoulder-hand syndrome: combined ultrasonic application to stellate ganglion and physical medicine. N.Y. State J. Med., 71:559, 1971.

Gracely, R. H., Dubner, R., Wolskee, P. J., and Deeter, W. R.: Placebo and naloxone can alter post-surgical pain by separate mechanisms. Nature 306:264, 1983.

Granit, R., Leksell, L., and Skoglund, C. R.: Fiber interaction in injured or compressed region of nerve. Brain, 67:125, 1944.

Greenberg, R. P., Price, D. D., and Becker, D. P.: Complications of persistent postoperative pain. In Green-field, L. J. (Ed.): Complications in Surgery and Trauma. Philadelphia, J. B. Lippincott Company, 1983, p. 709.

Grevert, P., Albert, L. H., and Goldstein, A.: Partial antagonism of placebo analgesia by naloxone. Pain, 16:129, 1983.

Grunert, B. K., Devine, C. A., Smith, C. J., Matloub, H. S., Sanger, J. R., and Yousif, N. J.: Graded work exposure: psychological stragegy to promote return to work following hand trauma. Presented at the Seventeenth Annual Meeting of the American Association for Hand Surgery, Puerto Rico, Nov. 4–8, 1987.

Halpern, L.: Drugs in the management of pain. Adv. Pain Res. Ther., 7:147, 1984.

Hannington-Kiff, J. G.: Intravenous regional sympathetic block with guanethidine. Lancet, 1:1019, 1974.

Hannington-Kiff, J. G.: Pain Relief. London, William Heinemann, 1975.

Hannington-Kiff, J. G.: Relief of Sudeck's atrophy by regional intravenous guanethidine. Lancet, 1:1132, 1977.

Hannington-Kiff, J. G.: Relief of causalgia in limbs by regional intravenous guanethidine. Br. Med. J., 2:367, 1979.

Hannington-Kiff, J. G.: Hyperadrenergic-effected limb causalgia: relief by I.V. pharmacologic norepinephrine blockade. Am. Heart J., 103:152, 1982.

Hardy, M. A. and Merritt, W. H.: A model to study sympathetic dystrophy: psychological testing and biofeedback results. Presented at The Plastic Surgery Research Council Annual Meeting, Hershey, Pennsylvania, 1982.

Hardy, M. A., and Merritt, W. H.: Psychological evaluation and pain assessment in patients with reflex sympathetic dystrophy. Am. J. Hand Ther., 1:155, 1988.

Hardy, M. A., Moran, C. A., and Merritt, W. H.: Desensitization of the traumatized hand. Va. Med. J., 109:134, 1982.

Hartley, J.: Reflex hyperemic deossification (Sudeck's atrophy). J. Mt. Sinai Hosp., 22:268, 1955.

Hartung, H. P., and Toyka, K. V.: Activation of macrophages by substance P: induction of oxidative burst and thromboxane release. J. Pharmacol., 89:301, 1983.

Hendler, N., Uematesu, S., Long, D.: Thermographic validation of physical complaints in "psychogenic pain" patients. Psychosomatics, 23:283, 1982.

Holden, W. D.: Sympathetic dystrophy. Arch. Surg., 57:373, 1948.

Hollister, L.: Tricyclic anti-depressants. N. Engl. J. Med., 99:106, 1978.

Horowitz, S. H.: Brachial plexus injuries with causalgia resulting from transaxillary rib resection. Arch. Surg., 120:1189, 1985.

Horowitz, S. H.: Iatrogenic causalgia; classification, clinical findings, and legal ramifications. Arch. Neurol., 41:821, 1984.

Houston, B.: Control over stress, locus of control and response to stress. J. Pers. Social Psych., 21:249, 1972.

Howell, J., Roseman, G., and Merritt, W.: Association of myofascial dysfunction with reflex sympathetic dystrophy. Submitted for presentation at the American Association for Hand Surgery Annual Meeting, Toronto, 1988 (unpublished data).

Hughes, J., Smith, T. W., Kosterliz, H. W., et al.: Identification of two related pentapeptides from the brain with potent opiate agonist activity. Nature, 258:577, 1975.

Imanuel, H. M., Levy, F. L., and Geldwert, J. J.: Sudeck's

atrophy: a review of the literature. J. Foot Surg., 20:243, 1981.

Jaeger, B., Singer, E., and Kroening, R.: Reflex sympathetic dystrophy of the face. Report of two cases and a review of the literature. Arch. Neurol., 43:693, 1986a.

Jaeger, S. H., Singer, D. I., and Whitenack, S. H.: Nerve injury complications: management of neurogenic pain syndromes. Hand Clin., 2:217, 1986b.

Jansco, N., Jansco-Gabor, A., and Szolesanyi, J.: Direct evidence for direct neurogenic inflammation and its prevention by denervation and by pre-treatment with capsaicin. Brit. Pharmacol. Chemother., 31:138, 1967.

Jebara, V. A., and Saade, B.: Causalgia: a wartime experience—report of twenty treated cases. J. Trauma, 27:519, 1987.

Johnson, E. W., and Pannozzo, A. N.: Management of shoulder-hand syndrome. J.A.M.A., 195:108, 1966.

Kellgren, J. H.: Observations on referred pain arising from muscle. Clin. Science, 3:175, 1938.

Kelly, M.: The nature of fibrositis. I. The myalgic lesion and its secondary effects: a reflex theory. Ann. Rheum. Dis., 5:1, 1945.

Kelly, M.: The relief of facial pain by procaine (Novocaine) injections. J. Am. Geriatr. Soc., 11:586, 1963.

Khayutin, V. M., Barazla, Lukoshkona, E. V., et al.: Chemosensitive spinal afferents: thresholds of specific and nociceptive reflexes as compared with thresholds of excitation for receptors in axons. Prog. Brain Res., 43:293, 1976.

Khoury, R., Kennedy, S. F., and McNamara, T. E.: Facial causalgia: report of case. J. Oral Surg., 38:782, 1980.

Kienböck, R.: Über akute Knochenatrophie bei Entzundung-processen an den Extremataten (falchlich sagenannate inactivitats atrophie der Knochen) und ihre Diagnose nach dem Roetgen-Bilds. Wien. Med. Wochenschr, 5:1345, 1901.

Kirklin, J., Chenoweth, A., and Murphy, F.: Causalgia: a review of its characteristics, diagnosis and treatment. Surgery, 21:321, 1947.

Kleinert, H., Cole, N., Wayne, L., Harvey, R., Kutz, J., and Atasoy, E.: Post-traumatic sympathetic dystrophy. Orthop. Clin. North Am., 4:917, 1973.

Kocher, R.: Use of psychotrophic drugs for the relief of chronic severe pain. Adv. Pain Res. Ther. 1:579, 1976.

Kozin, F.: The painful shoulder in reflex sympathetic dystrophy syndrome. In McCarty, D. J. (Ed.): Arthritis and Allied Conditions. 10th Ed. Philadelphia, Lea & Febiger, 1985, p. 1322.

Kozin, F.: Reflex sympathetic dystrophy syndrome. Bull. Rheum. Dis., 36:1, 1986.

Kozin, F., Genant, H., Bekerman, C., and McCarty, D.: The reflex sympathetic dystrophy syndrome. II. Roentgenographic and scintigraphic evidence of bilaterality and of periarticular accentuation. Am. J. Med., 60:332, 1976a.

Kozin, F., McCarty, D. J., Simms, J., and Fenant, H.: The reflex sympathetic dystrophy syndrome. I. Clinical and histological studies: evidence for bilaterality, response to corticosteroids and articular involvement. Am. J. Med., 60:321, 1976b.

Kozin, F., Soin, J. S., Ryan, L. M., Carrera, G. F., and Wortmann, R. L.: Bone scintigraphy in reflex sympathetic dystrophy syndrome. Radiology, 138:437, 1981.

Lader, M., and Marks, I.: Clinical Anxiety. London, Heinemann, 1971, p. 31.

Lankford, L. L.: Reflex sympathetic dystrophy. In Green, D. P. (Ed.): Operative Hand Surgery. Vol. 1. New York, Churchill Livingstone, 1982, p. 539.

Lee, K. H.: Transcutaneous nerve stimulators inhibit

spinothalamic tract cells. Adv. Pain Res. Ther., 9:203, 1985.

Leeman, S. E., Gamse, R., Lackner, D., and Gamse, G.: Effect of capsaicin pretreatment on capsaicin-evoked release of immunoreactive somatostatin and substance P from primary sensory neurons. Naunyn-Schmiedebergs-Arch-Pharmacol., 316:38, 1981.

Lehman, E. J. P.: Traumatic vasospasm: a study of four cases of vasospasm in the upper extremity. Arch. Surg. 29:92, 1934.

Lembeck, F., Gamse, R., and Juan, H.: Substance P in sensory nerve endings. In VonEuler, U. S., Pernow, B. (Eds.): Substance P (Thirty-Seventh Nobel Symposium, Stockholm, 1976). New York, Raven Press, 1977, p. 169.

Leriche, R.: De la causalgie envisagée comme une nérvite du sympathique et son traitement par la dénudation et l'excision des plexus nerveux péri-artériels. Presse Med., 24:178, 1916.

Leriche, R.: La Chirurgie de la Douleur. Paris, Masson et Cie, 1949.

Levine, J. D., Goetzl, E. J., and Basbaum, A. I.: Contribution of the nervous system to the pathophysiology of rhematoid arthritis and other polyarthritides. Rheum. Dis. Clin. North Am., 13:369, 1987.

Lewis, R.: Pain. New York, Macmillan Company, 1942, p. 124.

Lewis, T.: The Blood Vessels of the Human Skin and Their Responses. London, Shaw, 1927.

Lichtman, D. M., Florio, R. L., and Mack, G. E.: Carpal tunnel release under local anesthesia: evaluation of the out-patient procedure. J. Hand Surg., 4:544, 1979.

Lidz, T., and Payne, R. L.: Causalgia: report of recovery following relief of emotional stress. Arch. Neurol. Psych., 53:222, 1945.

Linson, M. A., Leffert, R., and Todd, D. P.: The treatment of upper extremity reflex sympathetic dystrophy with prolonged continuous stellate ganglion blockade. J. Hand Surg., Vol. 8:153, 1983.

Livingston, W. K.: Pain mechanisms. New York, Macmillan Company, 1943.

Loewenstein, W. R., and Altamirano-Orrega, R.: Enhancement of activity in a pacinian corpuscle by sympathomimetic agents. Nature, 178:1292, 1956.

Lorente de No, R.: Analysis of the activity of the chains of internuncial neurons. J. Neurophysiol., 1:207, 1938.

MacDonald, R. I., Lichtman, D. M., Hanlon, J. J., and Wilson, J. N.: Complications of surgical release for carpal tunnel syndrome. J. Hand Surg., 3:70, 1978.

MacKinnon, S. E., and Holder, L. E.: The use of three-phase radionuclide bone scanning in the diagnosis of reflex sympathetic dystrophy. J. Hand Surg., 9:556, 1984a.

MacKinnon, S. E., and Holder, L. E.: Reflex sympathetic dystrophy in the hands: clinical and scintigraphic criteria. Radiology, 152:517, 1984b.

Madden, J. W., Carlson, E. C., and Hines, J.: Presence of modified fibroblasts in ischemic contracture of the intrinsic musculature of the hand. Surg. Gynecol. Obstet., 140:509, 1975.

Manart, F. D., Sadler, T. R., Jr., Schmitt, E. A., and Rainer, W. G.: Upper dorsal sympathectomy. Am. J. Surg., 150:762, 1985.

Mankeltow, R. T., and McKee, N. H.: Free muscle transplantation to provide active finger flexion. J. Hand Surg., 3:416, 1976.

Markoff, M., and Farole, A.: Reflex sympathetic dystrophy syndrome; case report with review of the literature. Oral Surg., 661:23, 1986.

Massler, M.: Dental causalgia. Quintessence Int., *12*:341, 1981.

Mayer, D. J., and Liebeskind, J. C.: Pain reduction by focal electrical stimulation of the brain: an anatomical and behavioral analysis. Brain Res., *68*:73, 1974.

Mayer, D. J., Price, D. D., and Rafii, A.: Antagonism of acupuncture analgesia in man by the narcotic antagonist naloxone. Brain Res., *121*:36, 1977.

Mayfield, F. H.: Causalgia. Springfield, IL, Charles C Thomas, 1951.

Mayfield, F. H., and Devine, J. W.: Causalgia. Surg. Gynecol. Obstet., *80*:631, 1945.

Mays, K. S., North, W. C., and Schnapp, M.: Stellage ganglion "blocks" with morphine in sympathetic type pain. J. Neurol. Neurosurg. Psychiatry, *44*:189, 1981.

McCarty, D. J.: Arthritis and Allied Conditions. 9th Ed. Philadelphia, Lea & Febiger, 1979, p. 1111.

McLelland, J., and Ellis, S. J.: Causalgia as a complication of meningococcal meningitis. Br. Med. J., *292*:1710, 1986.

Medsger, T. A., Jr., Dixon, J. A., and Garwood, V. F.: Palmar fasciitis and polyarthritis associated with ovarian carcinoma. Ann. Intern. Med., *96*:424, 1982.

Melzak, R., and Wall, P. D.: Pain mechanisms: a new theory. Science *150*:971, 1965.

Merritt, W. H.: Complications of hand surgery and trauma. *In* Greenfield, L. J. (Ed.): Complications in Surgery and Trauma. Philadelphia, J. B. Lippincott Company, 1984, p. 852.

Merskey, H.: Psychological aspects of pain relief: hypnotherapy, psychotrophic drugs. *In* Swerdlow, M. (Ed.): Relief of Intractable Pain. New York, Excerpta Medica Foundation, 1978, p. 21.

Meyer, G. A., and Fields, H. L.: Causalgia treated by selective large fiber stimulation of peripheral nerve. Brain, *95*:163, 1972.

Michaels, R. M., and Sorber, J. A.: Reflex sympathetic dystrophy as a probable paraneoplastic syndrome: case report and literature review. Arthritis Rheum., *27*:1183, 1984.

Miehlke, K., Schulze, G., and Eger, W.: Klinische und experimentalle untersuchungen zum fibrositis-syndrom. Z. Rheumaforsch., *19*:310, 1960.

Miller, D. S., and DeTakats, G.: Post-traumatic dystrophy of the extremities: Sudeck's extremity. Surg. Gynecol. Obstet., *125*:558, 1941.

Mindham, R. H. S.: Tricyclic antidepressants and amine precursors. *In* Paykel, E. S. (Ed.): Handbook of Affective Disorders. New York, Oxford University Press, 1982, p. 231.

Mitchell, J. K.: Remote Consequences of Injuries of Nerves, and their Treatment. Philadelphia, Lea, 1895.

Mitchell, S. W.: Contributions relating to the causation and prevention of disease and to camp diseases. *In* Flint, A. (Ed.): United States Sanitary Commission Memoirs. New York, 1867, p. 412.

Mitchell, S. W.: Causalgia. *In* Injuries of Nerves and Their Consequences. Philadelphia, Lea Brothers & Company, Philadelphia, 1872, p. 292.

Mitchell, S. W., Moorehouse, G. R., and Keen, W. W.: Gunshot Wounds and Other Injuries of Nerves. Philadelphia, J. B. Lippincott Company, 1864.

Modell, W., and Travell, J.: Treatment of painful disorders of skeletal muscle. N.Y. State J. Med., *48*:2050, 1948.

Morettin, L. B., and Wilson, M.: Severe reflex algodystrophy (Sudeck's atrophy) as a complication of myelography: report of two cases. Am. J. Roentgenol. *110*:156, 1970.

Moruzzi, G.: Sistema nervoso vegetativo e sistema nervoso autonomo. Rass. Clin. Sci., *44*:239, 1968.

Neumann, M. M.: Non-surgical management of pain secondary to peripheral nerve injuries. Orthop. Clin. North Am., *19*:165, 1988.

Nilsson, J., von Euler, A. M., and Dalsgaard, C. J.: Stimulation of connective tissue cell growth by substance P and substance K. Nature, *315*:61, 1985.

Nuti, R., Vattimo, A., Martini, G., Turchetti, V., and Righi, G. A.: Carbocalcitonin treatment in Sudeck's atrophy. Clin. Orthop. Rel. Res., *215*:217, 1987.

Omer, G.: Management of pain syndromes in the upper extremity. *In* Hunter, J. M. (Ed.): Rehabilitation of the Hand. St. Louis, C. V. Mosby Company, 1978, p. 43.

Omer, G., and Thomas, S.: Treatment of causalgia: review of cases at Brook General Hospital. Tex. Med., *67*:93, 1971.

Pak, J. J., Martin, G. M., Magness, J. L., and Kavanaugh, G. J.: Reflex sympathetic dystrophy: review of one hundred and forty cases. Minn. Med., *53*:507, 1970.

Paré, A.: Les Oeuvres d'Ambroise Paré. Paris, Gabrien Buon, 1968, p. 401.

Payan, D. G., and Goetzl, E. J.: Modulation of lymphocyte function by sensory neuropeptides. J. Immunol., *135*:783S, 1985.

Peacock, E. E., Jr.: Wound Repair. 3rd Ed. Philadelphia, W. B. Saunders Company, 1984.

Peets, J. M., and Pomeranz, B.: Acupuncture-like transcutaneous electrical nerve stimulation analgesia is influenced by spinal cord endorphins but not serotonin: an intrathecal pharmacological study. Adv. Pain Res. Ther., *9*:519, 1985.

Plewes, L. W.: Sudeck's atrophy in the hand. J. Bone Joint Surg., *B38*:195, 1956.

Pollock, L. J., and Davis, L.: Peripheral Nerve Injuries. New York, Paul B. Hoeber, 1933.

Popelianskii, I. I., Zaslavskii, E. S., and Veselovskii, V. P.: [The medicosocial significance, etiology, pathogenesis, and diagnosis of nonarticular disease of soft tissue of the limbs and back.] (Russian) Vopr. Revm. *3*:38, 1976.

Poplawski, Z., Wiley, A., and Murry, J.: Post-traumatic dystrophy of the extremities. J. Bone Joint Surg., *65A*:642, 1983.

Portwood, M. M., Lieberman, J. S., and Taylor, R. G.: Ultrasound treatment of reflex sympathetic dystrophy. Arch. Phys. Med. Rehab., *68*:116, 1987.

Procacci, P., and Maresca, M.: Reflex sympathetic dystrophies and algodystrophies: historical and pathologic considerations. Pain, *31*:137, 1987.

Prough, D. S., McLeskey, C. H., Poehling, G. G., Koman, L. A., Weeks, D. B., et al.: Efficacy of oral nifedipine in the treatment of reflex sympathetic dystrophy. Anesthesiology, *62*:796, 1985.

Prudden, B.: Pain Erasure: the Bonnie Prudden Way. New York, M. Evans & Company, 1980.

Pulvertaft, R. G.: Psychological aspects of hand injuries. Hand, *7*:93, 1975.

Revill, S. I., Robinson, J. O., Rosen, M., and Hogg, M.: The reliability of a linear analogue scale for evaluating pain. Anaesthesia, *31*:1191, 1976.

Reynolds, D. V.: Surgery in the rat during electrical analgesia induced by focal brain stimulation. Science, *164*:444, 1969.

Richlin, D. M., Carron, H., Rowlingson, J. C., Sussman, M. D., Baugher, W. H., and Goldner, R. D.: Reflex sympathetic dystrophy: successful treatment by transcutaneous nerve stimulation. J. Pediatr., *93*:84, 1978.

Roberts, W. J.: A hypothesis on the physiological basis for causalgia and related pains. Pain, *24*:297, 1986.

Roberts, W. J., and Elardo, S. M.: Sympathetic activation of unmyelinated mechanoreceptors in cat skin. Brain Res., *339*:123, 1985a.

Roberts, W. J., and Elardo, S. M.: Sympathetic activation of A-delta nociceptors. Somatosens. Res., *3*:33, 1985b.

Rosen, P. S., and Graham, W.: The shoulder-hand syndrome: historical review with observations on seventy-three patients. Canad. Med. Assoc. J., *77*:86, 1957.

Rosen, P. S., and Graham, W.: Shoulder-hand syndrome in coronary disease. Geriatrics *18*:525, 1963.

Roth, M., and Mountjoy, C. Q.: The distinction between anxiety states and depressive disorders. *In* Paykel, E. S. (Ed.): Handbook of Affective Disorders. New York, Oxford University Press, 1982, p. 70.

Rowlingson, J. C.: The sympathetic dystrophies. Int. Anesthiol. Clin., *21*:117, 1983.

Ruff, M. R., Wahl, S. M., and Pert, C. B.: Substance P receptor–mediated chemotaxis of human monocytes. Peptides, *6*(Suppl.):107, 1985.

Schott, G. D.: Mechanisms of causalgia and related clinical conditions. The role of the central and of the sympathetic nervous systems. Brain, *109*:771, 1986.

Schultzberg, M., Hökfelt, T., Terenius, L., Elfvin, L. G., Lundberg, J. M., et al.: Enkephalin immunoreactive nerve fibers and cell bodies in sympathetic ganglia of the guinea-pig and rat. Neuroscience, *4*:249, 1979.

Secretan, H.: Oedme dur et hyperplasie traumatique du métacarpe dorsal. Rev. Med. Suisse Romande, *21*:409, 1901.

Shumacker, H. B., Jr.: Causalgia: a general discussion. Surgery, *28*:485, 1948.

Shumacker, H. B., Jr.: A personal overview of causalgia and other reflex dystrophies. Ann. Surg., *201*:278, 1985.

Shumacker, H. B., Jr., Speigel, I. J., and Upjohn, R. H.: Causalgia. II. The signs and symptoms with particular reference to vasomotor disturbances. Surg. Gynecol. Obstet., *86*:452, 1948a.

Shumacker, H. B., Jr., Speigel, I. J., and Upjohn, R. H.: Causalgia: the role of sympathetic interruption in treatment. Surg. Gynecol. Obstet., *86*:76, 1948b.

Silverman, S.: Psychological Aspects of Physical Symptoms. East Norwalk, CT, Appleton-Century-Crofts, 1968.

Simmons, B. P., and Vasile, R. G.: The clenched fist syndrome. J. Hand Surg., *5*:420, 1980.

Simson, G.: Propranolol for causalgia and Sudeck's atrophy. J.A.M.A., *227*:327, 1974.

Snyder, S. H., and Matthysse, S. (Eds.): Opiate receptor mechanisms. Neurosci. Res. Progr. Bull., *13*:1, 1975.

Spebar, M. J., Rosenthal, D., Collins, G. J., Jr., Jarstfer, B. S., and Walters, M. J.: Changing tends in causalgia. Am. J. Surg., *142*:744, 1981.

Spray, D. C.: Characteristics, specificity and efferent control of frog cutaneous cold receptors. J. Physiol. (Lond.), *237*:15, 1974.

Spurling, R. G.: Causalgia of the upper extremity: treatment by dorsal sympathetic ganglionectomy. Arch. Neurol. Psychol., *23*:784, 1930.

Stanisz, A. M., Befus, D., and Bienenstock, J.: Differential effects of vasoactive intestinal peptides, substance P, and somatostatin on immunoglobulin synthesis and proliferation of lymphocytes from Peyer's patches, mesenteric lymph nodes and spleen. J. Immunol., *136*:152, 1986.

Steinbrocker, O.: Shoulder-hand syndrome: present perspective. Arch. Phys. Med. Rehabil., *49*:388, 1968.

Steinbrocker, O., Spitzer, N., and Friedman, H. H.: The shoulder-hand syndrome in reflex dystrophy of the upper extremity. Ann. Intern. Med., *29*:22, 1948.

Sternbach, R. A.: Recent advances in psychologic pain therapy. Adv. Pain Res. Ther., *7*:251, 1984.

Sternbach, R. A., Murphy, R., Timmermans, G., Greenhoot, J., and Akeson, W.: Measuring the severity of clinical pain. Adv. Neurol., *4*:281, 1974.

Stilz, R. J., Carron, H., and Saunders, D. B.: Case history number 96: reflex sympathetic dystrophy in a six year old: successful treatment by transcutaneous nerve stimulation. Anesth. Analg., *56*:438, 1977.

Stjarne, L., and Brundin, J.: Beta-2 adrenoceptors facilitating noradrenaline secretion from human vasoconstrictor nerves. Acta Physiol. Scand., *97*:88, 1978.

Subbarao, J., and Stillwell, G. K.: Reflex sympathetic dystrophy syndrome of the upper extremity: analysis of total outcome of management in one hundred and twenty-five cases. Arch. Phys. Med. Rehab., *62*:549, 1981.

Sudeck, P.: Ueber die akute entzundliche Knochenatrophie. Arch. Klin. Chir., *62*:147, 1900.

Sunderland, S.: Pain mechanisms in causalgia. J. Neurol. Neurosurg. Psychiatry, *39*:471, 1976.

Tabira, T., Shibasaki, H., and Kuroiwa, Y.: Reflex sympathetic dystrophy (causalgia): treatment with guanethidine. Arch. Neurol., *40*:430, 1983.

Tahmoush, A. J.: Causalgia: redefinition as a clinical pain syndrome. Pain, *10*:187, 1981.

Tahmoush, A. J., Malley, J., and Jennings, J. R.: Skin conductance, temperature, and blood flow in causalgia. Neurology, *33*:1483, 1983.

Tasker, R. R., Organ, L. W., and Hawrylyshyn, P.: Deafferentation and causalgia. *In* Bonica, J. J. (Ed.): Pain. New York, Raven Press, 1980.

Taub, A., and Collins, W. F., Jr.: Observations on treatment of denervation dyesthesia with psychotropic drugs: post-herpetic neuralgia, anesthesia dolorosa, peripheral neuropathy. Adv. Neurol., *4*:309, 1974.

Thompson, J. E.: The diagnosis and management of post-traumatic pain syndromes (causalgia). Austr. N.Z. J. Surg., *49*:299, 1979.

Travell, J. G., and Simmons, D. G.: Myofascial Pain and Dysfunction—the Trigger Point Manual. Baltimore, Williams & Wilkins Company, 1983.

Tryor, F. J.: Anxiety states: symptoms and assessment of depression. *In* Paykel, E. S. (Ed.): Handbook of Affective Disorders. New York, Oxford University Press, 1982, p. 59.

Tsuge, K.: Management of established Volkmann's contracture. *In* Green, D. P. (Ed.): Operative Hand Surgery. New York, Churchill Livingstone, 1982, p. 499.

Turf, R. M., and Bacardi, B. E.: Causalgia: clarifications in terminology and a case presentation. J. of Foot Surg., *25*:284, 1986.

Uematsu, S., Hendler, N., Hungerford, D., Long, D., and Ono, N.: Thermography and electromyography in differential diagnosis of chronic pain syndromes and reflex sympathetic dystrophy. Electromyogr. Clin. Neurophysiol, *21*:165, 1982.

Vattimo, A., Nuti, R., Lore, F., and Canniggia, A.: Human calcitonin therapy of Sudeck's atrophy: pathophysiological aspects. *In* Caniggia, A. (Ed.): Human Calcitonin. Proceedings of the International Workshop on Human Calcitonin. Stresa Milano, Ciba-Geigy, 1982, p. 127.

Virchow, R.: Ueber parenchymatose entzundung. Arch. Pathol. Anat., *4*:261, 1852.

Visitsunthorn, U., and Prete, P.: Reflex sympathetic

dystrophy of the lower extremity: a complication of herpes zoster with dramatic response to propranolol. West. J. Med., *135*:62, 1981.

Volkmann, R.: Die ischaemishchen Muskellah-mungen und Kontracturen. Zentralbl. Chir., *8*:801, 1881.

Wall, P. D., and Gutnick, M.: Ongoing activity in peripheral nerves: the physiology and pharmacology of impulses originating from a neuroma. Exper. Neurol., *43*:580, 1981.

Wall, P. D., and Sweet, W. H.: Temporary abolition of pain in man. Science, *155*:108, 1977.

Wang, G. H.: The galvanic skin reflex. A review of old and recent works from a physiologic point of view. Am. J. Phys. Med., *36/37*:35, 1957–58.

Wang, J. K., Johnson, K. A., and Ilstrup, D. M.: Sympathetic blocks for reflex sympathetic dystrophy. Pain, *23*:13, 1985.

Watson, H. K., and Carlson, L.: Treatment of reflex sympathetic dystrophy of the hand with an active "stress loading" program. J. Hand Surg., *12A*:779, 1987.

Waylett, J.: Behavioral patterns in reflex sympathetic dystrophy. *In* Hunter, J. M. (Ed).: Rehabilitation of the Hand. St. Louis, C. V. Mosby Company, 1978.

Williams, H. L., and Elkins, E. C.: Myalgia of the head. Arch. Phys. Ther., *23*:14, 1942.

Woosley, R. L., and Niews, A. S.: Drug therapy—guanethidine. N. Engl. J. Med., *295*:1053, 1976.

Zimmerman, M.: Peripheral and central nervous mechanisms of nociception. Pain and pain therapy: facts and hypotheses. Adv. Pain Res. Ther. *3*:3, 1979.

Zohn, D. A., and Mennell, J.: Musculoskeletal Pain: Principles of Physical Diagnosis and Physical Treatment. Boston, Little, Brown & Company, 1976, p. 126.

Index

Index

Note: Page numbers in *italics* refer to illustrations; page number followed by *t* refer to tables.

Hemangiomas *(Continued)*
  capillary-cavernous
    argon laser therapy for, 3668, *3668*
    carbon dioxide laser therapy for, 3670
  carbon dioxide laser therapy for, 3669–3670, *3670, 3671*
  cavernous, 3583–3584, *3583*
  classification of, 3193, *3193t*
  clinical presentation of, in hand, 5315–5316
  complication of, in proliferation phase, *3206–3209,* 3206–3210
  cutaneous-visceral, with congestive heart failure, 3217–3219, *3218*
  differential diagnosis of
    by clinical methods, 3201, 3203, *3202*
    by radiographic methods, *3203,* 3203–3204, *3204*
    pyogenic granuloma and, 3204–3206, *3205*
  differentiation from vascular malformations, 3193–3194
  incidence of, 3199–3200
  involution phase of, 3210–3212, *3210–3212*
  multiple, 3200–3201, *3201*
  of hand, 5501, 5502, *5502t*
  of jaw, 3352–3353, *3354–3355*
  of orbit, 1653, 1655, *1655*
  pathogenesis of, 3194–3199, *3195–3198*
    angiogenesis dependency and, 3199
    animal models of, 3194–3195
    hormones and, 3199
    involution, light and electron microscopy of, 3197, *3198*
    proliferation
      electron microscopy of, 3196–3197, *3197*
      light microscopy of, 3195–3196, *3195–3196*
  pathology of, 3584
  port-wine. *See* Port-wine stains.
  signs of, first, 3200, *3200*
  treatment of
    by laser therapy, 3219
    by operative methods, 3219–3220, *3220–3224,* 3221–3222
    chemotherapy for, 3215–3216
    for emergent problems in proliferation phase, 3216–3219, *3217*
    for Kasabach-Merritt syndrome, 3219
    for local complications of bleeding and ulceration, 3214
    historical aspects of, 3212–3213
    in hand, 5316, *5317*
    in salivary glands, 3299–3300, *3300*
    in subglottic region, 3216–3217
    primum non nocere, 3213–3214
    steroid therapy for, 3214–3215, *3215*
  with thrombocytopenia, 3584
Hemangiopericytoma
  in children, 3187
  of head and neck, 3369–3371, *3370*
Hemangiosarcomas, of hand, 5505
Hematocrit, blood flow and, 448, *448*
Hematologic disorders, craniosynostosis of, *99,* 99–100
Hematomas
  after blepharoplasty, 2350–2351
  after facialplasty, of male, 2393–2396
  after forehead-brow lift, 2406
  after orbital or nasoethmoido-orbital fractures, 1105–1106
  from augmentation mammoplasty, 3885

Hematomas *(Continued)*
  from orthognathic surgery, 1404
  retrobulbar, after orbital and nasoethmoido-orbital fractures, 1103
Hemifacial hyperplasia, *1298–1299,* 1300–1301
Hemifacial microsomia, pathogenesis of, 2491, *2492,* 2493
Hemihypertrophy, gigantism of, 5365, 5371, *5370–5371*
Hemimandibular transplants, 201–203, *202*
Hemocoagulation, 178
Hemodynamic theories, of vascular malformation pathogenesis, 3226–3227
Hemodynamics, normal control of blood flow, 447–449, *448, 449*
Hemoglobin absorption curve, *3664*
Hemorrhage
  in facial wounds, emergency treatment for, 876–877, *878*
  in mandibular fracture treatment, 975
  postoperative, 1881
Hemostasis, 48
Heparin
  anticoagulation by, 458
  for treatment of cold injury, 857
  topical, 459
Hereditary hemorrhagic telangiectasia, 3227, 3238–3239, *3238*
Hereditary progressive arthro-ophthalmopathy, 73, 93, 3129
Heredity, in causation of craniofacial clefts, 2931
Hernias, abdominal, abdominal wall reconstruction for, *3761,* 3770–3772
Herpes simplex infections
  of hand, 5553, *5554*
  oral cancer and, 3418
Heterotopic ossification, in hand burns, 5473, 5476, *5477*
hGH. *See* Human growth hormone.
Hidden penis, 4177–4179, *4178, 4179*
Hidradenoma papilliferum, 3577
High density polyethylene (HDPE), 711–712
Hips
  contour deformities of
    classification of, *3999,* 4000
    suctioning techniques for, 4004, 4015, 4017
    type IV, 4002, *4009, 4010*
    type V, suction-lipectomy of, 4002, 4004, *4013*
    type VI, suction-assisted lipectomy for, 4004, *4014*
    type VII, suction-assisted lipectomy for, 4004, *4015*
  suction-assisted lipectomy of, complications of, 3978
Histiocytoma, 3578–3579, *3579*
Histiocytosis X, disorders of, 3351–3352
Histocompatibility antigens (HLA)
  genetics of, 187, 187–188, *188*
  keloid formation and, 735
  testing of, 188–189
  transplant rejection and, 190
  transplantation and, 187
History of plastic surgery, 2–22
  during early twentieth century, 8–18
  during first half of nineteenth century, 7
  during Renaissance, 3–4
  during World War II and postwar era, 18–20
  in ancient times, 2–3
  in seventeenth and eighteenth centuries, 4
  rebirth of, 4–7, *7*
  skin grafting, 7–8

Tibial grafts, 605, *605*
Tip-columellar angle, 1788, *1788, 1797*
Tissue expansion
  biology of, 477–478, *477–479*
  complications of, 504–506
  for breast reconstruction, 482–491, *484–490*
  for ear reconstruction, 501–502
  for extremities, 503–504, *504*
  for face reconstruction, 496, *497–500*, 501
  for nasal reconstruction, 1974–1975
  for scalp alopecia, 2224–2226, *2227, 2228*
  for scalp reconstruction, 491–496, *492, 493, 494, 495*
  for trunk, *502*, 502–503
  historical aspects of, 181, 475–476, *476*
  implant choice and placement in, 481
  inflation of implant in, 481–482
  patient selection for, 480–481
  source of increased tissue surface, 479–480, *480*
  types of implants for, 476–477
Titanium, for alloplastic implants, 705*t*, 705–706
Titterington position, for plain films, 886, *888*
Tobacco
  risks of, 3412
  smokeless, oral cancer and, 3418
Toe(s)
  microvascular transfer to hand, 5178, *5179*
    historical aspects of, 5153–5154
    indications for, 5154–5156
  mucous cysts of, 3581
  second, autotransplantation of. *See* Second toe auto-
    transplantation.
  transposition of, for correction of transverse absence
    of carpals or metacarpals, 5248, *5250–5251*, 5252
TONAR, 2912
Tongue
  anatomy of, 3478–3480, *3479*
  displacement of, in Robin sequence, 3128
  embryologic development of, 2468, *2469*, 2470
  flaps of. *See* Lingual flap.
  hypotonia of, corrective surgery for, in Down syn-
    drome, 3164–3165, *3165*
  posterior, cancers of, 3457, *3458*
  squamous cell carcinoma of, management of, 3450–
    3451, *3451*
Tongue flap
  for cheek reconstruction, 2049
  for intraoral reconstruction, 3438, *3440*
Tongue reduction, for open bite correction, 1360
Tongue-to-lip adhesion, 3134
  modified Routledge procedure, 3131, *3132*, 3133
Tonsillectomy
  for obstructive sleep apnea, 3150
  velopharyngeal closure and, 2729
Tonsils
  cancers of, 3455–3457, *3456*
  enlarged, velopharyngeal incompetence from, 2906
Torticollis, congenital muscular, 2085, 2087–2090,
  2086, 2089
Toxicity, of alloplastic implants, 701–702
Toxoplasmosis, craniofacial cleft formation and, 2928
Tracheal intubation, of retrognathia infant, 3130, 3131
Tracheostomy, for obstructive sleep apnea, 3150
Tracheotomy
  complications of, 876
  elective, 872–873, *873, 874, 875*, 875–876
  emergency low, 872, 873, *873*

Tracheotomy *(Continued)*
  indications for, 873
  techniques of, 873, 875–876, *873–875*
Traction devices, external, 1288
Tragion, 28, *28*
TRAM flap, 3908
  anatomy of, 3918–3919, *3918, 3920*
  for breast reconstruction, 3916–3920, 3922, *3917–
    3921*, 3925
  for genital reconstructive surgery, 4139, *4139, 4141,
    4142, 4143*
  limitations to usage of, 3917–3918
  postoperative abdominal hernia and, 3771–3772
Tranquilizers, craniofacial cleft formation and, 2929
Transcarpal amputation, 4340
Transcutaneous electrical nerve stimulation (TENS),
  for reflex sympathetic dystrophy, 4911–4912
Transcutaneous pO$_2$, as index of flap perfusion, 319*t*,
  320
Transfixion incision
  for rhinoplasty, 1818, *1820, 1821, 1821*
  transseptal, 1853
  variations in, 1842–1843, *1843*
Transforming growth factor (TGF-beta), 179
Translation, 2498, *2499*. *See also* Displacement.
Transplantation
  allograft reaction and, 187
  allograft rejection mechanism, modification of, 193–
    196
  general aspects of, 54–55
  histocompatibility antigens and, 187
  histocompatibility genetics of, 187
  historical background of, 186–187
  immediate, 55
  lymphoid system and, 189–190
  macrophage system and, 190
  mediate, 55
  of composite tissue, 196–203, *197*
  of craniofacial modules, 201–203, *202*
  rejection mechanism of
    afferent limb of, 190–191, *191*
    efferent limb of, 191–192, *192*
  success of, 196
Transposition flap
  design of, 289–290, *290*
  for coverage of soft tissues of hand, 4449–4450,
    4450–4451
  of scalp, 1527–1528
  Z-plasties, 4445, 4447–4448, *4446, 4447*
Transsexualism
  etiology of, 4239–4241
  hormonal therapy for, 4240–4241
  psychosocial aspects of, 129–131
  vaginoplasty for, *4241, 4241–4243, 4242*
Transverse rectus abdominis musculocutaneous flap.
  See TRAM flap.
Trapdoor effect, on scars, 742, *743, 744*
Trapezius flap
  for acquired mandibular defect, 1440, *1442*
  for cheek reconstruction, 2046–2047, *2047*, 2049
  for head and neck reconstructions, 386–387
  for intraoral and external reconstructions, 3444,
    3447–3448, *3447, 3448*
Trauma
  basal cell carcinoma and, 3619
  Dupuytren's disease and, 5055–5056

PLASTIC SURGERY

Editor
JOSEPH G. McCARTHY, M.D.
Lawrence D. Bell Professor of Plastic Surgery and
Director of the Institute of Reconstructive Plastic Surgery
New York University Medical Center
New York, New York

Editors, Hand Surgery Volumes
JAMES W. MAY, JR., M.D.
Director of Plastic Surgery and Hand Surgery Service
Massachusetts General Hospital
Associate Clinical Professor of Surgery
Harvard Medical School
Boston, Massachusetts

J. WILLIAM LITTLER, M.D.
Past Professor of Clinical Surgery
College of Physicians and Surgeons
Columbia University, New York
Senior Attending Surgeon
The St. Luke's–Roosevelt Hospital Center
New York, New York